1650

Dr. C. M. Wormington

OCULAR
DIFFERENTIAL
DIAGNOSIS

OCULAR
DIFFERENTIAL
DIAGNOSIS

Frederick Hampton Roy, M.D., F.A.C.S.

Department of Ophthalmology
University of Arkansas Medical Center
Little Rock, Arkansas
Little Rock Veterans Administration
Arkansas Children's Hospital

SECOND EDITION

Lea & Febiger   Philadelphia

Library of Congress Cataloging in Publication Data

Roy, Frederick Hampton.
  Ocular differential diagnosis.

  1. Eye—Diseases and defects—Diagnosis. 2. Diagnosis,
Differential. I. Title. [DNLM: 1. Diagnosis, Differential. 2.
Eye diseases—Diagnosis. WW141 R888o 1974]
RE76.R68   1974   617.7′1   73–19625
ISBN 0-8121-0479-X

Published in Great Britain by Henry Kimpton Publishers, London
Library of Congress Catalog Card Number: 73–19625
Printed in the United States of America

Print Number: 4   3

To my wife Nancy.

To all my children.

To Dr. Arlington Krause,
molder and questioner
in my early formative academic life.

To Dr. Philip Lewis
and Dr. Roger Hiatt
for guidance and direction.

PREFACE

It is a rather short time to have a second edition of a book. However, as deficiencies in the first edition were pointed out to me and because additional knowledge was available, I felt a revision was imperative. Several individuals mentioned the advantage of having a blank space at the end of each topic so that they could add additional references and material to keep their own copy up to date. I again urge you to write to me if you find omissions or errors in this edition.

In addition to the individuals mentioned in the Preface to First Edition, others have assisted in the preparation of the text by giving suggestions: Doctors P. Wilson, J. Massey, J. McDonald, J. Landers, A. Thomas, J. McNair, R. E. Hardberger, E. C. Clifton, J. Williamson, A. Woods, F. Boozeman, T. Grizzard, T. Wallace, R. S. Herrick, R. Kastelic, and B. Hoff.

This revision was made possible by the superb secretarial efforts of Mrs. Diane Butler, Mr. Steve Elrod, Mrs. Pat Baxter, and Mrs. Renee Massey.

Little Rock, Arkansas   FREDERICK HAMPTON ROY

PREFACE TO FIRST EDITION

The purpose of this book is threefold: (1) to aid the busy ophthalmologist in making a diagnosis by allowing him to quickly reduce the number of possibilities to a relatively small list; (2) to prevent the oversight of important considerations; and (3) to promote greater observance of the characteristics of the signs and symptoms of disease.

The book is not designed for study, but for quick reference while the patient's eyes are being dilated or immediately following his examination. Practicality is its objective; conciseness, arrangement, and authenticity its main features.

I have endeavored to present signs and symptoms in the most practical way for making a diagnosis. Some are grouped according to a particular portion of the eye, while others that cannot be said to belong to any region are designated as general symptoms. The signs and symptoms cover both medical and surgical ophthalmic conditions. The definition of each is followed by a list of the common and uncommon causes and by sources of reference. Each symptom is dealt with as completely as space and practicality will allow.

If any conditions for consideration in the differential diagnosis have been omitted, I urge that I be made aware of the omissions so that they may be included in a future edition. Laboratory findings have not been considered, since the book is designed to serve as the ophthalmologist's primary aid to diagnosis.

I am indebted to a number of published works for many of the charts and outlines used throughout the text. Thus, although much of the material is not my own, its arrangement and presentation are. I am grateful for permission for its use.

Many individuals, including Doctors S. Wilson, J. Fulmer, J. Watkins, M. Baldridge, C. Hanna, R. Lovell, J. Magie, J. Sanchez, G. Johnston, J. Parker, D. Meyer, M. Parker, J. Lyford, and G. Schroeder, have aided substantially in the preparation of the text by giving suggestions. My thanks are especially due to Doctor Fritz Fraunfelder, Chief of Ophthalmology, University of Arkansas Medical Center, for his suggestions and encouragement.

This book would not have been a reality without the persistent and meticulous secretarial and proofreading efforts of Miss Mary Kelly.

Little Rock, Arkansas   FREDERICK HAMPTON ROY

CONTENTS

HOW TO USE THIS BOOK

This book can be used easily and quickly by following the directions presented below

1. If the sign or symptom relates to a particular region of the eye, turn to the table of contents preceding this page to find the number of the page on which listings of the signs and symptoms pertaining to the specific region begins. This latter page (or those immediately following) will refer the user to that (or those) on which the various causes of the condition are listed. For example, let us assume that the patient has *pigmentation of the cornea.* The table of contents on page xi shows that the *cornea* section begins on page 215. Turning to page 215, the user finds reference to pages 221–224 on which the causes of corneal pigmentation are listed according to type. In the Index, this topic is listed as Cornea, pigmentation of, 221, and as Pigmentation of the cornea, 221.

2. If the symptom, such as *binocular diplopia* or *night blindness,* does not relate to a particular region of the eye, look for it either in the "Index" at the back of the book or under "General Symptoms and Signs" beginning on page 513.

Various features of a disease may be cross checked. For instance, a "pulsating exophthalmos with orbital bruit and conjunctival edema" may be sought under *orbit,* page 3, where the user of the book is referred to *exophthalmos,* pages 6–17, and *orbital bruit,* pages 20–21; and under *conjunctiva,* page 157, where the user is referred to *conjunctival edema,* page 178. The terms "exophthalmos," "orbital bruit" (under *orbit, bruit of,* as well as *bruit, orbital*), and "conjunctival edema" (under *conjunctiva, edema of,* and *edema, conjunctival*) may also be found in the Index. Terms such as "secondary glaucoma" are indexed under the noun, e.g. *glaucoma, secondary.*

REGIONAL
SIGNS AND SYMPTOMS

ORBIT

Contents

Pseudoproptosis (appearance of exophthalmos)

1. Unilateral high axial myopia

2. Unilateral congenital glaucoma

3. Unilateral secondary glaucoma resulting from ocular trauma during childhood

4. Congenital cystic eyeball

5. Retraction of upper lid as with thyroid disease (see lid retraction, p. 58)

6. Slight blepharoptosis as with Horner's syndrome (see blepharoptosis, p. 46)

7. Shallow orbit as in Crouzon's disease (craniofacial dysostosis)

8. Hypoplastic supraorbital ridges as in trisomy 18

9. Harlequin orbit (shallow orbit with arched superior and lateral wall) as with hypophosphatasia

10. Asymmetry of bony orbits

11. A relaxation of one or more of the rectus muscles, due either to a paralysis or to a previous operation during which one or more muscles were unduly recessed

12. Facial asymmetry

13. Contralateral enophthalmos (page 17)

Dollfus, M. A., et al.: Congenital Cystic Eyeball. Amer. J. Ophthal. 66:504–509, 1968.

Gitter, K., Meyer, D., Goldberg, R., and Sarin, L. K.: Ultrasonography in Unilateral Proptosis. Arch. Opthal. 79:370, 1968.

Howard, G. M., et al.: Orbital Growth after Unilateral Enucleation in Childhood. Arch. Ophthal. 73:80–83, 1965.

Johnson, R. V., and Kennedy, W. R.: Progressive Facial Hemiatrophy (Parry-Romberg Syndrome). Amer. J. Ophthal. 67:561, 1969.

Newell, F. W.: Ophthalmology, Principles and Concepts. St. Louis, C. V. Mosby Co., 1969, pp. 191–193.

Wright, J. E.: Proptosis. Ophthal. Surg. 2:62–69, 1971.

Exophthalmos (proptosis of orbital contents)

* = Most important

1. Inflammation
    A. Acute—orbital cellulitis
    B. Acute suppurative—mucormycosis (diabetic or debility)
    *C. Chronic (non-granulomatous)—pseudotumor
    D. Chronic (granulomatous)—tuberculosis, sarcoid, syphilis, parasites, aspergillosis
    E. Benign lymphoepithelial lesion (Mikulicz's disease)

2. Injuries
    A. Foreign body
    B. Orbital hemorrhage

3. Vascular disorders
    A. Collagen disease—lupus erythematosus or periarteritis nodosa
    B. Cranial arteritis
    C. Allergic vasculitis
    D. Thrombophlebitis
    E. Arteriovenous aneurysm or varices

4. Systemic disease
    *A. Thyroid disorder
    B. Myasthenia gravis

5. Tumors
    A. Primary in orbit
        *(1) Dermoid
        *(2) Hemangioma
        *(3) Lymphangioma
        *(4) Phakomatoses
            a. Neurofibromatosis (von Recklinghausen's syndrome)
            b. Sturge-Weber disease (encephalotrigeminal angiomatosis)
            c. Bourneville's disease (tuberous sclerosis)
            d. von Hippel-Lindau disease (retinocerebral angiomatosis)

     (5) Lipoma
   *(6) Fibrous xanthoma
   *(7) Rhabdomyosarcoma
     (8) Amputation neuroma
     (9) Neurilemmoma
  *(10) Glioma of optic nerve
  *(11) Meningioma
  *(12) Lacrimal gland lesions

        a. Epithelial tumor   50%
        b. Lymphoma   20%
        c. Pseudotumor   30%

  *(13) Inflammatory pseudotumor of orbit

        a. Systemic, such as sarcoid or collagen disease
        b. Local, such as fungus or foreign body
        c. Unknown cause

  *(14) Lymphoma and leukemia
   (15) Hand-Schüller-Christian disease (xanthomatous granuloma syndrome)
   (16) Juvenile xanthogranuloma (nevoxanthoendothelioma)
   (17) Aberrant lacrimal gland

B. Secondary orbital tumors

    (1) Direct extension from:

        a. Intraocular region: malignant melanoma, retinoblastoma, diktyoma
        b. Eyelid: basal cell carcinoma, squamous cell carcinoma, malignant melanoma; mucoepidermoid carcinoma
        c. Conjunctiva: squamous cell carcinoma, malignant melanoma; mucoepidermoid carcinoma
        d. Intracranium: meningioma
        e. Sinus: frontal, ethmoid, or maxillary (as nasopharyngeal carcinoma)

    (2) Metastatic lesions

        a. Neuroblastoma (child)
        b. Primary in lung (adult male)
        c. Primary in breast (adult female)
        d. Malignant melanoma of skin
        e. Other site

Baldridge, M.: Aberrant Lacrimal Gland in the Orbit. Arch. Ophthal. *84*:758–759, 1970.

Brenner, E. H., and Shock, J. P.: Proptosis Secondary to Systemic Lupus Erythematosus. Arch. Ophthal. *19*:81–82, 1974.

Collum, L. M. T., and Graham, M. V.: Orbital Pseudotumor. Ophthal. Surg. *2*:173–176, 1971.

Font, R. L., Naumann, G., and Zimmerman, L. E.: Primary Malignant Melanoma of the Skin Metastatic to the Eye and Orbit. Amer. J. Ophthal. *63*:738, 1967.

Green, W. R., Font, R. L., and Zimmerman, L. E.: Aspergillosis of the Orbit. Arch. Ophthal. *82*:302, 1969

Hogan, M. J., and Zimmerman, L. E.: Ophthalmic Pathology: An Atlas and Textbook. Philadelphia, W. B. Saunders Co., 1962.

Wadsworth, J. A. C.: Pathology of Orbital Tumors. Symposium on Surgery of the Ocular Adnexa. Transactions of New Orleans Academy of Ophthalmology. St. Louis, C. V. Mosby Co., 1966, pp. 137–158.

Syndromes Associated with Exophthalmos*

1. Albright's disease (polyostotic fibrous dysplasia): **unilateral proptosis, visual field defect, optic disc changes—osteitis fibrosa, skin pigmentations, endocrine dysfunction**

2. Apert's syndrome (acrocephalosyndactylia): **craniostenosis, facial dysostosis, hypoplasia of maxilla**

3. Bloch-Sulzberger disease (incontinentia pigmenti): **orbital mass, nystagmus, squint, cataract, disc changes, retinal pseudoglioma—bulbous skin eruptions and pigmentations**

4. Carotid artery-cavernous sinus fistula: **progressive exophthalmos, ophthalmoplegia, secondary glaucoma, disc changes, retinal edema and hemorrhages—unilateral headache, subjective buzzing or intracranial noise**

5. Congenital hydrocephalus: **increased head size, mental retardation, protruding eyes with deficiency in upward gaze, poor motor development**

*This section from Geeraets (pp. 238–239), with modifications.

6. Crouzon's disease (craniofacial dysostosis): bilateral exophthalmos, wide pupillary distance, oblique palpebral fissure, nystagmus, squint, visual loss, visual field defects, bluish sclera—prognathism, maxillary atrophy, deformity of anterior fontanel

7. Dejean's sign (orbital floor fracture): exophthalmos, diplopia—superior maxillary pain, numbness in region of first and second branch of fifth nerve

8. Feer's disease (infantile acrodynia): exophthalmos (rare), lacrimation, photophobia, injection of conjunctiva, dilated pupil, keratitis, optic disc changes—hypotonia of muscles, irritability, skin exfoliation on palms and soles

9. Foix's syndrome (cavernous sinus syndrome): proptosis, lid edema, paresis of third, fourth, and sixth nerves, chemosis, optic atrophy—jugular vein less distended on affected side, postauricular edema

10. Hand-Schüller-Christian disease (xanthomatous granuloma syndrome): exophthalmos, xanthelasma, ophthalmoplegia, corneal degeneration, optic nerve and retinal involvement—skin xanthomas, diabetes insipidus, skull defects

11. Hutchinson's disease (adrenal cortex neuroblastoma with orbital metastasis): exophthalmos, lid hematoma, subconjunctival hemorrhage, papilledema—anemia, increased sedimentation rate, occasional abdominal tumor

12. Jansen's disease: metaphyseal dysostosis

13. Kleeblattschadel syndrome (cloverleaf skull): trilobed skull from premature synostosis of coronal and lambdoidal sutures with severe exophthalmos, mental retardation

14. Leprechaunism

15. Möbius' disease (congenital paralysis of sixth and seventh nerves): proptosis, ptosis, disturbance in motility—facial diplegia, deafness, digital defects

16. Osteopetrosis

17. Progeria (Hutchinson-Gilford syndrome): small facies, exophthalmos, baldness, prominent scalp veins, beak-like nose, growth retardation

18. Pycnodysostosis

19. von Recklinghausen's disease: proptosis, ptosis, muscle palsies, glaucoma, anterior segment involvement, fundal changes—café-au-lait spots, nodular swelling, fibromas, spontaneous fractures

20. Rollet's syndrome (orbital apex-sphenoidal syndrome): exophthalmos, ptosis, diplopia, visual field changes, optic nerve involvement—hyperesthesias, vasomotor disturbances

21. Seckel's syndrome: bird-headed dwarf

22. Siegrist's sign (pigmented choroidal vessels): exophthalmos, choroidal changes—hypertension, albuminuria

23. Sphenocavernous syndrome: proptosis, external ophthalmoplegia—paresis of fifth nerve

24. Turner's syndrome (gonadal dysgenesis): exophthalmos, ptosis, squint, retinal involvement—webbed neck, deafness, diminished growth

Aita, J. A.: Congenital Facial Anomalies with Neurologic Defects. Springfield, Ill., Charles C Thomas, 1969, p. 261.

Geeraets, W. J.: Ocular Syndromes. Philadelphia, Lea & Febiger, 1969, pp. 238–239.

Gellis, S. S., and Feingold, M.: Atlas of Mental Retardation. Washington, D.C., U.S. Government Printing Office, 1968.

Goodman, R. M., and Gorlin, R. J.: The Face in Genetic Disorders. St. Louis, C. V. Mosby Co., 1970, p. 136.

Specific Exophthalmos

* = Most important

1. Age
   A. Newborn—most common
      (1) Orbital sepsis
      (2) Orbital neoplasm

B. Neonatal—osteomyelitis of the maxilla
C. Early childhood (up to one year of age)—most common
    *(1) Dermoid
    *(2) Hemangioma
    (3) Dermolipoma
    (4) Hand-Schüller-Christian disease (xanthomatous granuloma syndrome)
    (5) Letterer-Siewe disease
    *(6) Orbital extension of retinoblastoma
D. One to five years—most common
    *(1) Dermoid
    (2) Metastatic neuroblastoma
    (3) Rhabdomyosarcoma
    (4) Epithelial cyst, such as sebaceous cyst and epithelial inclusion cyst
    (5) Glioma of optic nerve
    (6) Sphenoid wing meningioma
    *(7) Orbital extension of retinoblastoma
    (8) Fibrous dysplasia
    (9) Metastatic embryonal sarcoma
    *(10) Hemangioma
E. Five to ten years—most common
    (1) Pseudotumor
    (2) Orbital extension of retinoblastoma
    (3) Malignant lymphomas and leukemias
    *(4) Dermoid
    *(5) Hemangioma
    (6) Meningioma
    (7) Fibrous dysplasia
    (8) Rhabdomyosarcoma
    (9) Orbital hematoma
    (10) Glioma of optic nerve
F. Ten to thirty years—most common
    *(1) Pseudotumor
    (2) Mucocele
    (3) Meningioma
    *(4) Thyroid ophthalmopathy
    (5) Lacrimal gland tumor
    (6) Malignant lymphomas and leukemias

11

(7) Dermoid

(8) Hemangioma

(9) Peripheral nerve tumors

(10) Undifferentiated sarcomas

(11) Osteoma

(12) Fibrous dysplasia

(13) Rhabdomyosarcoma

(14) Glioma of optic nerve

G. Thirty to fifty years—most common

*(1) Pseudotumor

(2) Mucocele

(3) Malignant lymphomas and leukemias

(4) Hemangioma

*(5) Endocrine ophthalmopathy

(6) Lacrimal gland tumors

(7) Rhinogenic carcinoma

(8) Malignant melanoma

(9) Osteosarcoma

(10) Fibrosarcoma

(11) Metastatic carcinoma

(12) Meningioma

(13) Dermoid

H. Fifty to seventy years—most common

*(1) Pseudotumor

*(2) Mucocele

*(3) Malignant lymphomas and leukemias

(4) Dermoid

(5) Carcinoma of palpebral or epibulbar origin

*(6) Meningioma

(7) Endocrine ophthalmopathy

(8) Lacrimal gland tumor

(9) Osteosarcoma

(10) Fibrosarcoma

(11) Undifferentiated sarcoma

(12) Metastatic carcinoma

(13) Osteoma

(14) Fibrous dysplasia

(15) Neurofibroma

(16) Hemangioma

I. Over seventy years—most common

      (1) Melanoma
      (2) Pseudotumor
      (3) Lymphoma
      (4) Metastatic tumor
      (5) Basal cell carcinoma
      (6) Mucocele

2. Unilateral exophthalmos—most common
   A. Anatomical conditions
      (1) Unilateral myopia of high degree
      (2) Defects in the vault of the orbit: meningocele, encephalocele, hydrencephalocele
      (3) Exophthalmos associated with arterial hypertension
      (4) Recurrent exophthalmos from retrobulbar hemorrhage, lymphangioma
      (5) Intermittent exophthalmos associated with venous anomalies within the cranium
      (6) Disease of the pituitary gland; meningiomas involving sphenoid
    *(7) Unilateral exophthalmos associated with toxic goiter
   B. Traumatic conditions
      (1) Fracture of the orbit with retrobulbar hemorrhage
      (2) Laceration and rupture of the tissues of the orbit and the extraocular muscles
      (3) Intracranial trauma sustained at birth; aneurysm in orbit
      (4) Pulsating exophthalmos from carotid-cavernous aneurysm
      (5) Spontaneous retrobulbar hemorrhage as seen in whooping cough
      (6) Chronic subdural hematoma bulging into orbit
   C. Inflammatory conditions
      (1) Retrobulbar abscess and cellulitis
      (2) Thrombophlebitis of the orbital veins
      (3) Cavernous sinus thrombosis
      (4) Erysipelas
      (5) Tenonitis
      (6) Periostitis (syphilitic or tuberculous)

   (7) Orbital mucocele, pyocele; cholesteatoma
   (8) Orbital exostosis
   (9) Paget's disease, with hyperostosis
   (10) Actinomycosis; trichinosis; mycotic pseudotumor
  D. Diseases of blood, lymph, and hematopoietic system
   (1) Rickets; scurvy; hemophilia
   (2) Lymphosarcoma
   (3) Chloroma
   (4) Hodgkin's disease
  E. Space-taking lesions
   (1) Vascular anomalies
    a. Congenital orbital varix (young patient with systemic abnormalities)
    b. Cavernous hemangioma (middle age)
    c. Capillary hemangioma (young children)
   (2) Orbital tumors: pseudotumors; orbital cysts; meningocele; lymphangioma; orbital meningioma; lacrimal gland tumor; sarcoma; metastatic carcinoma; metastatic adrenal tumors; osteomas arising in the accessory nasal sinuses; tumors of the nasopharynx, benign and malignant

3. Bilateral exophthalmos—most common
 A. Thyroid disorder
 B. Orbital myositis (due to causes other than thyroid dysfunction)
 C. Cavernous sinus thrombosis
 D. Metastatic neuroblastoma
 E. Hand-Schüller-Christian disease
 F. Crouzon's disease (craniofacial dysostosis)
 G. Paget's disease

4. Type proptosis—most common
 A. Straight forward—glioma of optic nerve
 B. Down and temporal—mucocele of frontal sinus
 C. Down and nasal—lacrimal gland lesion
 D. Downward—tumor of roof of orbit
 E. Upward—tumor of floor of orbit

5. Transient exophthalmos
 A. Orbital varices
 B. Orbital varices with intracranial extension

C. Arteriovenous malformations

D. Cavernous hemangioma

6. Pulsating exophthalmos—most common
    A. Carotidocavernous aneurysm
    B. von Recklinghausen's disease associated with bony defect of skull
    C. Large frontal mucocele
    D. Meningoencephalocele of posterior part of orbit
    E. Blow-out fracture of roof of orbit

7. Recurrent exophthalmos
    A. Recurrent ocular inflammation or hemorrhage
    B. Orbital cysts that rupture
    C. Lymphangioma
    D. Syndrome of intermittent exophthalmos—congenital venous malformations of the orbit: venous angioma and orbital varix
    E. Temporal lobe tumor with orbital extension
    F. Neurofibromatosis
    G. Vascular neoplasm

8. Intermittent exophthalmos
    A. Orbital varices
    B. Recurrent hemorrhage
    C. Vascular neoplasm
    D. Lymphangioma

9. Exophthalmos associated with conjunctival chemosis and restricted movement of eyes due to pain—trichinosis

10. Exophthalmos in an acutely ill patient—cavernous sinus thrombosis

11. Exophthalmos associated with engorged conjunctival episcleral vessels
    A. Nonpulsating—cerebral arteriovenous angioma, ophthalmic vein thrombosis, or cavernous sinus thrombosis
    B. Pulsating—carotidocavernous fistula

12. Exophthalmos associated with a palpable mass in region of the lacrimal gland
    A. Primary inflammatory exophthalmos

B. Neoplasm

C. Sarcoid

D. Hodgkin's disease

13. Exophthalmos in patient with uncontrolled diabetes, usually with acidosis, who develops unilateral lid edema, ptosis, internal and external ophthalmoplegia, proptosis, and severe vision loss—orbital mucormycosis

14. Exophthalmos in an infant with ecchymosis of the eyelids

A. Metastatic neuroblastoma

B. Orbital leukemia infiltration

Abboud, I. A., and Hanna, L. J.: Intermittent Exophthalmos. Brit. J. Ophthal. 55:628–632, 1971.

Baum, J. L.: Rhino-Orbital Mucormycosis. Amer. J. Ophthal. 63:335, 1967.

Bernasconi, V., et al.: Meningo-encephalocele of Posterior Part of Orbit. Neurochirurgia 11:19–29, 1968.

Boniuk, M.: The Ocular Manifestations of Ophthalmic Vein and Aseptic Cavernous Sinus Thrombosis. Trans. Amer. Acad. Ophthal. Otolaryng. 76:1519–1534, 1972.

Brauston, B. B., and Norton, E. W. D.: Intermittent Exophthalmos. Amer. J. Ophthal. 55:701–708, 1963.

Ferry, A. P.: Metastatic Carcinoma of the Eye and Ocular Adnexa. Int. Ophthal. Clin. 7:615–658, 1968.

Hou, P. K., and Garg, M. P.: Tumors of the Orbit. In Current Concepts in Ophthalmology, Vol. III. St. Louis, C. V. Mosby Co., 1972, pp. 176–185.

Iliff, C. E.: Mucoceles in the Orbit. Arch. Ophthal. 89:392–395, 1973.

Ingalls, R. G.: Tumors of the Orbit and Allied Pseudotumors. An Analysis of 216 Case Histories. Springfield, Ill., Charles C Thomas, 1953.

Jarrett, W. H., and Gutman, F. A.: Ocular Complications in the Paranasal Sinuses. Arch. Ophthal. 81:683, 1969.

Mortada, A.: Clinical Characteristics of Early Orbital Metastatic Neuroblastoma. Amer. J. Ophthal. 63:1787, 1967.

Mortada, A.: Pulsating Frontocele and Exophthalmos. Amer. J. Ophthal. 66:425–427, 1968.

Raaf, E. L.: Intraorbital Amyloid. Brit. J. Ophthal. 54:445–449, 1970.

Sanchez, J. J.: Exophthalmos from Chronic Frontal Epidural Hematoma. Rev. Esp. Otoneurooftal. 28:229–234, 1970.

Schub, M.: Corneal Opacities in Down's Syndrome with Thyrotoxicosis. Arch. Ophthal. 80:618–621, 1968.

Silva, D.: Orbital Tumors. Amer. J. Ophthal. 65:318, 1968.

Smith, M. F.: The Differential Diagnosis of Unilateral Exophthalmos. Int. Ophthal. Clin. 7:911–933, 1967.

Smith, R. R., and Blount, R. L.: Blow-out Fracture of the Orbital Roof with Pulsating Exophthalmos and Superior Gaze Paresis. Amer. J. Ophthal. 71:1052–1054, 1971.

Walsh, F. B., and Hoyt, W. F.: Clinical Neuro-ophthalmology, 3rd ed. Baltimore, Williams & Wilkins Co., 1969, pp. 1694–1697, 2008.

Walsh, W. B., and Dandy, W. E.: Pathogenesis of Intermittent Exophthalmos. Trans. Amer. Ophthal. Soc. 42:334–354, 1944.

Youssefi, B.: Orbital Tumors in Children. J. Pedit. Ophthal. 6:177, 1969.

Zizmor, J., et al.: Roentgenographic Diagnosis of Unilateral Exophthalmos. J.A.M.A. 197:121–124, 1966.

Enophthalmos (recession of the eyeball into the orbit)

1. Senility (common)

2. Wasting diseases—loss of orbital fat

3. Injury—blow-out fracture of floor of orbit (most common)

4. Orbital varices—transient exophthalmos with fat atrophy

5. Chronic or severe liver or gallbladder disease (usually in right eye owing to increased tone of orbicularis muscle and extraocular muscles)

6. Associated syndromes:*
   A. Arthrogryposis (amyoplasia congenita): joint immobility, ptosis, blepharophimosis
   B. Babinski-Nageotte syndrome (medullary tegmental paralysis): enophthalmos, ptosis, miosis, nystagmus—cerebellar ataxia, hemiparesis
   C. Cestan-Chenais syndrome: enophthalmos, ptosis, nystagmus, miosis—flaccid paralysis of soft palate and vocal cord, ataxia, contralateral hemiplegia

*From Geeraets (p. 238), with modifications.

D. Déjerine-Klumpke syndrome (thalamic hyperesthetic anesthesia): enophthalmos, ptosis, miosis—paralysis and atrophy of small muscles of upper extremities

E. Greig's syndrome (ocular hypertelorism syndrome): enophthalmos, wide interpupillary distance, epicanthus, sixth nerve palsy, astigmatism, optic atrophy—mental deficiency, skull deformation

F. von Herrenschwand's syndrome: enophthalmos, ptosis, miosis, heterochromia—decreased sweating on ipsilateral side of face

G. Horner's syndrome (cervical sympathetic paralysis syndrome): enophthalmos, ptosis, lacrimation, hypotony, miosis—anhidrosis, facial hemiatrophy

H. Pancoast's syndrome (superior pulmonary sulcus syndrome): enophthalmos, ptosis, miosis—shoulder pain, paresthesia of arm and hand

I. Parry-Romberg syndrome (progressive facial hemiatrophy): enophthalmos, Horner's syndrome, ptosis, miosis—facial hemiatrophy (loss of subcutaneous tissue)

J. Raeder's syndrome (paratrigeminal paralysis): mild enophthalmos, ptosis, diplopia, epiphora, scotoma, hypotonia, miosis—facial pain

K. Wallenberg's syndrome (dorsolateral medullary syndrome): enophthalmos, ptosis, miosis—nausea, difficulty in swallowing and speaking

L. Maple syrup urine disease: nystagmus, enophthalmos, epicanthal folds, cataracts

7. Apparent enophthalmos with horizontal conjugate gaze (see p. 154)

8. Metastatic adenocarcinoma of orbit

9. Neurofibromatosis: pulsating enophthalmos

Geeraets, W. J.: Ocular Syndromes. Philadelphia, Lea & Febiger, 1969, p. 238.

Johnson, R. V., and Kennedy, W. R.: Progressive Facial Hemiatrophy (Parry-Romberg Syndrome). Amer. J. Ophthal. 67:561, 1969.

Marre, M., and Richwein, R.: Reflectory Enophthalmos Syndrome in Patients with Liver and Gall Bladder Disease. Klin. Mb. Augenheilk. 151:158, 1967.

McCord, C. D., and Spitalny, L. A.: Localized Orbital Varices. Arch. Ophthal. *80*:455, 1968.

Roy, F. H., and Kelly, M. L.: Maple Syrup Urine Disease. J. Pediat. Ophthal. *10*: 70–73, 1973.

Sacks, J. G., and O'Grady, R. B.: Painful Ophthalmoplegia and Enophthalmos Due to Metastatic Carcinoma. Trans. Amer. Acad. Ophthal. Otolaryng. *75*:351–354, 1971.

Intraorbital Calcifications

1. Orbital phleboliths—helical form in veins—smooth, round, or oval

2. Chronic inflammatory and parasitic disease of the orbit

3. Organized hematomas of the orbit

4. Retinoblastoma

5. Retrolental fibroplasia

6. Myositis ossificans

7. Intraocular sarcoma

8. Mucocele

9. Calcification of orbital vessels
   A. Due to atheromatous plaque
   B. Monckeberg's sclerosis
   C. Secondary to metabolic-endocrine disturbances such as hyperparathyroidism or hypervitaminosis D (see band-shaped keratopathy p. 229)

10. Calcifications of more irregular configuration and texture
    A. Plexiform neurofibroma
    B. Tuberculosis
    C. Toxoplasmosis
    D. Cysticercosis
    E. Orbital hematoma

11. Sites of intraocular calcification
    A. Posterior pole to ora serrata in region of choroid and pigment epithelium
    B. Cyclitic membrane
    C. Peripapillary choroid
    D. Lens
    E. Retina
    F. Vitreous

12. Intraocular calcifications following:
    A. Trauma (perforating, non-perforating, or surgical)
    B. Congenital deformity
    C. Recurrent iritis and keratitis
    D. Retinal detachment

Alfano, J. E.: Orbital Intracranial Calcifications. Int. Ophthal. Clin. *3*:725–727, 1961.

Finkelstein, E. M., and Boniuk, M.: Intraocular Ossification and Hematopoiesis. Amer. J. Ophthal. *68*:683, 1969.

Hartman, E., and Gilles, E.: Roentgenologic Diagnosis in Ophthalmology. Philadelphia, J. B. Lippincott Co., 1958, pp. 126–127.

Henkind, P., and Morris, P. A.: Calcification of Orbital Vessels. Amer. J. Ophthal. *70*:321–326, 1970.

McCord, C. D., and Spitalny, L. A.: Localized Orbital Varices. Arch. Ophthal. *80*:455, 1968.

Zizmor, J.: Orbital Radiology in Unilateral Exophthalmos. *In* Turtz, A. I. (Ed.): Proceedings of the Centennial Symposium Manhattan Eye, Ear and Throat Hospital, Vol. I. St. Louis, C. V. Mosby Co., 1969, pp. 266–279.

Orbital Bruit (noise heard over orbit with stethoscope)

1. Bilateral
    A. Hyperthyroidism
    B. Severe anemias

2. Unilateral
    A. Arteriovenous aneurysm

B. Stenosis of carotid artery including thrombosis, sclerosis, or external pressure such as that due to an outerridge meningioma

C. Aneurysmal angioma of orbit or fundus such as in Wayburn Mason's syndrome

D. Abnormal communication in the cavernous sinus

E. Intermittent or pulsating exophthalmos (see pulsating exophthalmos, p. 15)

Cohen, J. H., and Miller, S.: Eyeball Bruits. New Eng. J. Med. *255*:459–464, 1956.

Malzone, W. F., and Gonyea, E. F.: Exophthalmos with Intracranial Arteriovenous Malformations. Neurology *23*:534–538, 1973.

Orbital Emphysema (air found in orbital tissues and adnexa usually demonstrable by palpation)

1. Due to fracture of ethmoid sinuses or orbital floor

2. Following forceful blowing of nose

3. Resulting from use of high-speed dental drill and air-water spray during oral operation

4. Orbital cellulitis and abscess with gas formation by infecting organism

5. Osteomyelitis and infected sinus with fistulous communication with gas formation by infecting organism

6. Injury from compressed air

Alexander, C. U., and Owens, T. F.: Periorbital Emphysema Related to Oral Surgery. Amer. J. Ophthal. *66*:1166–1167, 1968.

Kaplan, K., et al.: Orbital Emphysema from Nose Blowing. New Eng. J. Med. *278*:1234, 1968.

Walsh, M. A.: Orbitopalpebral Emphysema and Traumatic Uveitis from Compressed Air Injury. Arch. Ophthal. *87*:228–229, 1972.

Zizmor, J.: Orbital Radiology in Unilateral Exophthalmos. *In* Turtz, A. I. (Ed.): Proceedings of the Centennial Symposium Manhattan Eye, Ear and Throat Hospital, Vol. I. St. Louis, C. V. Mosby Co., 1969, pp. 266–279.

2

Orbital Pain

1. Retrobulbar neuritis

2. Orbital cellulitis or abscess

3. Orbital periostitis—due to injury, tuberculosis, syphilis, extension of sinus disease, or other condition

4. Myositis
   A. Collagen diseases
   B. Infectious myositis
   C. Trichinosis

5. Acute dacryoadenitis (see p. 86)

6. Pseudotumor or tumor of the orbit—pain infrequently present

7. Eye strain—from uncorrected errors of refraction

8. Break-bone fever (dengue fever)

9. Amputation neuroma of the orbit

10. Tumors of cerebellopontine angle, frequent lesion of seventh nerve

11. Status after trauma

12. Associated syndromes*:
    A. Charlin's syndrome (nasal nerve syndrome): severe orbital pain, pseudopurulent conjunctivitis, keratitis, anterior uveitis—rhinorrhea
    B. Ophthalmoplegic migraine: unilateral supraorbital pain, transitory oculomotor paralysis—migraine headache possible
    C. Tolosa-Hunt syndrome (painful ophthalmoplegia): retro-orbital pain, ptosis, ophthalmoplegia, scotoma, visual loss depending on optic nerve involvement, sluggish pupil reaction
    D. Raeder's syndrome (paratrigeminal syndrome)

*From Geeraets (p. 239), with modifications.

Geeraets, W. J.: Ocular Syndromes. Philadelphia, Lea & Febiger, 1969, p. 239.

Jampel, R. S., and Fells, P.: Monocular Elevation Paresis Caused by a Central Nervous System Lesion. Arch. Ophthal. *80*:45, 1968.

O'Brien, C. S.: Ophthalmology, Notes for Students. Iowa City, Athens Press, 1930, p. 336.

Tost, M., Knolle, H., and Krause, A. R.: The Place of Amputation Neuroma in the Differential Diagnosis of Orbital Pain. Z. Aerztl. Fortbild. *65*:96–99, 1971.

Shallow Orbits or Diminished Orbital Volume (illusion of proptosis or glaucoma)

1. Trisomy 13-15 (trisomy D)

2. Trisomy 18 (E syndrome)

3. Apert's syndrome (acrocephalosyndactyly)

4. Hypophosphatasia—harlequin orbit (shallow orbit with arched superior and lateral wall)

5. Crouzon's disease (craniofacial dysostosis)

6. Hyperostosis (hypertrophy of orbital bones)

7. Secondary to fracture

8. Early enucleation of eye

9. Radiation injury of bone

10. Craniostenosis

11. Osteogenesis imperfecta

12. Lateral displacement of the medial orbital wall by hypertrophic polypoid nasal sinus disease

13. Diseases of nasal passages and sinuses
    A. Fibrous dysplasia
    B. Rhinoscleroma
    C. Dentigenous cysts
    D. Hypoplasia of maxilla associated with chronic maxillary sinusitis

14. Aminopterin-induced syndrome—cranial dysplasia, broad nasal bridge, low-set ears

15. Cerebrohepatorenal syndrome—hypotonia, high forehead with flat facies

16. Stanesco's dysostosis syndrome—thick cortical bone, brachycephalic thin skull, relatively short upper arm, proportionally short fingers

17. Frontometaphyseal dysplasia—agenesis of frontal sinuses, hypoplastic mandible, metaphyseal splaying of tubular bones, conductive deafness, hirsutism

18. Oculoauriculovertebral dysplasia (Goldenhar's syndrome)

Bowen, D. I., Collum, L. M. T., and Rees, D. O.: Clinical Aspects of Oculo-auricular-vertebral Dysplasia. Acta Ophthal. 55:145–154, 1971.

Brenner, R. L., et. al.: Eye Signs of Hypophosphatasia. Arch. Ophthal. 81:614, 1969.

Cogan, D. G., and Kuwabara, T.: Ocular Pathology of the 13–15 Trisomy Syndrome. Arch. Ophthal. 72:246, 1964.

Ginsbert, J., Perrin, E. V., and Sueoka, W. T.: Ocular Manifestations of Trisomy 18. Amer. J. Ophthal. 66:59–67, 1968.

Smith, D. W.: Recognizable Patterns of Human Malformation. Philadelphia, W. B. Saunders Co., 1970, p. 279.

Stern, S. D., et al.: The Ocular and Cosmetic Problems in Frontometaphyseal Dysplasia. J. Pediat. Ophthal. 9:151–161, 1972.

Zizmor, J.: Orbital Radiology in Unilateral Exophthalmos. In Turtz, A. I. (Ed.): Proceedings of the Centennial Symposium Manhattan Eye, Ear and Throat Hospital, Vol. I. St. Louis, C. V. Mosby Co., 1969, pp. 266–279.

Pseudohypertelorism (illusion of increased distance between bony orbits and increased interpupillary distance)

1. Flat nasal bridge of nose

2. Epicanthal skin folds

3. Exotropia

4. Widely spaced eyebrows

5. Blepharophimosis

6. Increased distance between the inner canthi-telecanthus

DeMyer, W.: The Median Cleft Face Syndrome. Neurology *17*:961, 1967.

Hypertelorism (increased distance between bony orbits and increased interpupillary distance)

1. Myelomeningocele—Chiari malformations

2. Hydrocephalus

3. Frontal encephaloceles

4. Apert's syndrome (acrocephalosyndactylia)—craniostenosis, facial dysostosis, hypoplasia of maxilla

5. Cerebral gigantism—mental retardation, prognathism, and dolichocephalic skull

6. Cerebrohepatorenal syndrome (Lowe's syndrome)—hypotonia, hepatomegaly, cortical renal cysts, high-arched palate

7. Chondrodystrophia calcificans congenita (Conradi)—stippled epiphyses, contractures, shortening of proximal long bones, rhinomelia, cataracts, and optic atrophy

8. Cri du chat syndrome (cry of the cat syndrome)—microcephaly, rounded facies, mental/motor retardation, and a typical cat-like cry

9. Crouzon's disease (craniofacial dysostosis)—craniostenosis resulting in an abnormally shaped head; hypoplasia of the maxilla with prognathism; exophthalmos and a beaked nose

10. Hurler's syndrome (generalized gangliosidosis)—mental retardation, deposits of ganglioside within visceral organs and neurons

11. Infantile hypercalcemia with mental retardation (supravalvular aortic stenosis syndrome)

12. Ocular hypertelorism of Greig

13. Kleeblattschadel syndrome (cloverleaf skull)—trilobed skull from premature synostosis of coronal and lambdoidal sutures with severe exophthalmos, mental retardation

14. Median cleft face syndrome—cranium bifidum occultum, and median cleft nose, lip, and palate

15. Familial metaphyseal dysplasia (Pyle's disease)—bony abnormalities, macrocephaly, hypertelorism, bony prominence of the glabella, and prognathism

16. Nevoid basal cell carcinoma syndrome (basal cell nevus syndrome)—jaw cysts, ectopic calcificans

17. Oral-facial-digital syndrome—cleft lip and tongue, lobulated tongue, dental abnormalities, brachydactylia, syndactylia

18. Otopalatodigital syndrome—mental retardation, cleft palate, digital abnormalities, and conductive hearing loss

19. Ring chromosome 18—mental retardation, microcephaly, strabismus, ptosis, deafness

20. Familial characteristic

21. Infantile gigantism—dolichocephaly, high prominent forehead, hypertelorism, depressed nasal bridge, prognathism, high-arched palate

22. Ichthyosis

23. Klippel-Feil syndrome (synostosis of cervical vertebrae)—platybasia, brevicollis, low posterior hairline

24. Sprengel's syndrome

25. Larsen's syndrome—frontal bossing, depressed nasal bridge, flat face, flat and broad thumbs

26

26. Turner-Bonnevie-Ullrich-Nielsen syndrome (pterygolymphangiectasia syndrome)—hyperelastic skin, facial paralysis, cubitus valgus

27. Albers-Schönberg disease—broad skull, prominent eyes, depressed nasal bridge, short stature, small face

28. Potter's syndrome (bilateral renal agenesis)—oligohydramnios, flat spade-like hands, mermaid-form lower extremities, conspicuous crease below lower lip

29. Morquio-Ullrich syndrome

30. Multiple lentigenes syndrome (leopard syndrome)—EKG abnormalities, pulmonary stenosis, deafness, growth retardation

31. Association of hypertelorism, microtia, and facial clefting

32. Trisomy 13-15

33. Leprechaunism—large prominent eyes, flaring and upturned nostrils, prominent lips, mental retardation, dwarfism

34. Marfan's syndrome—dolichocephaly, myopia, long nose with flat bridge, long and narrow face, high-arched palate, large ears

35. Craniocarpotarsal syndrome (whistling face)—deep-set eyes, epicanthus, flat face with full cheeks, high-arched palate

36. Lissencephalia—microcephaly, narrow face, low-set malformed ears, prominent frontal and occipital regions

37. Metaphyseal dysostosis (Jansen)—muscular atrophy, exophthalmos, flat nose, large mouth, mental retardation

38. Waardenburg's syndrome—heterochromia or pale blue irides, broad nasal base, absent uvula, full lips, protruding lower lip, partial or spotted albinism

39. Mandibulofacial dysostosis (Treacher Collins)—poorly developed supraorbital ridges, small nose, large and fish-like mouth, hair growth extending toward cheek, eyelid colobomas

40. Oculomandibulodyscephaly (Hallermann-Streiff)—microbrachycephaly, cataract, nystagmus, high-arched palate, small mouth, thin lips, small face

41. Osteogenesis imperfecta—basilar invagination, blue sclera, small triangular face, hypotonia, short stature

42. Ehlers-Danlos syndrome—frontal bossing, epicanthus, prominent ears, muscle and joint hypotonia, hyperelastic skin

43. Congenital hemihypertrophy (Silver)—broad forehead, small triangular face, inverted V-shaped mouth, genitourinary abnormalities, café-au-lait spots, precocious puberty

44. Klinefelter XXXXY syndrome—dolichocephaly, epicanthus, prognathism, large mouth, mental retardation

45. Cretinism (hypothyroidism)—low wrinkled forehead, optic atrophy, short nose, "pig-like" facies, broad flat palate, thick lips

46. Multiple basal cell nevi—large cranium with broad nasal bridge, relative prognathism

47. Traumatic naso-orbital fracture

48. Aminopterin-induced syndrome—cranial dysplasia, broad nasal bridge, low-set ears

49. Rieger's syndrome—hypoplasia of the anterior stromal leaf of iris, iridotrabecular adhesions, posterior embryotoxon

50. Chromosome 18 partial short arm deletion syndrome (Wolf's syndrome)—iris and/or retinal coloboma, hypertelorism, epicanthus, strabismus, microcephaly, hydrocephalus, seizures

51. Chromosome 18 partial long arm deletion syndrome—microcephaly, hypertelorism, retraction of middle face, prominent chin, carp-like mouth

52. Carpenter's syndrome—acrocephaly, polydactyly and syndactyly of feet, lateral displacement of inner canthi

53. Noonan's syndrome (male Turner's syndrome)—antimon-goloid slant, epicanthal folds, exophthalmos, high myopia, keratoconus, posterior embryotoxon, strabismus

54. Cerebrohepatorenal syndrome (Zellweger's syndrome)—high-arched forehead, hypertelorism, marked muscular hypotonia, hepatomegaly, albuminuria

55. Sjögren-Larsson syndrome—congenital ichthyosis, spastic paralysis, mental retardation, degenerative retinitis

56. Hunter's syndrome (mucopolysaccharidosis II)—dwarfism, mental retardation, clouding of the cornea, X-linked recessive

57. Cherubism—fullness of cheeks, hypertelorism, mandibular lesions from molar area to rames angle

58. Chromosome 18 short arm deletion—webbed neck, ptosis, cataracts, hypertelorism, strabismus

59. Maple syrup urine disease—ptosis, strabismus, nystagmus

Aita, J. A.: Congenital Facial Anomalies with Neurologic Defects. Springfield, Ill., Charles C Thomas, 1969, pp. 28, 42, 47, 66, 82, 106, 114, 120, 146, 148, 215, 230, 241–242, 259–260.

Bixler, D., Christian, J. C., and Garlin, R. L.: Hypertelorism, Microtia, and Facial Clefting. Amer. J. Dis. Child. 118:495–500, 1969.

DeMyer, W.: The Median Cleft Face Syndrome. Neurology 17:961, 1967.

Geeraets, W. J.: Ocular Syndromes. Philadelphia, Lea & Febiger, 1969.

Gellis, S. S., and Feingold, M.: Atlas of Mental Retardation. Washington, D.C., Government Printing Office, 1968.

Golin, R., Anderson, R., and Blow, M.: Multiple Lentigenes Syndrome. Amer. J. Dis. Child. 117:652–662, 1969.

Goodman, R. M., and Gorlin, R. J.: The Face in Genetic Disorders. St. Louis, C. V. Mosby Co., 1970, pp. 32, 82, 150.

Levenson, J. E., Crandall, B. F., and Sparkes, R. S.: Partial Deletion Syndromes of Chromosome 18. Ann Ophthal. 3:756–760, 1971.

Lyford, J. H., and Roy, F. H.: Arhinencephaly Unilateralis, Uveal Coloboma, and Lens Reduplication. Amer. J. Ophthal. 77:315–318, 1974.

Roy, F. H., Dungan, T., and Inlow, C.: Infantile Hypercalcemia and Supravalvular Stenosis. J. Pediat. Ophthal. 8:188–194, 1971.

Roy, F. H., and Kelly, M. L.: Maple Syrup Urine Disease. J. Pediat. Ophthal. *10*:70–73, 1973.

Schwartz, D. E.: Noonan's Syndrome Associated with Ocular Abnormalities. Amer. J. Ophthal. *73*:955–960, 1972.

Stanescu, B., and Drolands, C.: Cerebro-hepato-renal (Zellweger's) Syndrome. Arch. Ophthal. *87*:590–592, 1972.

Zagora, E.: Eye Injuries. Springfield, Ill., Charles C Thomas, 1970, p. 157.

Hypotelorism (decreased distance between bony orbits and decreased interpupillary distance)

1. Cebocephalia—flat rudimentary nose, holoprosencephaly (incompletely developed forebrain)

2. Ocular-dental-digital dysplasia (dysplasia oculodentodigitalis)—hypoplastic enamel, syndactylia of the fourth and fifth fingers, microphthalmia and a thin nose with small alae nasi and anteverted nostrils

3. Trisomy 13-15—large broad nose, microphthalmia, low-set ears and micrognathia

4. Ethmocephalus—microcephaly and alobar holoprosencephaly

5. Median cleft lip—microcephaly, flat nose, and alobar holoprosencephaly

6. Median philtrum-premaxilla anlage—bilateral lateral cleft lip, flat nose, microcephaly, and alobar holoprosencephaly

7. Cockayne's syndrome—microcephaly, degenerative retinal pigmentation, senile facies, progressive deafness, mental retardation

8. Trisomy 21 (mongolism)—short, round cranium with flat occiput, epicanthus, relative prognathism, protruding tongue, externally defective ears, short stature

9. Mesodermal dysmorphodystrophy (Marchesani)—glaucoma, myopia, high-arched palate, relative prognathism, brachycephaly

10. Goldenhar's syndrome (oculoauriculovertebral dysplasia)— high-arched palate, ear abnormalities, dermoid, anophthalmos

11. Francois' diencephalic syndrome—dental anomalies, dwarfism, hypotrichosis, skin atrophy, microphthalmos, cataracts

12. Arhinencephaly

13. Trigonocephaly (triangular head) with small, narrow, and pointed frontal bone

14. Familial

Aita, J. A.: Congenital Facial Anomalies with Neurologic Defects. Springfield, Ill., Charles C Thomas, 1969, pp. 65, 155, 212, 260.

Bowen, D. I., Collum, L. M. T., and Rees, D. O.: Clinical Aspects of Oculo-auriculo-vertebral Dysplasia. Acta Ophthal. 55:145–154, 1971.

Currarino, G., and Silverman, F. C.: Orbital Hypotelorism, Arhinencephaly and Trigonocephaly. Radiology 74:206–217, 1960.

DeMyer, W., Zeman, W., and Palmer, C.: The Face Predicts the Brain: Diagnostic Significance of Median Facial Anomalies for Holoprosencephaly (Arhinencephaly). Pediatrics 34:256, 1964.

Francois, J., and Pieroid, J.: The Francois Dysencephalic Syndrome and Skin Manifestations. Amer. J. Ophthal. 71:1241–1250, 1971.

Gellis, S. S., and Feingold, M.: Atlas of Mental Retardation. Washington, D.C., U.S. Government Printing Office, 1968.

Deep-Set Eyes

1. Marfan's syndrome—prominent supraorbital ridges, long narrow face, high-arched palate, large ears, muscular hypotonia

2. Mesodermal dysmorphodystrophy (Marchesani)—brachycephaly, hypotelorism, glaucoma, high-arched palate, heavy musculature

3. Cockayne's syndrome—microcephaly, senile facies, prognathism, high-arched palate, cataracts, degenerative retinal pigmentation

4. Craniocarpotarsal syndrome—straight-up forehead, stiff and immobile facies, high-arched palate, microstomia

5. Oculocerebrorenal syndrome (Lowe)—cataracts, glaucoma, large low-set ears, pale skin, hypotonia, shrill cry

6. Syndrome of blepharophimosis with myopathy—depressed nasal bridge, fixed immobile facies, small face, pursed lips, multiple irregular rows of eyelashes

7. Pycnodysostosis (occasionally)—large head, blue sclera, beak-like nose, large and low-set ears, small mouth

8. Familial

Aita, J. A.: Congenital Facial Anomalies with Neurologic Defects. Springfield, Ill., Charles C Thomas, 1969, pp. 47, 58, 65, 121, 139, 150, 212, 261.

Prominent Supraorbital Ridges

1. Hurler's syndrome—large skull, heavy eyebrows, small and upturned nose, high-arched palate, low-set ears, hirsutism

2. Congenital lipodystrophy—dolichocephaly, thick lips, corneal opacities, acromegaloid features, brownish skin

3. Cleidocranial dysostosis—brachycephaly, hypertelorism, small triangular face, large forehead, high-arched palate, pronounced nasolabial folds

4. Marfan's syndrome—dolichocephaly, sunken orbits, blue sclera, long narrow face, high-arched palate

5. Apert's syndrome (acrocephalosyndactylia)—brachycephaly, exophthalmos, large ears, high-arched or cleft palate, mental retardation

6. Basal cell nevus—large cranium, hypertelorism, broad nasal bridge, prognathism, skin lesions

7. Ectodermal dysplasia—usually sex-linked, rare autosomal dominant, hypohidrosis, hypotrichosis, hypodentia

8. Congenital syphilis—depression of base of nose, corneal involvement, frontal bossing

9. Frontometaphyseal dysplasia—agenesis of frontal sinuses, hypoplastic mandible, metaphyseal splaying of tubular bones, conductive deafness, hirsutism

Aita, J. A.: Congenital Facial Anomalies with Neurologic Defects. Springfield, Ill., Charles C Thomas, 1969, pp. 39, 62, 132, 139, 144, 233, 261.
Stern, S. D., et al.: The Ocular and Cosmetic Problems in Frontometaphyseal Dysplasia. J. Pediat. Ophthal. 9:151–161, 1972.
Wilson, F. M., Grayson, M., and Pieroni, D.: Corneal Changes in Ectodermal Dysplasia: Case Report, Histopathology, and Differential Diagnosis. Amer. J. Ophthal. 75:17–27, 1973.

Osteolysis of Bony Orbit

1. Primary orbital disease
   A. Infectious, including tuberculosis and syphilis
   B. Neoplastic, including neurofibroma and lacrimal gland tumor
   C. Cystic, including dermoid and epidermoid cyst

2. Hyperparathyroidism

3. Reticuloendotheliosis
   A. Hand-Schüller-Christian disease

B. Eosinophilic granuloma

C. Letterer-Siewe disease

4. Secondary extension of infectious or neoplastic disease from adjacent sinuses, brain, skin, bone, and nasopharynx

5. Metastasis from remote primary neoplasms

6. Autoimmune diseases, such as Wegener's granulomatosis

7. Injury, such as blow-out fracture of orbital floor

8. Meningocele and encephalocele of orbit

9. Sinus disease including mucoceles

10. Congenital

Lombardi, G.: Radiology in Neuro-ophthalmology. Baltimore, Williams & Wilkins Co., 1967.

Zizmor, J.: Orbital Radiology in Unilateral Exophthalmos. *In*: Turtz, A. I. (Ed.): Proceedings of the Centennial Symposium Manhattan Eye, Ear and Throat Hospital, Vol. I. St. Louis, C. V. Mosby Co., 1969, pp. 266–279.

Fossa Formation of the Orbit (local expansion of the bony orbital wall caused by persistent pressure; bony cortex is intact)

1. Orbital dermoid

2. Encapsulated benign lacrimal gland tumor

3. Encapsulated malignant lacrimal gland tumor

Zizmor, J.: Orbital Radiology in Unilateral Exophthalmos. *In* Turtz, A. I. (Ed.): Proceedings of the Centennial Symposium Manhattan Eye, Ear, and Throat Hospital, Vol. I. St. Louis, C. V. Mosby Co., 1969, pp. 266–279.

Expansion of Orbital Margins (usually associated with benign tumors of the orbit)

1. Hemangioma

2. Neurofibroma

3. Lacrimal gland tumors

4. Dermoid

5. Meningioma

Zizmor, J.: Orbital Radiology in Unilateral Exophthalmos. *In* Turtz, A. I. (Ed.): Proceedings of the Centennial Symposium Manhattan Eye, Ear, and Throat Hospital, Vol. I. St. Louis, C. V. Mosby Co., 1969, pp. 266–279.

Hypertrophy of Orbital Bones (hyperostosis and/or sclerosis)

1. Acromegaly

2. Anemias of childhood (severe: Cooley's, sickle cell, spherocytosis, iron deficiency)

3. Cerebral atrophy (childhood)

4. Craniostenosis

5. Engelmann's disease (hereditary diaphyseal dysplasia)

6. Hyperostosis frontalis interna

7. Infantile cortical hyperostosis (Caffey's disease)

8. Microcephaly

9. Myotonia atrophica

10. Osteopetrosis

11. Paget's disease

12. Tumors of orbit, including osteoma, fibrous dysplasia, meningioma, metastatic neuroblastoma, mixed tumors of lacrimal gland, transitional cell carcinomas of the nasopharynx

13. Idiopathic

Lombardi, G.: Radiology in Neuro-ophthalmology. Baltimore, Williams & Wilkins Co., 1967.

Minton, L. R., and Elliott, J. H.: Ocular Manifestations of Infantile Cortical Hyperostosis. Amer. J. Ophthal. *64*:902, 1967.

Morse, P. H., Walsh, F. B., and McCormick, J. R.: Ocular Findings in Hereditary Diaphyseal Dysplasia (Engelmann's Disease). Amer. J. Ophthal. *68*:100–104, 1969.

Teplick, J. G., and Haskin, M. E.: Roentgenologic Diagnosis, Vol. 1, 2nd ed. Philadelphia, W. B. Saunders Co., 1971, p. xxxvi.

Expansion of Optic Canal

1. Glioma of optic nerve

2. Neurofibroma of optic nerve

3. Meningioma of optic nerve

4. Retinoblastoma extension

5. Sarcoma extension

6. Congenital asymmetry between canals

Zizmor, J.: Orbital Radiology in Unilateral Exophthalmos. *In* Turtz, A. I. (Ed.): Proceedings of the Centennial Symposium Manhattan Eye, Ear, and Throat Hospital, Vol. I. St. Louis, C. V. Mosby, Co., 1969, pp. 266–279.

Erosion of Optic Canal

1. Aneurysm of ophthalmic artery
2. Aneurysm of internal carotid artery
3. Arteriovenous aneurysms
4. Pituitary adenoma and carcinoma
5. Mucocele of sphenoid
6. Carcinoma of sphenoid

Zizmor, J.: Orbital Radiology in Unilateral Exophthalmos. *In* Turtz, A. I. (Ed.): Proceedings of the Centennial Symposium Manhattan Eye, Ear, and Throat Hospital, Vol. I. St. Louis, C. V. Mosby Co., 1969, pp. 266–279.

A–Scan Ultrasonography of the Orbit

See foldout on preceding page.

Standardized A–scan instruments are used. Orbital mass lesions are detected or ruled out with A–scan echography with an accuracy of 98%. An echographic differential diagnosis is possible in approximately 84% of patients, with an accuracy of more than 87%. Sinusoidal amplification of 36 decibels dynamic range with 8 megahertz probes that produce parallel non-focused beams, using the contact method at tissue sensibility, is required.

*Numbers in parentheses indicate the number of histologically examined or otherwise verified cases

From Ossoing, K. C.: Personal communication.

B-Scan Ultrasonography of the Orbit

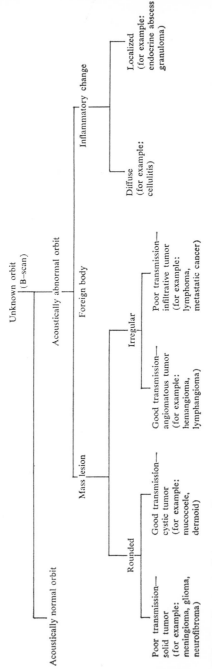

Coleman, D. J.: Reliability of Ocular and Orbital Diagnosis with B-scan Ultrasound. Amer. J. Ophthal. *74*:704–718, 1972.

LIDS

Contents

Mongoloid Obliquity (temporal canthus is higher than nasal canthus)

1. Orientals

2. Mongoloid (trisomy 21 or Down's syndrome)—epicanthus, thin cranial bones, high-arched palate, protruding and fissured tongue, general hyperflexibility, small brain

3. V esotropia and V exotropia

4. Cebocephalia—flat rudimentary nose, ocular hypotelorism and holoprosencephaly (incompletely developed forebrain)

5. Laurence-Moon-Biedl syndrome—mental retardation, obesity, hypogenitalism, polydactylia and retinitis pigmentosa

6. Pleonostenosis (Leri)—mongoloid facies, thick and stubby long bones, enlarged thumbs and great toes, short stature

7. Anhidrotic ectodermal dysplasia—overhanging brow, depressed nasal bridge, partial or complete anodontia, protruding lips

8. Chondrodystrophia (Conradi)—large skull, flat nasal bridge, cataracts, optic atrophy

9. Klinefelter's XXXXY syndrome—prognathism, flat and wide nasal bridge, epicanthus, hypertelorism, mental retardation

10. Bilateral renal agenesis—hypertelorism, prognathism; low-set, large, soft, floppy ears; anorectal malformations; flat and spade-like hands

11. Chromosome 18 short arm deletion—webbed neck, ptosis, cataracts, hypertelorism, strabismus

Aita, J. A.: Congenital Facial Anomalies with Neurologic Defects. Springfield, Ill., Charles C Thomas, 1969, pp. 126, 148, 155, 177, 221, 241, 260.

Gellis, S. S., and Feingold, M.: Atlas of Mental Retardation. Washington, D.C., U.S. Government Printing Office, 1968.

Ginsberg, J., Perrin, E. V., and Sueoka, W. T.: Ocular Manifestations of Trisomy 18. Amer. J. Ophthal. 66:59, 1968.

Levenson, J. E., Crandall, B. F., and Sparkes, R. S.: Partial Deletion Syndromes of Chromosome 18. Ann. Ophthal. 3:756–760, 1971.

Antimongoloid Obliquity (downward displacement of temporal canthus)

1. Mandibulofacial dysostosis (Franceschetti and Treacher Collins)—poorly developed supraorbital ridges, absent meibomian glands, large fish-like mouth, external ear deformities

2. Craniofacial dysostosis (Crouzon)—prominent frontal bosses, exophthalmos, external strabismus, beaked nose, high-arched palate

3. Acrocephalosyndactylia (Apert)—brachycephaly, exophthalmos, hypertelorism, strabismus, high-arched palate, large ears

4. Congenital facial hemiatrophy

5. Rubinstein-Taybi syndrome—prominent forehead, epicanthus, broad or flat nasal base, high-arched palate, dysphasia, broad thumbs and toes

6. A esotropia and A exotropia

7. De Lange's syndrome (congenital muscular hypertrophy-cerebral syndrome)—microbrachycephaly, optic atrophy, ptosis, telecanthus, thin lips and low-set ears

8. Cri du chat syndrome (cat cry syndrome)—microcephaly, epicanthus, broad nasal base, low-set ears, severe mental retardation

9. Trisomy 18 (E syndrome)—prominent occiput, microcephaly, irregular and eccentric pupils, high-arched palate, microstomia, low-set and malformed ears

10. Turner's syndrome (gonadal dysgenesis)—epicanthus, ptosis, increased difference between nose and mouth, low-set ears, webbed neck

11. Linear sebaceous nevi—convulsions and mental retardation, large cranium, hypertelorism, broad nasal bridge

12. Cerebral gigantism

13. Otopalatodigital syndrome (OPD)—cleft palate, digital abnormalities, conductive hearing loss, prominent frontal and occipital eminences, prominent supraorbital ridges, absent frontal and sphenoid sinuses, small facial bones

14. Bird-headed dwarf (Seckel)—microcephaly, large eyes, narrow beaked nose, narrow face, mental retardation

15. Mesodermal dysmorphodystrophy (Marchesani)—brachycephaly, low hairline, hypertelorism, myopia, glaucoma, high-arched palate

16. Maxillofacial dysostosis

17. Oculoauriculovertebral syndrome (Goldenhar)—high-arched palate; coloboma of upper lid, iris, choroid; microtia; microphthalmos

18. Pycnodysostosis—large head, prominent or deep-set eyes, beak-like nose, high-arched palate, large low-set ears, small mouth

19. Oculomandibulodyscephaly (Hallermann-Streiff)—microbrachycephaly, microphthalmia, cataract, nystagmus, high-arched palate

20. Cloverleaf cranium—massive bulges in both temporal regions and midline frontoparietal region, acrocephaly, massive cheeks, anteverted nostrils, shallow orbits, cleft palate

21. Noonan's syndrome (male Turner's syndrome)—hypertelorism, epicanthal folds, exophthalmos, high myopia, keratoconus, posterior embrytoxon, strabismus

22. Craniocarpotarsal dysplasia (Freeman-Sheldon syndrome; whistling face syndrome)—antimongoloid lid fissures, esotropia, mild ptosis, high-arched skull, protruding lips as in whistling, receding chin, high-arched palate

23. Chromosome 18 short arm deletion—webbed neck, ptosis, cataracts, hypertelorism, strabismus

Aita, J. A.: Congenital Facial Anomalies with Neurologic Defects. Springfield, Ill., Charles C Thomas, 1969, pp. 6, 35, 39, 65, 74, 80, 82, 92, 121, 166, 171, 179, 194, 199, 233, 260.

Gellis, S. S., and Feingold M.: Atlas of Mental Retardation. Washington, D.C., U.S. Government Printing Office, 1968.

Ginsbert, J., Perrin, E. V., and Sueoka, W. T.: Ocular Manifestations of Trisomy 18. Amer. J. Ophthal. *66*:59, 1968.

Goodman, R. M., and Gorlin, R. J.: The Face in Genetic Disorders. St. Louis, C. V. Mosby Co., 1970, p. 46.

Lessell, S., and Forbes, A. P.: Eye Signs in Turner's Syndrome. Arch. Ophthal. *76*:211–213, 1966.

Levenson, J. E., Crandall, B. F., and Sparkes, R. S.: Partial Deletion Syndromes of Chromosome 18. Ann. Ophthal. *3*:756–760, 1971.

Lund, O. E.: Combinations of Ocular and Cerebral Malformations with Cranio-facial Dysplasia. Ophthalmologica *152*:13–36, 1966.

Roy, F. H., et al.: Ocular Manifestations of the Rubinstein-Taybi Syndrome. Arch. Ophthal. *79*:272, 1968.

Schwartz, D. E.: Noonan's Syndrome Associated with Ocular Abnormalities. Amer. J. Ophthal. *73*:955–960, 1972.

Pseudoptosis (conditions simulating ptosis but the lid droop is not the result of levator malfunction, and the ptosis is usually corrected when the causative factors are cleared up or removed)

1. Due to globe displacement
    A. Anophthalmia including poorly fitting prosthesis
    B. Enophthalmos such as that resulting from blow-out fracture of the floor of the orbit or atrophy of orbital fat (see enophthalmos p. 17)
    C. Microphthalmia
    D. Phthisis bulbi
    E. Hypotonia and inward collapse of eye
    F. Cornea plana
    G. Hypotropia of that eye or hypertropia of the other eye

2. Due to mechanical displacement of the lid
   A. Inflammation
      (1) Trachoma—thick, heavy lid
      (2) Chalazion or hordeolum
      (3) Elephantiasis
      (4) Chronic conjunctivitis—conjunctival thickening
      (5) Traumatic or infectious edema involving the lid
   B. Tumors, especially fibromas or lipomas
   C. Scar tissue due to burns, physical trauma, and lacerations may bind the lid down
   D. Tumors of lacrimal gland—S-shaped lid

3. Dermachalasis (ptosis adiposa, baggy lids, "puffs")—senile atrophy of the lid skin

4. Blepharochalasis—rare condition occurring in young individuals, characterized by recurrent bouts of inflammatory lid edema with subsequent stretching of the skin

5. The oriental lid—the palpebral fissure is narrower than normal and the upper lid rarely has a furrow; hence the fold usually hangs down to or over the lid margin

6. Duane's retraction syndrome—narrowing of the lid fissure on adduction of the affected eye

7. Blepharospasm—eyebrow lower than normal

8. Contralateral widening of the lid fissure as pseudoproptosis (p. 5), exophthalmos (pp. 6–15), or lid retraction (pp. 58–61)

Beard, C.: Ptosis. St. Louis, C. V. Mosby Co., 1969, pp. 39–72.
Crawford, J. S.: Ptosis: Is It Correctable and How? Ann. Ophthal. 3:452–456, 1971.
Duke-Elder, S.: System of Ophthalmology, Vol. III, Part 2. St. Louis, C. V. Mosby Co., 1964, pp. 505–509.
Fox, S. A.: Surgery of Ptosis. New York, Grune & Stratton, Inc., 1968, pp. 214–230.
Hawkins, W. R.: Inward Collapse of an Eye. Arch. Ophthal. 84:385–386, 1970.
Huber, A.: Eye Symptoms in Brain Tumors, 2nd ed. St. Louis, C. V. Mosby Co., 1971, p. 13.

Blepharoptosis (ptosis, droopy upper lid) (weak levator palpebrae superioris muscle)

* = Most important

1. Congenital ptosis
   *A. Simple (75 to 80% of all congenital ptosis)—may be the result of autosomal dominant inheritance
   B. Complicated ptosis
      (1) Ptosis with ophthalmoplegia (10 to 15% of all congenital ptosis)—the most commonly involved muscle is the superior rectus
      (2) Ptosis with other lid deformities such as epicanthus, blepharophimosis, microphthalmia, and lid coloboma—may be hereditary
      (3) Synkinetic (paradoxical) ptosis—aberrant nervous connections from the other extrinsic muscles of the eye and jaw to the levator muscle
         a. Marcus Gunn phenomenon (jaw winking reflex)—motor root of the fifth cranial nerve to the muscle of mastication also is misdirected through the third nerve to the levator muscle
         b. Phenomenon of Marin Amat (reverse jaw winking reflex)
         c. Misdirected third nerve syndrome—bizarre eyelid movements that may accompany various eye movements; the ptotic eyelid may rise as the medial rectus, the inferior rectus, or the superior rectus muscle contracts

2. Acquired ptosis
   A. Traumatic ptosis
      (1) Eyelid laceration
      (2) Postsurgical ptosis
         a. Enucleation
         b. Orbital operation
         c. Cataract operation

(3) Foreign bodies lying in the roof of the orbit

(4) Fracture of orbital roof, also following contusion with resulting hematoma but without fracture

(5) Air blast injury

B. Neurogenic ptosis

   (1) Peripheral involvement of the third nerve (see p. 134)

   (2) Basilar, cortical, and nuclear lesions

   (3) Cerebral hemorrhages, tumors, or abscesses

   (4) Multiple neuritis, nerve syphilis, or multiple sclerosis

   (5) Horner's syndrome—lower lid higher than other lower lid

   (6) Familial dysautonomia (Riley-Day syndrome)

   (7) Misdirected third nerve syndrome—following third nerve palsy the fibers do not regrow into their respective muscles

   (8) Aseptic meningitis, transient

C. Myogenic ptosis

   (1) Primary muscular atrophy (late familial ptosis), in which ptosis is usually the only symptom

   (2) Dystrophia myotonia, in which there is dystrophia not only of the extraocular muscles but also of the face, neck, and extremities

   (3) Myasthenia gravis, non-familial acquired ptosis

   (4) The congenital fibrosis syndrome characterized by bilateral ptosis and gradual fibrosis of all the extraocular muscles

   (5) Oculopharyngeal muscular dystrophy characterized by dysplagia and progressive bilateral ptosis

   (6) Progressive familial myopathic ptosis and involvement of one, some, or all extraocular (and no other) muscles of one or both eyes

   (7) Late spontaneous unilateral ptosis

   (8) Amyloid degeneration with involvement of the levator muscle

   (9) Senility—loss of general muscle tone and atrophy of orbital fat

   (10) Ptosis and normal pregnancy

(11) Hyperthyroidism and ptosis—following active stages

(12) Corticosteroid ptosis—due to prolonged topical corticosteroid therapy

(13) Mascara ptosis—due to subconjunctival deposits of mascara

(14) Ptosis associated with chronic conjunctivitis and uveitis

(15) Guanethidine ptosis—topical use

D. Protective ptosis—following injury to the eye

E. Mechanical ptosis

    (1) Tumor

        a. Benign tumor—such as neurofibroma or hemangioma

        b. Malignant tumor—such as basal cell carcinoma, squamous cell carcinoma, malignant melanoma, or rhabdomyosarcoma

        c. Metastatic lesion—such as from breast or lung

        d. Sinus extension—such as mucocele of frontal sinus

    (2) Blepharochalasis—hereditary with recurrent attacks of severe edema and residual damage to the tissues

    (3) Cicatricial ptosis—such as that secondary to cicatricial conjunctivitis (see cicatricial conjunctivitis, p. 170) or surgical trauma to the superior fornix

    (4) Contact lens migration

    (5) Palpebral form of vernal conjunctivitis

Asregadoo, E. R.: Guanethidine Ophthalmic Solution 5%. Arch. Ophthal. *84*:21–24, 1970.

Beard, C.: Ptosis. St. Louis, C. V. Mosby Co., 1969, pp. 39–72.

Boniuk, V.: An Unusual Case of Blepharoptosis. Ann. Ophthal. *6*: 373–374, 1974.

Fox, S. A.: Surgery of Ptosis. New York, Grune & Stratton, 1968, pp. 20–25.

Fox, S. A.: Lid Surgery, Current Concepts. New York, Grune & Stratton, 1972, pp. 58–63.

Gilkes, M. J.: Hyaline Degeneration of the Conjunctiva. Trans. Ophthal. Soc. U.K. *81*:299, 1961.

Goldberg, M. F., Payne, J. W., and Brunt, P. W.: Ophthalmologic Studies of Familial Dysautonomia. Arch. Ophthal. 80:732, 1968.

Huber, A.: Eye Symptoms in Brain Tumors, 2nd ed. St. Louis, C. V. Mosby Co., 1971, p. 13.

King, Y. Y.: Ocular Changes Following Air Blast Injury. Arch. Ophthal. 86:125–126, 1971.

Paris, G. L., and Beard, C.: Blepharoptosis Following Dermolipoma Surgery. Ann. Ophthal. 5:697–699, 1973.

Wand, O.: Ptosis Associated with Aseptic Meningitis. Arch. Ophthal. 88:334–335, 1972.

Yassin, J. G., White, R. H., and Shannon, G. M.: Blepharoptosis as a Complication of Contact Lens Migration. Amer. J. Ophthal. 72:536–537, 1971.

Syndromes Associated with Ptosis*

1. Addison's disease (idiopathic hypoparathyroidism): ptosis, blepharospasm, keratoconjunctivitis, cataract, retinopathy, papilledema—moniliasis, tetany, weakness, skin pigmentation, seizures

2. Apert's syndrome (acrocephalosyndactylia syndrome): ptosis, slant canthus, exophthalmos, squint, field defects, keratitis, optic atrophy—syndactylia

3. Babinski-Nageotte syndrome (medullary tegmental paralysis): ptosis, enophthalmos, nystagmus, miosis—cerebellar hemiataxia, hemiparesis

4. Bing's syndrome: bilateral ptosis, chorioretinitis, glaucoma, paralysis of extraocular muscles

5. Cestan-Chenais syndrome: ptosis, enophthalmos, nystagmus, miosis—flaccid paralysis of soft palate and vocal cord, contralateral hemiplegia, ataxia

6. Cushing's syndrome (2) (cerebellopontine angle syndrome): pareses VII and VI, nystagmus, decreased corneal reflex, tinnitus, deafness, defect in labyrinth function

*This section from Geeraets (pp. 232–234), with modification.

7. Dandy-Walker syndrome (atresia of foramen Magendie): ptosis, sixth nerve palsy, optic nerve involvement—hydrocephalus

8. Déjerine-Klumpke syndrome: ptosis, enophthalmos, miosis —paralysis and atrophy of small muscles of upper extremities

9. Ehlers-Danlos syndrome (fibrodysplasia elastica generalisata): hyperelasticity of palpebral skin, ptosis, epicanthus, hypotony of extraocular muscles, glaucoma, thin sclera and cornea, keratoconus, subluxated lens, retinopathy—cutaneous hyperelasticity, atrophic skin, excessive articular laxity

10. Erb-Goldflam syndrome (myasthenia gravis): ptosis, strabismus, diplopia—myasthenia gravis, muscle weakness

11. von Herrenschwand's syndrome (sympathetic heterochromia): ptosis (sympathetic), enophthalmos, miosis, heterochromia—decreased sweating on ipsilateral side of face

12. Horner's syndrome (cervical sympathetic paralysis): ptosis, enophthalmos, lacrimation, miosis—anhidrosis, facial hemiatrophy

13. Hurler's disease (mucopolysaccharides type I [MPS I]): ptosis, squint, corneal involvement, optic nerve involvement—retarded development, dorsolumbar kyphosis, head deformities

14. Marcus Gunn syndrome (jaw winking and inverse jaw winking syndrome): ptosis, lid elevates with movement of the mandible

15. Möbius' syndrome (congenital paralysis of the sixth and seventh nerves): ptosis, proptosis, muscle involvement— facial diplegia, deafness, digital defects

16. Naffziger's syndrome (scalenus anticus syndrome): ptosis, miosis—reduced strength of hand grip

17. Noonan's syndrome (male Turner's syndrome): ptosis, hypertelorism, exophthalmos—valvular pulmonary stenosis, short stature, webbed neck, cubitus valgus, micrognathia

18. Ophthalmoplegic-retinal degeneration (Kearns-Sayre syndrome): ptosis, ocular myopathy, retinitis pigmentosa—progressive muscular dystrophy (possible)

19. Pancoast's syndrome (superior pulmonary sulcus syndrome): ptosis, enophthalmos, miosis—shoulder pain, paresthesia of arm and hand

20. Parinaud's syndrome (paralysis of vertical movements): ptosis, diplopia, mydriatic pupils, papilledema—vertigo

21. Parry-Romberg syndrome (progressive facial hemiatrophy): ptosis, enophthalmos, keratitis, iritis, Horner's syndrome, miosis—facial hemiatrophy (loss of subcutaneous tissue), neuralgia of fifth nerve, seizures

22. Raeder's syndrome (paratrigeminal paralysis): ptosis, enophthalmos, diplopia, scotoma, miosis, facial pain

23. von Recklinghausen's syndrome (neurofibromatosis): ptosis, proptosis, muscle palsies, hydrophthalmos, anterior segment and uveal involvement, optic nerve involvement—nodular swellings, café-au-lait spots, spontaneous fractures, fibromas

24. Rollet's syndrome (orbital apex-sphenoidal syndrome): ptosis, exophthalmos, diplopia, optic nerve involvement—vasomotor disturbances, hyperesthesias

25. Tolosa-Hunt syndrome (painful ophthalmoplegia): ptosis, ophthalmoplegia, retro-orbital pain, scotomas, visual loss, sluggish pupil reaction

26. Trisomy-18 (E syndrome): unilateral ptosis, narrow palpebral fissures, epicanthus, hypoplastic supraorbital ridges, corneal opacities—mental retardation, facial anomalies, failure of flexion of fingers

27. Turner's syndrome (gonadal dysgenesis): ptosis, exophthalmos, squint, retinal involvement—webbed neck, deafness, diminished growth

28. Wallenberg's syndrome (dorsolateral medullary syndrome): ptosis, enophthalmos, diplopia, miosis—nausea, difficulty in speaking and swallowing

29. Weber's syndrome (cerebellar peduncle syndrome): ptosis, third nerve palsy, fixed pupil—hemiplegia, paralysis of face and tongue

30. Wernicke's syndrome (hemorrhagic polioencephalitis superior syndrome): ptosis, ophthalmoplegia—peripheral neuritis, ataxia, mental disturbances

31. Eaton-Lambert syndrome: ptosis, diplopia, weakness and prolonged muscle action

32. Rubinstein-Taybi syndrome: mental retardation, broad thumbs and toes, high-arched palate

33. De Lange dwarf: small, broad skull, optic atrophy, ptosis, high-arched palate, low-set ears, feeble growl cry

34. Smith's syndrome (facioskeletogenital dysplasia): microcephaly, ptosis, high-arched palate, large low-set ears, mental retardation

35. Craniocarpotarsal dysplasia (Freeman-Sheldon syndrome; whistling face syndrome): antimongoloid lid fissures, esotropia, mild ptosis, high-arched skull, protruding lips as in whistling, receding chin, high-arched palate

36. Cri du chat syndrome (crying cat syndrome): short arm deletion of chromosome 5, strabismus, decreased tearing, hypertelorism, tortuosity of retinal vessels

37. Smith-Lemli-Opitz syndrome: strabismus, ptosis, mental retardation, skeletal and genital abnormalities, epicanthal folds

38. Leigh's disease (subacute necrotizing encephalomyelopathy)

39. Pachydermoperiostosis (Touraine-Solente-Gole syndrome): furrowing of skin of face and scalp, clubbing of fingers, autosomal dominant

40. Progressive intracranial arterial occlusion syndrome: unilateral ptosis, adolescent bilateral amaurosis, persistent head turn

41. Chromosome 18 short arm deletion: webbed neck, ptosis, cataracts, hypertelorism, strabismus

42. Maple syrup urine disease: ptosis, nystagmus, esotropia, hypertelorism

Aita, J. A.: Congenital Facial Anomalies with Neurologic Defects. Springfield, Ill., Charles C Thomas, 1969, pp. 199, 246, 299.

Geeraets, W. J.: Ocular Syndromes. Philadelphia, Lea & Febiger, 1969, pp. 232–234.

Gellis, S. S., and Feingold, M.: Atlas of Mental Retardation. Washington, D.C., U.S. Government Printing Office, 1968.

Goodman, R. M., and Gorlin, R. J.: The Face in Genetic Disorders. St. Louis, C. V. Mosby Co., 1970, pp. 46, 132.

Howard, R. O.: Ocular Abnormalities in the Cri du Chat Syndrome. Amer. J. Ophthal. 73:949–954, 1973.

Howard, R. O., and Albert, D. H.: Ocular Manifestations of Subacute Necrotizing Encephalomyelopathy (Leigh's Disease). Arch. Ophthal. 74:386–393, 1972.

Kennedy, W. R., and Jimeney-Pabon, E.: The Myasthenic Syndrome Associated with Small Cell Carcinoma of the Lung (Eaton-Lambert Syndrome). Neurology 18:757–766, 1968.

Levenson, J. E., Crandall, B. F., and Sparkes, R. S.: Partial Deletion Syndromes of Chromosome 18. Ann. Ophthal. 3:756–760, 1972.

MacRae, D. W., et al.: Ocular Manifestations of the Meckel Syndrome. Arch. Ophthal. 88:106–113, 1972.

Perkins, E. S., and Dobree, J. H.: The Differential Diagnosis of Fundus Conditions. St. Louis, C. V. Mosby Co., 1972, pp. 170–171.

Roy, F. H., and Kelly, M. L.: Maple Syrup Urine Disease. J. Pediat. Ophthal. 10:70–73, 1973.

Zappia, R. J., et al.: Progressive Intracranial Arterial Occlusion Syndrome. Arch. Ophthal. 86:455–458, 1971.

Specific Blepharoptosis

1. Unilateral ptosis with dilated pupil—tumor or abscess of temporal lobe and third nerve palsy

2. Unilateral ptosis with miosis—midbrain lesion near the posterior commissure and Horner's syndrome

3. Ptosis with disturbance of integrated ocular movement—lesion near superior colliculus

3

53

4. Bilateral ptosis with small immobile pupils and loss of upward rotation of eyeballs—lesion near posterior commissure

5. Ptosis with loss of voluntary elevation but normal involuntary elevation of the lid when the eye looks up—supranuclear lesion

6. Ptosis in repose and normal elevation with active motion—hereditary cerebellar ataxia of Pierre-Marie

7. Ptosis onset in adolescent—familial chronic external ophthalmoplegia

8. Ptosis may be early and only sign of nuclear paralysis in:
   A. Hemorrhagic superior poliomyelitis of Wernicke
   B. Botulism
   C. Multiple sclerosis
   D. Tabes
   E. Vasospasm of ophthalmoplegic migraine

9. Ptosis with cranial nerve dysfunction suggests a basal lesion such as:
   A. Meningitis
   B. Herpes zoster
   C. Polyneuritis of cranial nerves
   D. Aneurysm
   E. Trauma
   F. Epidemic paralyzed vertigo (Gerlier's disease)

10. Transient ptosis
    A. Influenza
    B. Acute exanthema
    C. Acute infection such as erysipelas
    D. Eclampsia
    E. Scurvy
    F. Exogenous poisons such as those due to alcohol, lead, carbon monoxide, arsenic, snake venom

11. Ptosis with orbicularis weakness—muscle disease

Haessler, F. H.: Eye Signs in General Disease. Springfield, Ill., Charles C Thomas, 1960, pp. 46–47.

Horner's Syndrome (paralysis of sympathetic nerve supply with lid ptosis, miosis, apparent enophthalmos, frequently dilatation of the vessels, with absence of sweating [anhidrosis] on the homolateral side. This pupil demonstrates a decreased sensitivity to cocaine and a hypersensitivity to Adrenalin. Patient may have heterochromia with congenital Horner's.)

1. Region of first neuron—lesions of hypothalamus and diencephalic region also suggest diabetes insipidus, disturbed temperature regulation, adiposogenital syndrome, and autonomic epilepsy of Penfield
   A. Basal meningitis, such as in syphilis
   B. Pituitary tumor
   C. Tumor of third ventricle
   D. Midbrain, such as in syphilis
   E. Pons, such as in intrapontine hemorrhage
   F. Medulla, such as in Wallenberg's syndrome (lateral medullary syndrome)—thrombosis of posterior inferior cerebellar artery
   G. Cervical region
      (1) Syringomyelia
      (2) Tumor
      (3) Injury
      (4) Syphilis (tabes)
      (5) Poliomyelitis
      (6) Meningitis
      (7) Amyotrophic lateral sclerosis
      (8) Related to scleroderma and facial hemiatrophy
      (9) Vascular malformation

2. Region of second neuron
   A. Spinal birth injury—Klumpke's paralysis with injured lower brachial plexus
   B. Cervical rib
   C. Thoracic lesions
      (1) Pancoast's tumor—in apex of lung, such as carcinoma, or tuberculosis
      (2) Aneurysm of aorta, subclavian or carotid artery
      (3) Mediastinal tumors

    (4) Lymphadenopathy of Hodgkin's disease, leukemia, lymphosarcoma, or tuberculosis

  D. Neck

    (1) Enlarged lymph gland, tumors, aneurysm, and thyroid gland

    (2) Carcinoma of esophagus

    (3) Retropharyngeal tumors

    (4) Neuroma of sympathetic chain

    (5) Intraoral trauma with damage to internal carotid plexus

    (6) Thin intervertebral foramina of spinal cord, such as in pachymeningitis, hypertrophic spinal arthritis, ruptured intervertebral disc, and meningeal tumors

    (7) Traction of sternocleidomastoid muscle such as from positioning on operating table

    (8) Complications of tonsillectomy

    (9) Mandibular tooth abscess

    (10) Lesions of middle ear, such as in acute purulent otitis media and petromastoid operation

 3. Region of third neuron

  A. Aneurysm of internal carotid and its branches

  B. Paratrigeminal syndrome (Raeder's)

  C. Cavernous sinus syndrome (see p. 134)

  D. Tumors or cysts of orbit

  E. Use of guanethidine or reserpine, topical

  F. Cluster headaches (migranous neuralgia)

  G. Migraine

Giles, C. L., and Henderson, J. W.: Horner's Syndrome: An Analysis of 216 Cases. Amer. J. Ophthal. *46*:289, 1958.

Haessler, F. H.: Eye Signs in General Disease. Springfield, Ill., Charles C Thomas, 1960, pp. 48–50.

Lessell, S., et al.: Brain Stem Arteriovenous Malformations. Arch. Ophthal. *86*:255–259, 1971.

Pruett, R. C.: Horner's Syndrome Following Intra-oral Trauma. Arch. Ophthal. *78*:420, 1967.

Riley, F. C., and Moyer, N. J.: Experimental Horner's Syndrome: A Pupillographic Evaluation of Guanethidine-induced Adrenergic Blockade in Humans. Amer. J. Ophthal. *69*:442–447, 1970.

Sears, M. L., Kier, E. L., and Chavis, R. M.: Horner's Syndrome Caused by Occlusion of the Vascular Supply to Sympathetic Ganglia. Amer. J. Ophthal. *77*:717–724, 1974.

Walsh, F. B., and Hoyt, W. F.: Clinical Neuro-ophthalmology, 3rd ed. Baltimore, Williams & Wilkins Co., 1969, pp. 514–520.

Ptosis of Lower Lid (uncommon drooping of lower lid so that lid margin is adjacent to the globe but below the limbus)

1. Cicatricial with mechanical displacement by scar, tumor, or skin disease. May be associated with ectropion

2. Paralytic due to lower lid lagophthalmos

3. Pseudoptosis such as in exophthalmos and higher degrees of myopia

4. Idiopathic

Fox, S. A.: Idiopathic Blepharoptosis of Lower Eyelid. Amer. J. Ophthal. 74:330–331, 1972.
Fox, S. A.: Lid Surgery, Current Concepts. New York, Grune & Stratton, 1972, pp. 122–124.

Inability to Voluntarily Close the Eyelids

1. Failure to comprehend the command

2. Unwillingness to comply

3. Lesions of facial nerves, facial nuclei, orbicularis oculi muscle (see p. 63)

4. Lesions of cerebral cortex and its projections, including bilateral frontal lesions

Lessell, S.: Supranuclear Paralysis of Voluntary Lid Closure. Arch. Ophthal. 88:241–244, 1972.

Pseudo-lid Retraction

1. Exophthalmos (see pp. 6–15)

2. Unilateral high axial myopia

3. Unilateral congenital glaucoma

4. Congenital cystic eyeball

5. Abnormalities of orbit
   A. Asymmetry
   B. Shallow, such as in Crouzon's disease
   C. Harlequin (shallow orbit with arched superior and lateral wall), such as in hypophosphatasia

6. Ptosis of other eyelid

Fox, S. A.: The Palpebral Fissure. Amer. J. Ophthal. *62*:73–78, 1966.
Walsh, F. B., and Hoyt, W. F.: Clinical Neuro-ophthalmology, 3rd ed. Baltimore, Williams & Wilkins Co., 1969, pp. 257–263, 305–317.

Lid Retraction (normally over 85% of vertical palpebral fissures 10 mm or less with the eyelids just concealing the corneoscleral limbus at the 12 and 6 o'clock meridians)

1. Lid retraction with upward movement of eye
   A. Congestive dysthyroid disease
   B. Levator muscles receive excessive stimuli from nerve fiber of superior rectus
   C. With excessive stimulation of levator muscles in Bell's phenomenon with seventh nerve palsy

D. Deficiency in upward gaze—following rectus operation or weakness of superior rectus

E. Pretectal or peri-aqueductal lesions in midbrain

2. Lid retraction with downward movement of eye
   A. Non-congestive type of dysthyroid exophthalmos (Graefe's sign)—lid lag in downward gaze
   B. Aberrant regeneration of third nerve of inferior rectus to levator (pseudo-Graefe's phenomenon)—elevation of lid in downward gaze
   C. Extrapyramidal syndrome of postencephalitic parkinsonism and progressive supranuclear palsy
   D. Failure of levator to relax on downward movement of eye
      (1) Secondary neuromuscular
      (2) Mechanical, such as from a scar

3. Lid retraction with horizontal gaze
   A. Duane's retraction syndrome—retraction on attempted abduction
   B. Underaction of lateral rectus muscle and spillover to levator causing widening

4. Lid retraction due to supranuclear lesions—usually bilateral when due to lesion in or about posterior commissure (Collier's sign, tucked lids, posterior fossa stare)
   A. Malingering
   B. Hysteria
   C. Epidemic encephalitis
   D. Tumors of midbrain; meningiomas of sphenoid wing; sellar, parasellar, and suprasellar tumors; and frontal or temporal lobe tumors
   E. Bulbar poliomyelitis
   F. Chronic multiple sclerosis
   G. Hydrocephalic infants
   H. Sylvian aqueduct syndrome (Koeber-Solus-Elschnig syndrome)
   I. Closed head injury associated with defective adduction of eyes, coarse nystagmus, nuclear palsy, pyramidal signs
   J. Coma due to disease of ventral midbrain and pons
   K. Syphilis (tabes)

L. Meningitis

M. Parkinson's disease

N. Craniostenosis, such as in hypophosphatasia

O. Parinaud's syndrome

5. Lid retraction due to neuromuscular disease—commonly asymmetric or unilateral
    A. Drugs
        (1) Phenylephrine and other sympathomimetics
        (2) Prostigmin and Tensilon, especially with myosthenic levator involvement
        (3) Succinylcholine, subparalytic doses
        (4) Excess thyroid extract
    B. Mechanical suspension of lid such as that due to scar, tumor, surgical attachment to frontalis muscle, or shortening of levator muscle
    C. Infant lid retraction—transient due to maternal hyperthyroidism
    D. Irritation of cervical sympathetic nerve (Horner's syndrome) (see p. 55)
    E. Fuch's phenomenon—healing of injured third nerve, previously ptotic lid has involuntary spastic raising with movement of eyes
    F. Peripheral seventh nerve paresis with loss of orbicularis oculi muscle tone

6. Lid retraction with myopathic disease
    A. Thyroid myopathy
        (1) Stellwag's sign—retraction of upper lid associated with infrequent or incomplete blinking
        (2) Dalrymple's sign—widening of palpebral fissure
    B. Associated with hepatic cirrhosis

7. Lid retraction following operations on vertical muscles such as recession of superior rectus muscle or simultaneous recession and restriction of the levator by common fascial check ligament between the two muscles

8. Paradoxical lid retraction due to paradoxical levator innervation
    A. Movement of lower jaw
        (1) Contraction of external pterygoid muscle by opening mouth (Marcus Gunn)

(2) Contraction of internal pterygoid muscle by closing mouth
  B. Defective ocular abduction with abducens palsy
  C. Misdirection of third nerve axons (following acquired or congenital lesions)—occurs on attempt to adduct, elevate, or depress eye
  D. Lid retraction associated with ptosis of the opposite eyelid (levator denervation supersensitivity)

9. Physiologic
  A. Act of surprise
  B. Time of attention
  C. Slow onset of blindness, such as that secondary to glaucoma and optic atrophy

Brenner, R. L., Smith, J. L., Cleveland, W. W., Bejar. R. L., and Lockhart, W. S.: Eye Signs of Hypophosphatasia. Arch. Ophthal. *81*:614, 1969.

Cogan, D. G.: Neurology of the Ocular Muscles. Springfield, Ill., Charles C Thomas, 1969, pp. 47, 71, 139–147, 166.

Fox, S. A.: The Palpebral Fissure. Amer. J. Ophthal. *62*:73–78, 1966.

Haessler, F. H.: Eye Signs in General Disease. Springfield, Ill., Charles C Thomas, 1960, p. 52.

Huber, A.: Eye Symptoms in Brain Tumors, 2nd ed. St. Louis, C. V. Mosby Co., 1971, pp. 13–15.

Manley, D. R.: Symposium on Horizontal Ocular Deviations. St. Louis, C. V. Mosby Co., 1971, pp. 13–14.

Parker, M., and Roy, F. H.: Lid Elevation: An Unusual Case. J. Pediat. Ophthal. *9*:183–186, 1972.

Walsh, F. B., and Hoyt, W. F.: Clinical Neuro-ophthalmology, Vol. I, 3rd ed. Baltimore, Williams & Wilkins Co., 1969, pp. 257–263, 305–317.

Lid Lag (when patient looks down the eyelids lag behind briefly)

* = Most important

1. Lid lag of supranuclear origin—extrapyramidal syndromes have defective inhibition of lids in downward gaze
  A. Postencephalitic parkinsonism

B. Progressive supranuclear palsy

C. Congenital supranuclear lid lag

2. Lid lag associated with neuromuscular disease
   A. Physiologic lagophthalmos—short upper tarsus in Chinese and some Caucasians with incomplete descent of the lid during sleep
   B. Excessive intake of thyroid extract

3. Lid lag with myopathic disease
   *A. Thyroid myopathy—Graefe's sign—the upper lid pauses and then follows the eye downward
   B. Myotonic dystrophia
   C. Periodic myotonic lid lag—familial (hyperkalemic) myotonic periodic paralysis

Walsh, F. B., and Hoyt, W. F.: Clinical Neuro-ophthalmology, Vol. I, 3rd ed. Baltimore, Williams & Wilkins Co., 1969, pp. 305–306.

Blepharospasm (spasmodic eyelid closure)

* = Most important

1. Hereditary reflex blepharospasm

*2. Psychogenic—onset commonly in children and young adults

3. Basal ganglion dysfunction—onset usually after middle age; including Parkinson's disease

4. Psychologic reflex blepharospasm——seen in premature infants with tactile stimulation of lids

5. Postencephalitic blepharospasm

6. Pain or light sensitivity following injury, inflammation, or foreign bodies of lids, conjunctiva, cornea, or iris

7. Cogan's syndrome (non-syphilitic interstitial keratitis) with vestibulo-auditory symptoms

8. Associated with syphilis, tetanus, and tetany

9. Idiopathic (essential)

Fox, S. A.: Essential (Idiopathic) Blepharospasm. Arch. Ophthal. 76:368, 1966.

Haidar, A., and Chaney, J.: Case Report of Successful Treatment of a Reflex Trigeminal Nerve Blepharospasm by Behavior Modification. Amer. J. Ophthal. 75:148–149, 1973.

Henderson, J. W.: Essential Blepharospasm. Trans. Amer. Ophthal. Soc. 54:453, 1956.

Irvin, A. R., Daroff, R. B., Sanders, M. D., and Hoyt, W. F.: Familial Reflex Blepharospasm. Amer. J. Ophthal. 65:889, 1968.

Facial Palsy (paralysis of the facial muscles supplied by the seventh nerve. Orbicularis oculi paralysis may result in epiphora and ectropion.)

* = Most important

1. Congenital

2. Birth injury with nerve crushed at exit of stylomastoid foramen

3. Myogenic paralysis
   A. Myotonic atrophia
   B. Facioscapulohumeral type of muscular dystrophy
   C. Myasthenia gravis
   D. Hypokalemia, periodic
   E. Curare poisoning
   F. Botulism
   G. Congenital facial diplegia
   H. Infants, from maternal ingestion of thalidomide

4. Neurologic paralysis
   A. Supranuclear paralysis—upper face including orbicularis relatively unaffected with affected lower face
      (1) Voluntary movement—pyramidal fibers involved, such as in Weber's syndrome, with contralateral hemiplegia of face and limbs and ipsilateral oculomotor paralysis
      (2) Weakness or abolition of the emotional movements of the face with retention of full voluntary activity, such as with lesion of anterior part of frontal lobe or near optic thalamus
   B. Peripheral paralysis—involvement of upper and lower face
      (1) Pontine lesion—associated structures involved include sixth nerve, conjugate ocular deviation to the same side, ipsilateral paralysis of jaw muscles and pyramidal tract in paralysis of limb of opposite side
         a. Tumors
         b. Syringobulbia
         c. Vascular lesions
         d. Acute nuclear lesions, such as with anterior poliomyelitis, Landry's paralysis, or degenerative conditions
         e. Progressive muscular atrophy
         f. Foville's syndrome—ipsilateral sixth nerve with loss of conjugate deviation to same side and hemiplegia of the opposite limbs
         g. Millard-Gubler syndrome—ipsilateral sixth nerve and hemiplegia of the opposite limbs
      (2) Posterior fossa—associated with nerve deafness, loss of taste on anterior two thirds of tongue, and occasionally diminution of tears
         a. Acoustic neuroma
         b. Meningitis, including syphilitic and tuberculous
         c. Fracture of the skull
         d. Tumors of facial nerve
         e. Facial neuritis due to polyneuritis cranialis,

beri-beri, encephalitis, diabetes, or intrathecal anesthesia
(3) Petrous temporal bone—associated with decreased lacrimation and salivary secretion, loss of taste on anterior two thirds of tongue, and intensified sensation of loud noises
  *a. Bell's palsy—inflammation of facial nerve of unknown etiology
  *b. Otitis media
  *c. Arteriosclerosis
  d. Hypertension
  e. Diabetes mellitus
  f. Fractures
  g. Herpes zoster, spread from geniculate ganglion
  h. Secondary syphilis
  i. Nerve leprosy
  j. Cephalic tetanus
(4) Facial lesions at or beyond the stylomastoid foramen
  a. Neoplasia or inflammatory swellings of the parotid such as in uveoparotid fever (Heerfordt's disease) and Mikulicz's disease
  b. Supporting lymph nodes behind the angle of the jaw
  c. Fracture of the ramus of the mandible
  d. Melkersson-Rosenthal syndrome—chronic swelling of face; bilateral, recurrent facial palsy; furrowing of the tongue

Duke-Elder, S., and Scott, G. I.: System of Ophthalmology, Vol. XII. St. Louis, C. V. Mosby Co., 1971, pp. 916–924.
Walsh, F. B., and Hoyt, W. F.: Clinical Neuro-ophthalmology, 3rd ed. Baltimore, Williams & Wilkins Co., 1969, pp. 330–339.

Infrequent Blinking

1. Thyrotoxicosis
2. Exophthalmic ophthalmoplegia (Stellwag's sign)
3. Mild postencephalitic states
4. Myostatic paresis of parkinsonism
5. Intake of ethanol
6. Wearing contact lens
7. Psychotic states
8. Infants in first few months of life
9. Progressive supranuclear palsy

Haessler, F. H.: Eye Signs in General Disease. Springfield, Ill., Charles C Thomas, 1960.

Pfaffenbach, D. D., Layton, D. D., and Kearns, T. P.: Ocular Manifestations in Progressive Supranuclear Palsy. Amer. J. Ophthal. 74:1179–1189, 1972.

Walsh, F. B., and Hoyt, W. F.: Clinical Neuro-ophthalmology, 3rd ed. Baltimore, Williams & Wilkins Co., 1969.

Frequent Blinking

1. Reflex—strong lights, sudden approach of objects toward eyes, loud noises, and touching the cornea. Reflex blinking common in albinos and light intolerance

2. Spontaneous—mental state and environment
   A. Children with habit spasm of facial tic
   B. Older persons with inadequate lacrimation and local irritation of the eyes

3. Disorders of central nervous system disease such as parkinsonism or various forms of pseudobulbar palsy

Adler, F. H.: Physiology of the Eye. St. Louis, C. V. Mosby Co., 1965, pp. 23–25.
Walsh, F. B., and Hoyt, W. F.: Clinical Neuro-ophthalmology, 3rd ed. Baltimore, Williams & Wilkins Co., 1969, p. 341.

Baggy Eyelids (puffiness or swelling of the eyelids)

1. Trichinosis

2. Stasis

3. Localized edema

4. Protrusion of fat through orbital fascia

5. Hyperthyroidism—adult or in newborn infant, myxedema and hypothyroidism

6. Nephrosis and acute glomerulonephritis—early morning edema

7. Angioneurotic edema

8. Premenstrual edema

9. Vasodilatation

10. Allergic gastroenteropathy with protein loss

11. Hodgkin's disease

12. Cavernous sinus thrombosis

13. Granulomatous ileocolitis

14. Chloromas such as myelogenous and lymphatic leukemia

15. Meningococcal meningitis

16. Orbital pseudotumor

17. Orbital tumor

18. Relapsing fever (tick fever)

19. Serum sickness—systemic reaction to foreign serum, serum products, vaccines, penicillin, and sulfa drugs

20. Tularemia

21. Meningiomas of sphenoid ridge with impediment of venous circulation of ophthalmic veins or cavernous sinus

22. Lymphogranuloma venereum

23. Associated syndromes:
     A. Foix's syndrome: lid edema, proptosis, paralysis of third, fourth, and sixth nerves, chemosis, optic atrophy —external jugular vein less distended on affected side, postauricular edema
     B. Hutchinson's syndrome: lid hematoma, subconjunctival hemorrhage, exophthalmos, papilledema—anemia, increased sedimentation rate, occasional abdominal tumor
     C. Melkersson-Rosenthal syndrome: recurrent facial paralysis, facial edema, furrowed tongue

Geeraets, W. J.: Ocular Syndromes. Philadelphia, Lea & Febiger, 1969.

Haessler, F. H.: Eye Signs in General Disease. Springfield, Ill., Charles C Thomas, 1960, p. 53.

Hallett, J. W., and Mitchell, B.: Melkersson-Rosenthal Syndrome. Amer. J. Ophthal. 65:542, 1968.

Huber, A.: Eye Symptoms in Brain Tumors, 2nd ed. St. Louis, C. V. Mosby Co., 1971, pp. 16–17.

Kirby, T. J., and Sorenson, J. U.: Swelling of the Eyelids. Amer. J. Ophthal. 52:408, 1961.

Macoul, K. L.: Ocular Changes in Granulomatous Ileocolitis. Arch. Ophthal. 84:95–97, 1970.

Newell, F.: Ophthalmology, Principles and Concepts. St. Louis, C. V. Mosby Co., 1969, p. 161.

Thygeson, P.: Historical Review of Oculogenital Disease. Amer. J. Ophthal. 71:975–985, 1971.

Waldmann, T. A., et al.: Allergic Gastroenteropathy: A Cause of Excessive Gastrointestinal Protein Loss. New Eng. J. Med. 276: 761–769, 1967.

Ectropion (lid margin turned outward from the eyeball)

1. Congenital ectropion
   A. With tight septum; microblepharon
   B. With partial coloboma
   C. With mandibulofacial dysostosis (Franceschetti's syndrome)
   D. With megaloblepharon (euryblepharon)
   E. With microphthalmos or buphthalmos

2. Acquired ectropion
   A. Spastic ectropion
      (1) Acute spastic ectropion
      (2) Chronic spastic ectropion becomes cicatricial ectropion
   B. Atonic ectropion
      (1) Senile ectropion—tissue relaxation
      (2) Paralytic ectropion—lagophthalmos such as in seventh nerve palsy (see p. 63)
   C. Cicatricial ectropion including scars and leprosy
   D. Allergic ectropion—anaphylactic, contact, and microbial (usually temporary)
   E. Myasthenia gravis—afternoon ectropion

Beard, C.: Affections of the Eyelids That Cause Tearing in the Lacrimal System. *In* Veirs, E. R., Ed.: Proceeding of the First International Symposium. St. Louis, C. V. Mosby Co., 1971, pp. 37–50.

Fox, S. A.: Lid Surgery, Current Concepts. New York, Grune & Stratton, 1972, pp. 79–94, 136.

Hill, J. C.: Ectropion. Int. Ophthal. Clin. *4*:95–112, 1964.

Orth, D. H., Fretzin, D. F., and Abramson, V.: Collodion Baby with Transient Bilateral Upper Lid Ectropion. Arch. Ophthal. *91*:206–207, 1974.

Shindle, R. D., and Leone, C. R., Jr.: Cicatricial Ectropion Associated with Lamellar Ichthyosis. Arch. Ophthal. *89*:62–64, 1973.

Slem, G.: Clinical Studies of Ocular Leprosy. Amer. J. Ophthal. *71*:431–434, 1971.

Walsh, F. B., and Hoyt, W. F.: Clinical Neuro-ophthalmology, 3rd ed. Baltimore, Williams & Wilkins Co., 1969, p. 339.

Entropion (inversion of lid margin)

1. Congenital, including congenital epiblepharon—inferior oblique insufficiency

2. Acquired
   A. Spastic entropion—acute, affecting lower lid, precipitated by acute inflammation or prolonged patching
   B. Mechanical entropion—anophthalmos, enophthalmos, or microphthalmos
   C. Senile entropion—relative enophthalmos secondary to fat atrophy
   D. Cicatricial entropion—physical and chemical burns of conjunctiva and cicatrizing diseases (see p. 170, cicatricial conjunctivitis) including trachoma and leprosy

Fox, S. A.: Entropion and Trichiasis. Int. Ophthal. Clin. *4*:113–123, 1964.
Fox, S. A.: Lid Surgery, Current Concepts. New York, Grune & Stratton, 1972, pp. 95–107, 136.
Slem, G.: Clinical Studies of Ocular Leprosy. Amer. J. Ophthal. *71*:431–434, 1971.

Epicanthus (fold of skin over the inner canthus of eye)

1. Types
   A. Epicanthus supraciliaris (unusual type)—epicanthal fold arises near brow and runs toward tear sac
   B. Epicanthus palpebralis (common type)—epicanthal fold arises from the upper lid above the tarsal region, and extends to the lower margin of the orbit
   C. Epicanthus tarsalis (Mongolian eye)—epicanthal fold arises from the tarsal (lid) fold and loses itself in the skin close to the inner canthus

D. Epicanthus inversus—fold arises in the lower lid and extends upward to a point slightly above the inner canthus; it is accompanied by long medial canthal tendons, blepharophimosis, and ptosis

2. Associated conditions:
   A. Chromosome 18 deletion (deletion 18)—mental retardation, hypoplastic mandible, low-set or malformed ears, hypertelorism
   B. Cri du chat (cry of the cat)—microcephaly, strabismus, "moon-face," high-arched palate, mental retardation
   C. Down's syndrome (trisomy 21, mongolism)—strabismus, nystagmus, protruding fissured tongue, short neck, high-arched palate
   D. Hurler's syndrome (MPS I)—large skull, heavy eyebrows, small and upturned nose, high-arched palate, thick lips
   E. Oculodentodigital dysplasia—hypotelorism, microphthalmia, iris defects, low-set ears, sunken orbits
   F. Ring chromosome 18—mental retardation, hypoplastic mandible, digital defects, hypertelorism
   G. Smith-Lemli-Opitz syndrome
   H. Turner's syndrome (gonadal dysgenesis)—hypoplastic mandible, shark-like mouth, high-arched palate, ptosis, short neck
   I. Turner's syndrome (in males) (Noonan's syndrome)—hypertelorism, webbed neck, micrognathia, low-set ears
   J. Rubinstein-Taybi syndrome—prominent forehead, strabismus, broad thumbs, broad great toes, high-arched palate
   K. Infantile hypercalcemia—large mouth and lips, blunt medial canthi, convergent strabismus, broad forehead, low-set ears
   L. Craniocarpotarsal syndrome (Freeman-Sheldon syndrome; whistling face syndrome)—deep-set eyes, stiff facies, high-arched palate, microstomia, thin and small upper lip
   M. Ehlers-Danlos syndrome—frontal bossing, prominent ears, hypertelorism, thin velvety skin

N. Congenital facial paralysis (Möbius' syndrome)—clubbed feet, syndactyly, high-arched palate, hypoplastic mandible

O. Bilateral renal agenesis—crease below lower lip; hypertelorism; low-set, large, soft, floppy ears; flat nose

P. Chondrodystrophia (Conradi's syndrome)—large cranium, flat nasal bridge, cataracts, anteverted nares

Q. Klinefelter's XXXXY syndrome—flat nasal bridge, prognathism, hypertelorism, frontal bossing, mental retardation

R. Oculocerebrorenal syndrome (Lowe's syndrome)—cataracts, glaucoma, large and low-set ears, hypoplastic mandible, pale skin, blond hair

S. Familial blepharophimosis—dysplasia of eyelids, strabismus, nystagmus, ptosis

T. Cerebrohepatorenal syndrome—hypotonia, high forehead, flat facies, hepatomegaly

U. Thalassemia

V. Leroy's syndrome—high narrow forehead, inner epicanthic folds, narrow nasal bridge, clear corneas

W. Aminopterin-induced syndrome—cranial dysplasia, broad nasal bridge, low-set ears

X. Basal cell nevus syndrome—broad facies, rib anomalies, mild mental deficiency, frontoparietal bossing

Y. Chromosome 18 short arm deletion—webbed neck, ptosis, cataracts, hypertelorism, strabismus

Z. Ring chromosome in the D group (13-15)—microphthalmos, epicanthus, blepharophimosis, cataracts

AA. Carpenter's syndrome—acrocephaly, polydactyly and syndactyly of feet, lateral displacement of inner canthi

BB. Chromosome 18 partial short arm deletion syndrome (Wolf's syndrome)—iris and/or retinal coloboma, hypertelorism, epicanthus, strabismus, microcephaly, hydrocephalus, seizures

Aita, J. A.: Congenital Facial Anomalies with Neurologic Defects. Springfield, Ill., Charles C Thomas, 1969, pp. 47, 71, 115, 126, 132, 150, 155, 171, 178, 179, 186, 230, 236, 241, 260, 261.
Bilchik, R. C., et al.: Anomalies with Ring D Chromosome. Amer. J. Ophthal. 73:83–89, 1972.

Gellis, S. S., and Feingold, M.: Atlas of Mental Retardation. Washington, D.C., U.S. Government Printing Office, 1968.

Goodman, R. M., and Gorlin, R. J.: The Face in Genetic Disorders. St. Louis, C. V. Mosby Co., 1970, pp. 32, 38.

Johnson, C. C.: Epicanthus. Amer. J. Ophthal. 66:939, 1968.

Levenson, J. E., Crandall, B. F., and Sparkes, R. S.: Partial Deletion Syndromes of Chromosome 18. Ann. Ophthal. 3:756–760, 1971.

McKusick, V. A.: Heritable Disorders of Connective Tissue, 3rd ed. St. Louis, C. V. Mosby Co., 1966, pp. 197–198.

Roy, F. H., Dungan, T., and Inlow, C.: Infantile Hypercalcemia and Supravalvular Aortic Stenosis. J. Pediat. Ophthal. 8:188–194, 1971.

Smith, D. W.: Recognizable Patterns of Human Malformation. Philadelphia, W. B. Saunders Co., 1970, pp. 92, 98, 114, 168, 232, 256, 279.

Depigmentation of Eyelid (hypopigmentation)

1. Chemical compounds
   A. Hydroquinone and its monobenzyl and monomethyl ether analogs
   B. Eserine
   C. Guanonitrofurazone
   D. Mercaptoethylamines
   E. Thio-tepa

2. Vitiligo
   A. Vogt-Koyanogi-Harada syndrome—alopecia, uveitis, poliosis, deafness, sterile meningitis
   B. Waardenburg's syndrome—lateral displacement of medial canthi, blepharophimosis, iris heterochromia, deafness, albinotic hair strain
   C. Kwashiorkor—malnutrition in children
   D. Lepromatous leprosy
   E. Pinta (etiologic agent is a spirochete, *Treponema carateum*), tertiary stage

73

F. Burns
G. Tuberous sclerosis

3. Albinism—usually generalized

Allen, A. C.: The Skin, a Clinicopathological Treatise, 2nd ed. New York, Grune & Stratton, Inc., 1967.
Berkow, J. W., Gill, J. P., and Wise, J. B.: Depigmentation of Eyelids after Topically Administered Thiotepa. Arch. Ophthal. *82*:415, 1969.

Tumors of the Lid

1. Molluscum contagiosum—small, greasy-appearing elevation that is usually umbilicated, or any other granuloma

2. Neoplasm
   A. Basal cell epithelioma—very common; may be no different in color from the surrounding area; may be a red, circumscribed, lobulated growth involving the lid margin, or may have an umbilicated center (rodent ulcer)
   B. Squamous cell or Zeis cell epithelioma—hard, pearly-appearing lesion, usually without increased vascularity
   C. Meibomian-gland carcinoma—resembles a chalazion
   D. Metastatic tumors of lid—respiratory tract, breast, skin (melanoma), gastrointestinal tract, or kidney
   E. Keratoacanthoma—benign, hemispherical, elevated tumor with a central keratin-filled crater; develops within several months
   F. Hemangioma—rubor of vascular tumor, usually having a smooth surface with tufts of vessels near the surface
   G. Benign mixed tumor of the lacrimal (palpebral) gland

3. Metaplasia or hyperplasia
   A. Trichoepithelioma
   B. Syringoma

74

C. Sebaceous adenoma

D. Papilloma—smooth, rounded, or pedunculated elevation

E. Nevus—usually pigmented, raised, and smooth surfaced; however, may be papillomatous or contain hair

F. Benign calcifying epithelioma

G. Inverted follicular keratosis

H. Blue nevus—blue-black and velvet-like in appearance

4. Cyst

A. Sebaceous

B. Sudoriferous

C. Traumatic

D. Congenital inclusion

5. Lipoid proteinosis—wax-like, pearly nodules

Aurora, A. L., and Blodi, F. C.: Reappraisal of Basal Cell Carcinoma of the Eyelids. Amer. J. Ophthal. 70:329–336, 1970.

Boniuk, M., and Zimmerman, L.: Eyelid Tumors with Reference to Lesions Confused with Squamous Cell Carcinoma. Part III, Keratoacanthoma. Arch. Ophthal. 77:29, 1967.

Jensen, A. D., Khododoust, A. A., and Emery, J. M.: Lipoid Proteinosis. Arch. Ophthal. 88:273–277, 1972.

Murphy, M. B., and Rodrigues, M. M.: Benign Mixed Tumo· of the (Palpebral) Lacrimal Gland Presenting as a Nodular Eyelid Lesion. Amer. J. Ophthal. 77:108–111, 1974.

Portney, G. L.: Meibomian Cell Adenocarcinoma. Ann. Ophthal. 4:193–196, 1973.

Riley, F. C.: Metastatic Tumors of the Eyelid. Amer. J. Ophthal. 69:259–264, 1970.

Wadsworth, J. A. C.: Pathology of Orbital Tumors. Symposium on Surgery of the Ocular Adnexa. Transactions of New Orleans Academy of Ophthalmology. St. Louis, C. V. Mosby Co., 1966, pp. 118–136.

Xanthelasma (smooth yellowish deposits in the eyelid, especially the superior nasal and inferior nasal areas)

1. Xanthelasma with hyperlipemia (primary or secondary)

A. Type II—familial hyper-β-lipoproteinemia (familial hypercholesterolemia): frequent

    B. Type III—familial hyper-β- and hyper-pre-β-lipoproteinemia (familial hyperlipemia with hypercholesterolemia) : frequent

    C. Other types infrequent, including type I, familial fat-induced hyperlipoproteinemia (hyperchylomicronemia); type IV, familial hyper-pre-β-lipoproteinemia (carbohydrate-induced hyperlipemia); type V, familial hyperchylomicronemia with hyper-pre-β-lipoproteinemia (mixed hyperlipemia)

2. Xanthelasma without hyperlipemia
    A. Local (no systemic disease)
    B. Generalized
    C. Xanthoma disseminatum
    D. Histiocytosis X
        (1) Letterer-Siewe disease
        (2) Hand-Schüller-Christian disease
        (3) Eosinophilic granuloma
    E. Reticulohistiocytoma cutis

Kahan, A., Kahan, I. L., and Timar, V.: Lipid Anomalies in Cases of Xanthelasma. Amer. J. Ophthal. *63*:320, 1967.

Pedace, F. J., and Winkelmann, R. K.: Xanthelasma Palpebrarum. J.A.M.A. *193*:893–894, 1965.

Roe, D. A.: Essential Hyperlipemia with Xanthomatosis. Arch. Dermatol. *97*:436, 1968.

Spaeth, G. L.: Ocular Manifestations of the Lipidoses. *In* Tassman, W. (Ed.): Retinal Diseases in Children. New York, Harper & Row, 1971, pp. 127–206.

Chronic Blepharitis (inflammation of lids)

1. Seborrheic—lid margin covered with small, white or gray scales
    A. Associated with seborrheic dermatitis of the scalp
    B. Aggravated by chemical fumes, smoke, and smog
    C. May be associated with uncorrected refractive errors

(especially hyperopia), myotonic dystrophy, or parkinsonism
   D. May be due to *Pityrosporon ovale*
   E. *Aspergillus fumigatus* may be its cause

2. Ulcerative-suppurative inflammation of the follicles of the lashes and the associated glands of Zeis and Moll
   A. *Staphylococcus aureus* or *S. albus* may be responsible
   B. Due to mixed infection of a staphylococcus and *P. ovale*
   C. Associated with vaccinia
   D. Due to *Blastomyces dermatitidis*
   E. Herpes simplex—vesicles at lash line then ulceration

3. Angular—inflammation of the angles of the lids, usually associated with an angular conjunctivitis
   A. Due to *Moraxella lacunata*
   B. Due to *Staphylococcus aureus*
   C. Due to *Candida albicans*

4. Other types
   A. Due to mites (*Demodex folliculorum*)
   B. Due to pubic lice (*Phthirus pubis*)

Ackerman, B. A.: Crabs. The Resurgence of Phthirus pubis. New Eng. J. Med. *278*:950, 1968.

Coston, T. O.: Demodex folliculorum Blepharitis. Trans. Amer. Ophthal. Soc. *65*:361, 1967.

Fedukowicz, H. B.: External Infections of the Eye. New York, Appleton-Century-Crofts, Inc., 1963.

Scheie, H. G., and Albert, D. M.: Adler's Textbook of Ophthalmology, 8th ed. Philadelphia, W. B. Saunders Co., 1969, pp. 257–258.

Thickened Eyelids

1. Trachoma

2. Multiple chalazia

3. Chronic conjunctivitis

4. Blepharitis—lid margins thickened (see p. 76)

5. Tarsitis—rare, such as in syphilis or tuberculosis

6. Trisomy 18 (E syndrome)

7. Congenital hypothyroidism

8. Pheochromocytoma, medullary thyroid carcinoma, and neurofibromatosis

Baum, J. L., and Adler, M. E.: Pheochromocytoma, Medullary Thyroid Carcinoma and Multiple Mucosal Neuroma. Arch. Ophthal. 87:574–584, 1972.

Gellis, S. S., and Feingold, M.: Atlas of Mental Retardation. Washington, D.C., U.S. Government Printing Office, 1968.

Ginsberg, J., Perrin, E. V., and Sueoka, W. T.: Ocular Manifestations of Trisomy 18. Amer. J. Ophthal. 66:59–67, 1968.

Blepharophimosis (short palpebral fissure)

1. Progeria—frontal and parietal bosses, beaked nose, small face, a high-arched palate, small ears without lobes

2. Craniocarpotarsal syndrome (Freeman-Sheldon syndrome; whistling face syndrome)—straight-up forehead, hypertelorism, broad nasal bridge, stiff facies, high-arched palate

3. Down's syndrome (trisomy 21, mongolism)—flat occiput, speckled iris, strabismus, high-arched palate, short maxillae, short nose with flat bridge

4. Microphthalmos—microcephaly, mental retardation, absent or defective optic nerves, epilepsy

5. Rieger's syndrome—hypoplasia of iris, broad face, hypoplastic maxillae, prognathism, peg-shaped teeth

6. Oculodentodigital syndrome—sunken orbits, hypotelorism, low-set ears, iris defects, epicanthus

7. Waardenburg's syndrome—heterochromia, absent uvula, full lips, hypertelorism, white forelock

8. Syndrome of blepharophimosis with myopathy—deep-set eyes, small face, pursed lips, fixed facies, high-arched palate

9. Traumatic

10. Trisomy 18 (E syndrome)—clenched hand, short sternum, low-arched dermal ridge, patterning on fingertips

11. Carpenter's syndrome—acrocephaly, polydactyly and syndactyly of feet, lateral displacement of inner canthi

12. Mohr's syndrome (orofaciodigital syndrome II)—cleft tongue, conductive deafness, low nasal bridge with lateral displacement of inner canthi

13. Ring chromosome in the D group (13-15)—microphthalmos, epicanthus, blepharophimosis, cataracts

Aita, J. A.: Congenital Facial Anomalies with Neurologic Defects. Springfield, Ill., Charles C Thomas, 1969, pp. 47, 58, 71, 155, 206, 238, 261.

Bilchik, R. C., et al.: Anomalies with Ring D Chromosome. Amer. J. Ophthal. 73:83–89, 1972.

Goodman, R. M., and Gorlin, R. J.: The Face in Genetic Disorders. St. Louis, C. V. Mosby Co., 1970, p. 150.

Mullaney, J.: Ocular Pathology in Trisomy 18 (Edward's Syndrome). Amer. J. Ophthal. 76:246–254, 1973.

Smith, W. D.: Recognizable Patterns of Human Malformation. Philadelphia, W. B. Saunders Co., 1970, pp. 38, 122, 228, 279.

Zagora, E.: Eye Injuries. Springfield, Ill., Charles C Thomas, 1970, p. 136.

Euryblepharon (horizontally elongated palpebral aperture [normal 28 to 30 mm]. May be associated with ectropion and present in other family members.)

1. Excessive tension of skin

2. Defective separation of the lids

3. Excessive pull of the platysma

4. Localized displacement of the lateral canthi

5. Hypoplasia of tarsus

Gupta, A. K., Ramamurthy, S., and Skukla, K. N.: Euryblepharon. J. Pediat. Ophthal. 9:173–174, 1972.
Wolter, J. R.: Familial Euryblepharon. J. Pediat. Ophthal. 9:175–176, 1972.

Lid Coloboma

1. Traumatic

2. Franceschetti's syndrome (mandibulofacial dysostosis)—fish-like face, high-arched palate, abnormal dentition, lack of cilia, microphthalmia

3. Goldenhar's syndrome (oculoauriculovertebral dysplasia)—epibulbar dermoid, micrognathia, preauricular fistulas, auricular appendages, vertebral anomalies

4. Treacher Collins syndrome (mandibulofacial dysostosis)

5. Nevus sebaceous of Jadassohn—antimongoloid lid; dermoid limbus; coloboma of iris-choroid; nystagmus; esotropia; external oculomotor palsy, unilateral; thickening of bones of orbit

Geeraets, W. J.: Ocular Syndromes, 2nd ed. Philadelphia, Lea & Febiger, 1969, pp. 231–232.
Haslam, R. H., and Wirtschafter, J. D.: Unilateral External Oculomotor Nerve Palsy and Nevus Sebaceous of Jadassohn. Arch. Ophthal. 87:293–300, 1972.

Poliosis (whitening of the hair and eyebrows and eyelashes)

1. Vogt-Koyanagi-Harada syndrome—uveitis, retinal detachment, vitiligo, poliosis, dysacousia

2. Waardenburg's syndrome—deafness, albinism, white forelock, hypertelorism, heterochromia iridis

3. Albino

4. Ageing

5. Leprosy

6. Werner's syndrome

Bullock, J. D., and Howard, R. O.: Werner's Syndrome. Arch. Ophthal. *90*:53–56, 1973.

Slem, G.: Clinical Studies of Ocular Leprosy. Amer. J. Ophthal. *71*:431–434, 1971.

Walsh, F. B., and Hoyt, W. F.: Clinical Neuro-ophthalmology, 3rd ed. Baltimore, Williams & Wilkins Co., 1969, pp. 1380–1385.

Trichomegaly (long lashes)

1. Normal

2. Ectodermal dysplasia

3. Congenital with pigmentary retinal degeneration, dwarfism, and mental retardation

4. Associated with cataract and hereditary spherocytosis

5. Isolated adrenal malfunction and ovarian atrophy

6. De Lange's syndrome—mental retardation; bushy, confluent eyebrows; wide upper lip; hirsutism

7. Rubinstein-Taybi syndrome—mental retardation, broad thumbs and toes, strabismus, elfin facies, high-arched palate

8. Noonan's syndrome

Gellis, S. S., and Feingold, M.: Atlas of Mental Retardation. Washington, D.C., U.S. Government Printing Office, 1968.
Goldstein, J. H., and Holt, A. E.: Trichomegaly, Cataract, and Hereditary Spherocytosis in Two Siblings. Amer. J. Ophthal. *73*:333–335, 1972.
Milot, J., and DeMay, F.: Ocular Anomalies in De Lange Syndrome. Amer. J. Ophthal. *74*:394–399, 1972.

Madarosis (loss of eyelashes)

1. Chronic epinephrine therapy

2. Vogt-Koyanagi-Harada disease

3. Endocrine disease, including hypothyroidism, hyperthyroidism, and pituitary insufficiency

4. Inflammation and infection of the lids, including seborrheic blepharitis, squamous blepharitis, herpes zoster, vaccinia, mycotic infection, furuncles, and erysipelas

5. Radiation

6. Severe debilitating systemic diseases, including tuberculosis, syphilis, and sickle cell anemia

7. Intoxication with arsenic, bismuth, thallium, barbiturates, propylthiouracil, gold, quinine, vitamin A, and antimetabolites

8. Chronic skin diseases, including psoriasis, neurodermatitis, exfoliative dermatitis, ichthyosis, alopecia areata, acne, lichen planus, epidermolysis bullosa, and lupus erythematosus

9. Trauma

10. Lipoid proteinosis (Urbach-Wiethe syndrome)—margin of lid has nodules with loss of cilia, facial nodules, hoarseness, cobblestone lips

Goodman, R. M., and Gorlin, R. J.: The Face in Genetic Disorders. St. Louis, C. V. Mosby Co., 1970, p. 88.
Kass, M. A., Stamper, R. L., and Becker, B.: Madarosis in Chronic Epinephrine Therapy. Arch. Ophthal. *88*:429–431, 1972.

Distichiasis (accessory row of lashes growing from openings of Meibomian gland)

1. Congenital

2. Hereditary—autosomal dominant

Deutsch, A. R.: Distichiasis and Epicanthus. Ann. Ophthal. *3*:168–173, 1971.

Coarse Eyebrows

1. Hurler's syndrome (MPS I)—mental retardation, coarse features, hirsutism, hepatomegaly, large tongue

2. Hunter's syndrome (MPS II)—mental retardation, coarse features, hirsutism, hepatomegaly, large tongue

3. Sanfilippo's syndrome (MPS III)—mental retardation, hirsutism, coarse features, hepatomegaly, large tongue

4. Rubinstein-Taybi syndrome—mental retardation, broad thumbs and toes, strabismus, coloboma of iris, high-arched palate

5. Congenital hypothyroidism (cretinism)—mental retardation, delayed skeletal maturation, dry and cold extremities, myxedema, and large tongue protruding from open mouth

6. Normal variation

Gellis, S. S., and Feingold, M.: Atlas of Mental Retardation. Washington, D.C., U.S. Government Printing Office, 1968.

Synophrys (confluent eyebrows extending to midline)

1. Cornelia de Lange's syndrome—synophrys of eyebrows; thin, downward turning upper lip; micromelia; mental retardation

2. Waardenburg's syndrome—lateral displacement of medial canthi, partial albinism, deafness, white forelock

3. Basal cell nevus syndrome—basal cell nevi, broad facies, rib anomalies, frontoparietal bossing

4. 13 Trisomy syndrome—severe mental defect; microphthalmia; cleft lip, cleft palate, or both; retinal dysplasia

5. No. 4 short arm deletion—ocular hypertelorism with broad or beaked nose; microcephaly and/or cranial asymmetry; low-set, simple ear with preauricular tag

6. Frontometaphyseal dysplasia—agenesis of frontal sinuses, hypoplastic mandible, metaphyseal splaying of tubular bones, conductive deafness, hirsutism

7. Normal variation

Milot, J., and DeMay, F.: Ocular Anomalies in De Lange Syndrome. Amer. J. Ophthal. 74:394–399, 1972.

Smith, D. W.: Recognizable Patterns of Human Malformation. Philadelphia, W. B. Saunders Co., 1970, pp. 279–280.

Stern, S. D., et al.: The Ocular and Cosmetic Problems in Frontometaphyseal Dysplasia. J. Pediat. Ophthal. 9:151–161, 1972.

LACRIMAL SYSTEM

Contents

4

Dacryoadenitis (inflammation of lacrimal gland)

1. Acute dacryoadenitis—rare catarrhal inflammation of the lacrimal gland that usually accompanies systemic disease
   A. In children—mumps, measles, influenza, scarlet fever, erysipelas, typhoid fever
   B. In adult—gonorrhea, endogenous conjunctivitis and uveitis, infectious mononucleosis, typhoid fever
   C. Secondary to inflammation from lids or conjunctiva, to include *Klebsiella pneumoniae,* coliform organisms, staphylococcus, streptococcus, *Diplococcus pneumoniae,* and *Neisseria gonorrhoeae*

2. Chronic dacryoadenitis—proliferative inflammation of the lacrimal gland, usually due to specific granulomatous disease
   A. Mikulicz's syndrome—dacryoadenitis and parotitis manifested by chronic bilateral swelling of the lacrimal and salivary glands
      (1) Tuberculosis
      (2) Leukemia
      (3) Lymphosarcoma
      (4) Sarcoidosis
      (5) Hodgkin's disease
      (6) Lymphoma
      (7) Reticuloendothelial disease
   B. Heerfordt's disease—chronic bilateral parotitis and uveitis, often associated with paresis of the cranial nerves, usually the seventh nerve, and other general symptoms
      (1) Sarcoidosis
      (2) Tuberculosis
   C. Miliary tuberculosis
   D. Syphilis (gumma)
   E. Pseudotumor
   F. Boeck's sarcoid

3. Painless enlargement of lacrimal gland
   A. Leukemia
   B. Mumps

4. Painful enlargement of lacrimal gland
    A. Lymphomatous disease (25%)
    B. Chronic enlargement arising from sarcoid or orbital pseudotumor (25%)
    C. Lacrimal gland neoplasm (50%)
        (1) Benign
            a. Mixed tumor
            b. Adenoma
        (2) Malignant
            a. Mixed tumor
            b. Carcinoma unrelated to mixed tumor
                1) Adenocarcinoma (adenoid cystic carcinoma)
                2) Mucoepidermoid carcinoma
                3) Squamous cell carcinoma

Bedrossian, E. H.: The Eye. Springfield, Ill., Charles C Thomas, 1958, p. 165.

Forrest, A. W.: Epithelial Tumors of the Lacrimal Gland. *In* Veirs, E. R., (Ed.): The Lacrimal System: Proceedings of the First International Symposium. St. Louis, C. V. Mosby Co., 1971, pp. 19–28.

Forrest, A. W.: Pathologic Criteria for Effective Management of Epithelial Lacrimal Gland Tumors. Amer. J. Ophthal. *71*:178, 1971.

Geeraets, W. J.: Ocular Syndromes. Philadelphia, Lea & Febiger, 1969, p. 139.

Newell, F. W.: Ophthalmology, Principles and Concepts. St. Louis, C. V. Mosby Co., 1969, pp. 182–183.

Bloody Tears

1. Conjunctival fibroma

2, Inflammatory granuloma of conjunctiva

3. Hemangioma of conjunctiva

4. Malignant melanoma

5. Hemophilia

6. Vicarious menstruation

7. Hysteria

8. Cachectic conjunctivitis

9. Trauma—local

10. Gross disturbance of autonomic nervous system

11. Advanced athrombia

12. Application of a drug such as silver nitrate

13. Severe conjunctivitis with marked hyperemia

14. Pathologic process of lacrimal gland

15. Jaundice

16. Severe epistaxis with regurgitation through the lacrimal passages

17. Subconjunctival hemorrhage following sudden venous congestion of head from stooping, coughing, or choking

18. Hereditary hemorrhagic telangiectasis (Rendu-Osler-Weber disease)

19. Associated with pubic lice and nits on the lashes

20. Pannus or other corneal vascular lesion

21. Focal dermal hypoplasia syndrome (Goltz's syndrome)— papilloma of the lips, strabismus, uveal colobomas, microphthalmia, usually in female

Banta, R. G., and Seltzer, J. L.: Bloody Tears from Epistaxis through the Nasolacrimal Duct. Amer. J. Ophthal. *75*:726–727, 1973.

Belau, P. G., and Rucker, C. W.: Bloody Tears. Proc. Mayo Clin. *36*:234, 1961.

Duke-Elder, S.: System of Ophthalmology, Vol. VII, Part 1. St. Louis, C. V. Mosby Co., 1962, pp. 37–39.

Goodman, R. M., and Gorlin, R. J.: The Face in Genetic Disorders. St. Louis, C. V. Mosby Co., 1970, p. 70.

Wolper, J., and Laibson, P. R.: Hereditary Hemorrhagic Telangiectasis (Rendu-Osler-Weber Disease) with Filamentary Keratitis. Arch. Ophthal. *81*:272, 1969.

1. Hypersecretion of tears—may be due to basic secretors (mucin, lacrimal, including secretion from glands of Kraus and Wolfring, and oil, including secretion from Zeis', Moll's, and Meibomian palpebral glands), or reflex secretors (main lacrimal glands and accessory palpebral glands)
   A. Primary (disturbance of lacrimal gland)
   B. Central or psychic
      (1) Emotional states
      (2) Physical pain
      (3) Voluntary lacrimation, such as when acting
      (4) Corticomeningeal lesions
      (5) Hysteria
   C. Neurogenic
      (1) Exposure to wind, cold, or bright light
      (2) Inflammation or infection of the conjunctiva, uvea, cornea, orbit, lids, sinuses, teeth, or ears
      (3) Lesions affecting the lids, such as trichiasis, entropion, ectropion, trachoma, and facial paralysis
      (4) Ametropia, tropia, or phoria, and eyestrain or fatigue
      (5) Glaucoma
      (6) Chemical and drug irritations, such as those due to eye medications, gases, and dust
      (7) Crocodile or alligator tears (gustolacrimal reflex)—unilateral profuse tearing when eating
         a. Congenital, often associated with ipsilateral paresis of lateral rectus muscle
         b. Acquired with onset in early stage of facial palsy (Bell's palsy) or sequela with parasympathetic fibers to the otic ganglion growing back into superficial petrosal nerve
         c. Section of the greater superficial petrosal nerve

        (8) Stimulation of some cortical areas—thalamus, hypothalamus, cervical sympathetic ganglia, or the lacrimal nucleus including pseudobulbar palsy from parkinsonism, various senile dementias, giant-cell arteritis, hypothalamic tumors, encephalitis, and meningitis

        (9) Horner's syndrome (cervical sympathetic paralysis syndrome)

      (10) Morquio-Brailsford syndrome (MPS IV)

      (11) Sjögren's syndrome (keratoconjunctivitis sicca)

      (12) Caloric lacrimo- and reflex-bilateral lacrimation when syringing the ear with warm or cold water

      (13) Ophthalmorhinostomatohygrosis syndrome

      (14) Reflex, such as vomiting or laughing

      (15) Myasthenia gravis—afternoon ectropion

   D. Symptomatic

      (1) Tabes

      (2) Thyrotoxicosis

2. Inadequacy of lacrimal drainage system

   A. Congenital anomalies of lacrimal apparatus

      (1) Unformed puncta

      (2) Absence or atresia of the canaliculi

      (3) Obstruction of nasolacrimal drainage system

      (4) Fistulas of lacrimal sac and nasolacrimal duct

      (5) Lateral displacement of medial canthi with lateral displacement of puncta and lengthening of canaliculi as in Waardenburg's syndrome

   B. Dacryocystitis

   C. Traumatic lesions of lacrimal drainage system

   D. Distended canaliculi with obstruction, such as from *Actinomyces israeli* (*Streptothrix foersteri*), papilloma, or dacryolith

   E. Obstruction caused by topical epinephrine

   F. Eversion of lower lacrimal punctum, including ectropion

   G. Tumor obstruction, including polyps, papillary hypertrophy, and neurofibromas

   H. Inadequacy of physiologic lacrimal pump

I. Complications from diseases such as pemphigus and Stevens-Johnson

J. Following use of strong miotics

3. Pseudoepiphora such as wound fistula following intraocular operation with leak of aqueous

Anderson, D. R.: Unilateral Epiphora Caused by Papilloma of the Lower Canaliculus. Arch. Ophthal. *78*:618, 1967.

Beard, C.: Affections of the Eyelids That Cause Tearing. *In* Veirs, E. R. (Ed.): The Lacrimal System: Proceedings of the First International Symposium. St. Louis, C. V. Mosby Co., 1971, pp. 37–50.

Duke-Elder, S., and Scott, G. I.: System of Ophthalmology, Vol. XII. St. Louis, C. V. Mosby Co., 1971, pp. 959–965.

Geeraets, W. J.: Ocular Syndromes. Philadelphia, Lea & Febiger, 1969, p. 231.

Howard, R. O., and Caldwell, J. B. H.: Congenital Fistula of the Lacrimal Sac. Amer. J. Ophthal. *67*:931, 1969.

Huber, A.: Eye Symptoms in Brain Tumors, 2nd ed. St. Louis, C. V. Mosby Co., 1971, pp. 11–12.

Jones, L. T.: Tear-Sac Foreign Bodies. Amer. J. Ophthal. *60*:111, 1965.

Jones, L. T.: The Lacrimal Secretory System and Its Treatment. Amer. J. Ophthal. *62*:47, 1966.

Jones, L. T., and Linn, M. L.: The Diagnosis of the Causes of Epiphoria. Amer. J. Ophthal. *67*:751, 1969.

La Piana, F. G.: Management of Occult Atretic Lacrimal Puncta. Amer. J. Ophthal. *74*:332–333, 1972.

Pico, G.: Congenital Anomalies of the Lacrimal System. *In* Veirs, E. R. (Ed.) Proceedings of the First International Symposium. St. Louis, C. V. Mosby Co., 1971, pp. 3–9.

Putterman, A. M.: Treatment of Epiphoria with Absent Lacrimal Puncta. Arch. Ophthal. *89*:125–127, 1973.

Richards, W. W.: Actinomycotic Lacrimal Canaliculitis. Amer. J. Ophthal. *75*:155–157, 1973.

Saunders, T. E.: The Lacrimal Gland. Symposium on Surgery of the Ocular Adnexa. Transactions of New Orleans Academy of Ophthalmology. St. Louis, C. V. Mosby Co., 1966, pp. 64–90.

Spaeth, G. L.: Nasolacrimal Duct Obstruction Caused by Topical Epinephrine. Arch. Ophthal. *77*:355, 1967.

Traisman, H. S., Alfano, J. E., and Salafsky, I.: Tear Duct Obstruction Associated with Malformations of the Hands and Feet. J. Pediat. Ophthal. *10*:200–203, 1973.

Walsh, F. B., and Hoyt, W. F.: Clinical Neuro-ophthalmology, 3rd ed. Baltimore, Williams & Wilkins Co., 1969, pp. 339, 555–562.

Dry Eye (paucity or absence of tears)

1. Xerosis—local tissue changes
   A. Cicatricial degeneration of conjunctiva and mucous tissues (see p. 170)
      (1) General: diphtheria
      (2) Upper lid: trachoma
      (3) Lower lid:
         a. Erythema multiforme (Stevens-Johnson syndrome)
         b. Reiter's syndrome
         c. Ocular pemphigoid
         d. Chemical irritation (especially due to alkali)
         e. Radium burns
         f. Vaccinia
         g. Dermatitis herpetiformis
         h. Epidermolysis bullosa
         i. Sjögren's syndrome
         j. Avitaminosis A
   B. Exposure keratitis
      (1) Ocular proptosis as in exophthalmos
      (2) Deficient lid closure as part of facial palsy
      (3) Levator spasm
      (4) Ectropion (see p. 69)
      (5) Lack of blinking as during coma
      (6) Rapid evaporation in hot, dry areas
      (7) Stiff, immobile, retracted lids, such as those occurring secondary to tuberculoid leprosy
      (8) Infrequent blinking such as with progressive supranuclear palsy
      (9) Melkersson-Rosenthal syndrome—recurrent facial paralysis, facial edema, furrowed tongue

2. Keratoconjunctivitis sicca—primary tear diminution of main and accessory lacrimal glands
   A. Congenital
      (1) Congenital absence of lacrimal gland as in Bonnevie-Ullrich syndrome
      (2) Neurogenic

       (3) Associated with generalized disturbance
          a. Anhidrotic type of ectodermal dysplasia
          b. Familial dysautonomia (Riley-Day syndrome)
          c. Cri du chat syndrome (crying cat syndrome)
             —short arm deletion of chromosome 5, strabismus, decreased tearing, hypertelorism, tortuosity of retinal vessels

B. Neurogenic hyposecretion
       (1) Central—aplasia of lacrimal nucleus or lesion of seventh nerve between nucleus and geniculate ganglion
          a. Pontine lesions
          b. Basal fractures
          c. Otitis media
       (2) Peripheral—greater superficial petrosal nerve, sphenopalatine ganglion, or lacrimal branch
          a. Skull fractures
          b. Associated with neoplasms
          c. Neurologic lesion of fifth nerve (neuroparalytic keratitis)
       (3) Herpes zoster of the geniculate ganglion (Ramsey Hunt syndrome)
       (4) Parasympathetic blocking drugs, such as atropine and scopolamine, may decrease an already barely adequate secretion
       (5) Botulism
       (6) Deep anesthesia
       (7) Debilitating diseases such as typhus and cholera, and high temperature
       (8) Allergy

C. Systemic disease
       (1) Gougerot-Sjögren syndrome—postmenopausal women, rheumatoid arthritis. May be associated with malignant lymphoma, chronic thyroiditis, familial amyloidosis, or pancreatitis
       (2) Rheumatoid arthritis
       (3) Mikulicz's syndrome—dacryoadenitis and parotitis (see p. 86)
          a. Tuberculosis
          b. Leukemia

       c. Lymphosarcoma

       d. Sarcoidosis

       e. Hodgkin's disease

       f. Lymphoma

   (4) Disseminated lupus erythematosus

   (5) Scleroderma

   (6) Polyarteritis nodosa

   (7) Pheochromocytoma, medullary thyroid carcinoma, and multiple mucosal neuromas

D. Toxic

   (1) Side effects of antihistamines and nasal decongestants

   (2) Deep anesthesia

   (3) Debilitating diseases

Barsam, P. C., Sampson, W. G., and Feldman, G. L.: Treatment of Dry Eye and Related Problems. Ann. Ophthal. *4*:122–133, 1972.

Baum, J. L., and Adler, M. E.: Pheochromocytoma, Medullary Thyroid Carcinoma and Multiple Mucosal Neuroma. Arch. Ophthal. *87*:574–584, 1972.

Duke-Elder, S.: System of Ophthalmology, Vol. VIII, Part 1. St. Louis, C. V. Mosby Co., 1965, pp. 128–138, 593.

Duke-Elder, S., and Leigh, A. G.: System of Ophthalmology, Vol. VIII, Part 2. St. Louis, C. V. Mosby Co., 1965, p. 802.

Duke-Elder, S., and Scott, G. I.: System of Ophthalmology, Vol. XII. St. Louis, C. V. Mosby Co., 1971, pp. 966–969.

Geeraets, W. J.: Ocular Syndromes. Philadelphia, Lea & Febiger, 1969, p. 139.

Hallett, J. W., and Mitchell, B.: Melkersson-Rosenthal Syndrome. Amer. J. Ophthal. *65*:542, 1968.

Howard, R. O.: Familial Dysautonomia (Riley-Day Syndrome). Amer. J. Ophthal. *64*:392, 1967.

Howard, R. O.: Ocular Abnormalities in the Cri du Chat Syndrome. Amer. J. Ophthal. *73*:949–954, 1973.

Jones, L. T.: The Lacrimal Secretory System and Its Treatment. Amer. J. Ophthal. *62*:47, 1966.

Kuming, B. S., and Politzer, W. M.: Xerophthalmia and Protein Malnutrition in Bantu Children. Brit J. Ophthal. *51*:649, 1967.

Newell, F. W.: Ophthalmology, Principles and Concepts. St. Louis, C. V. Mosby Co., 1969, p. 171.

Pfaffenbach, D. D., Layton, D. D., and Kearns, T. P.: Ocular Manifestations in Progressive Supranuclear Palsy. Amer. J. Ophthal. *74*:1179–1189, 1972.

Taylor, R.: Modern Treatment of Severe "Shrinkage of the Conjunctiva." Brit. J. Ophthal. *51*:31–43, 1967.

Dacryocystitis (infection of the lacrimal sac)

1. Acute dacryocystitis
   A. Beta-hemolytic streptococcus
   B. *Staphylococcus aureus*
   C. Pneumococcus
   D. Influenza
   E. Friedländer's bacillus
   F. *Pseudomonas aeruginosa*
   G. *Haemophilus aegyptius* (Koch-Weeks bacillus)
   H. *Neisseria catarrhalis*
   I. *Serratia marcescens*—gram-negative coccibacillus
   J. Other microorganisms

2. Chronic dacryocystitis
   A. Tuberculosis
   B. Syphilis
   C. Trachoma
   D. *Actinomyces israeli,* Aspergillus, *Candida albicans,* and *Nocardia asteroides*
   E. *Escherichia coli* and *Proteus vulgaris*
   F. *Bacillus fusiformis* and *Treponema vincenti*
   G. Systemic sarcoidosis
   H. Other microorganisms or disease

Bedrossian, E. H.: The Eye. Springfield, Ill., Charles C Thomas, 1958, p. 165.
Bigger, J. F., et al.: Serratia marcescens Endophthalmitis. Amer. J. Ophthal. 72:1102–1105, 1971.
Chatterjee, B. M., Chatterjee, S., and Barua, D.: Spirochetal Infection of the Canaliculus. Arch. Ophthal. 66:649, 1961.
Coleman, S. L., Brull, S., and Green, W. R.: Sarcoid of the Lacrimal Sac and Surrounding Area. Arch. Ophthal. 88:645–646, 1972.
Fedukowicz, H. B.: External Infections of the Eye. New York, Appleton-Century-Crofts, Inc., 1963.
Newton, J. C., and Tuleveck, C. B.: Lacrimal Canaliculitis Due to Candida albicans. Amer. J. Ophthal. 53:933, 1962.
Penikett, E. J. K., and Rees, D. L.: Nocardia asteroides Infection of the Nasolacrimal System. Amer. J. Ophthal. 53:1006, 1961.

EXTRAOCULAR MUSCLES

Contents

Pseudoesotropia (an ocular appearance of esotropia when no manifest deviation of the visual axis is present)

1. Prominent epicanthal fold
2. Negative angle kappa—pupillary light reflex displaced temporally
3. Telecanthus—the orbits are normally placed, but the medial canthi are far apart secondary to lateral displacement of the soft tissues
4. Abnormal shape of skull or abnormal thickness of skin surrounding the orbits
5. Lateral displacement of the concavity of the upper eyelid margin from the center of the pupil
6. Hypotelorism with narrow interpupillary distance
7. Entropion
8. Enophthalmos

Aita, J. A.: Congenital Facial Anomalies with Neurologic Defects. Springfield, Ill., Charles C Thomas, 1969.

Shaterian, E. T., and Weissman, I. L.: An Unusual Case of Pseudostrabismus. Amer. Orthopt. J. *23*:68–70, 1973.

Urist, M. J.: Pseudostrabismus Caused by Abnormal Configuration of the Upper Eyelid Margins. Amer. J. Ophthal. *75*:455–456, 1973.

Von Noorden, G. K., and Maumenee, A. E.: Atlas of Strabismus, 2nd ed. St. Louis, C. V. Mosby Co., 1973, pp. 29–36.

Eso- (visual axis deviated inward; may be latent or manifest)

1. Esophoria—tendency for one eye to turn inward
2. Esotropia—manifest inward deviation of an eye, "crossed eyes," convergent strabismus

3. Non-paralytic (comitant)—angle of deviation is constant in all directions of gaze
    A. Accommodative—hyperopic refractive error
    B. Non-accommodative—refractive error not cause of deviation
        (1) Anomalous insertion of horizontally acting muscles
        (2) Abnormal check ligaments
        (3) Faulty innervational development
        (4) Autosomal dominant trait
        (5) Idiopathic

4. Paralytic (non-comitant) abducens palsy—the angle of deviation varies in different directions of gaze (see sixth nerve palsy, p. 139)

5. V esotropia—deviation greater in downward gaze
    A. Underaction—superior oblique muscles
    B. May be associated with mongoloid obliquity to the lids

6. A esotropia
    A. Underaction—inferior oblique muscles
    B. May be associated with antimongoloid obliquity to the lids

7. Alternating esotropia—either eye may be used with facility

8. Monocular esotropia—one eye may be used to the exclusion of the other; amblyopia is usual in the deviating eye

9. High AC/A ratio—greater convergence for near than for distance, causing greater esodeviation for near than for distance
    A. Age—gradually improves after eighth birthday
    B. Optical corrections (ametropic lens correction, bifocals, and prisms within the spectacle lens)—do not permanently alter high AC/A ratio
    C. Orthoptics—do not alter ratio
    D. Parasympathomimetic drugs (miotics) improve ratio while the effect lasts
    E. Surgery—permanently alters ratio

10. Convergence excess—greater esodeviation for near than for distance

11. Divergence insufficiency—greater esodeviation for near than for distance

Parks, M. M.: Horizontal Deviations (Course 58, 1973). Instruction Section, American Academy of Ophthalmology and Otolaryngology.
Sears, M., and Guber, D.: The Change in the Stimulus AC/A Ratio after Surgery. Amer. J. Ophthal. 64:872–876, 1967.
Vaughan, D., Cook, R., and Asbury, T.: General Ophthalmology. Los Altos, Lange Medical Publications, 1971.
Von Noorden, G. K., and Maumenee, A. E.: Atlas of Strabismus, 2nd ed. St. Louis, C. V. Mosby Co., 1973, pp. 162–170.

Pseudoexotropia (an ocular appearance of exotropia when no manifest deviation of the visual axis is present)

1. Hypertelorism with wide interpupillary distance

2. Positive angle kappa—pupillary light reflex displaced nasally

3. Exophthalmos

4. Narrow lateral canthus

5. Wide palpebral fissure

6. Displaced macula which may be the result of retrolental fibroplasia

7. Heterochromia when the lighter colored eye appears to diverge

Lyle, T. K., and Wybar, K. C.: Lyle and Jackson's Practical Orthoptics in the Treatment of Squint. Springfield, Ill., Charles C Thomas, 1967, pp. 335–336.
Shaterian, E. T., and Weissman, I. L.: An Unusual Case of Pseudostrabismus. Amer. Orthopt. J. 23:68–70, 1973.
Von Noorden, G. K., and Maumenee, A. E.: Atlas of Strabismus, 2nd ed. St. Louis, C. V. Mosby Co., 1973, pp. 29–36.

Exo- (visual axis deviated outward—may be latent or manifest)

1. Exophoria—tendency for one eye to turn outward
2. Exotropia—manifest outward deviation of an eye, "wall eyes," divergent strabismus
3. Intermittent exotropia—alternates from exophoria to exotropia
4. Constant exotropia—deviation always present
5. Refractive—myopic refractive error cause of deviation
6. Non-refractive—refractive error not cause of deviation
   A. Anomalous insertion of horizontally acting muscles
   B. Abnormal check ligaments
   C. Faulty innervational development
   D. Autosomal dominant trait
   E. Idiopathic
7. V exotropia—deviation greater in upward than in downward gaze
   A. Underaction—superior oblique muscles
   B. Underaction—superior rectus muscle
   C. Inferior oblique muscle with short tendon sheath
   D. May be associated with mongoloid obliquity to the lids
8. A exotropia—deviation greater in downward than in upward gaze
   A. Underaction—inferior rectus muscles
   B. Underaction—inferior oblique muscles
   C. May be associated with antimongoloid obliquity to the lids
9. Low AC/A ratio—less convergence for near than for distance, causing greater exodeviation for near than for distance
   A. Myopic refractive error that is increasing—further lowers AC/A ratio; glasses help correct ratio
   B. Exodeviation in infants and children—further lowers AC/A ratio; operation helps to correct ratio
   C. Age—does not alter low AC/A ratio

D. Optical corrections (ametropic lens correction, bifocals, and prisms within the spectacle lens)—do not alter low AC/A ratio

E. Orthoptics—do not alter ratio

F. Parasympatholytic drugs (cycloplegics)—improve ratio while the effect lasts

G. Surgery—permanently alters ratio

10. Divergence excess—greater exodeviation for distance than for near

11. Convergence insufficiency—greater exodeviation for near than for distance

12. Internuclear ophthalmoplegia—paralysis of medial rectus muscles on attempted conjugate lateral gaze without evidence of third nerve paralysis due to involvement of medial longitudinal fasciculus (see ophthalmoplegia, p. 147)

13. Oculomotor palsy (see third nerve, p. 134)

Lyle, T. K., and Wybar, K. C.: Lyle and Jackson's Practical Orthoptics in the Treatment of Squint. Springfield, Ill., Charles C Thomas, 1967, pp. 335–336.

Parks, M. M.: Horizontal Deviations (Course 58, 1973). Instruction Section, American Academy of Ophthalmology and Otolaryngology.

Urist, M. J.: A- and V-Patterns in Isolated Vertical Muscle Palsies. Amer. J. Ophthal. *68*:1095, 1969.

Vaughan, D., Cook, R., and Asbury, T.: General Ophthalmology. Los Altos, Lange Medical Publications, 1971.

Von Noorden, G. K., and Maumenee, A. E.: Atlas of Strabismus, 2nd ed. St. Louis, C. V. Mosby Co., 1973, pp. 162–170.

Pseudohypertropia

1. Facial asymmetry with one eye placed higher than the other

2. Unilateral ptosis

3. Unilateral coloboma

Shaterian, E. T., and Weissman, I. L.: An Unusual Case of Pseudo-strabismus. Amer. Orthopt. J. *23*:68–70, 1973.

Hyper- (visual axis deviated upward, may be manifest or latent)

1. Hyperphoria—tendency for one eye to turn upward
2. Hypertropia—manifest upward deviation of an eye
3. Non-paralytic hypertropia
   A. Abnormal insertion of muscles
   B. Abnormal fascial attachments
   C. Complications of systemic diseases, such as myasthenia gravis, multiple sclerosis, thyrotoxicosis, orbital tumors, and brain stem disease
4. Paralytic hypertropia—isolated cyclovertical muscle palsy

Greater Vertical		Head Tilt	Under Action
Right Hypertropia	Right Gaze	Right greater	LIO
		Left greater	RIR
	Left Gaze	Right greater	RSO
		Left greater	LSR
Left Hypertropia	Right Gaze	Right greater	RSR
		Left greater	LSO
	Left Gaze	Right greater	LIR
		Left greater	RIO

5. Double hyperphoria (alternating sursumduction)—fuses but cover test shows alternating hyperphoria
6. Apparent paralysis of elevation of one eye
   A. Local neuromuscular and orbital causes
      (1) Dysthyroid ophthalmoplegia (non-congestive and congestive form)

105

(2) Myasthenia gravis
(3) Orbital floor fracture
(4) Abiotropic ophthalmoplegia (progressive nuclear ophthalmoplegia)
(5) Superior division, oculomotor nerve paresis
(6) Unilateral double elevator palsy, congenital absence of superior rectus and inferior oblique muscles
(7) Myositis
   a. "Collagen diseases"
   b. Infectious myositis
   c. Trichinosis
(8) Systemic amyloidosis with ocular muscle infiltration
(9) Vertical retraction syndrome
(10) Superior oblique tendon sheath syndrome (Brown's)

B. Skew deviation due to a central nervous system lesion —one eye is above the other; may be the same for all directions of gaze or vary in different directions of gaze
   (1) Unilateral labyrinthine disease
   (2) Cerebellar tumors, such as astrocytomas and medulloblastomas
   (3) Acoustic neuromas
   (4) Vascular accidents of pons and cerebellum, such as thrombosis of cerebellar and pontine arteries
   (5) Unilateral internuclear ophthalmoplegia (see internuclear ophthalmoplegia, p. 147) and less frequently bilateral internuclear ophthalmoplegia
   (6) Compressive lesions, such as platybasia and Arnold-Chiari malformation
   (7) Brain stem arteriovenous malformations

C. Central nervous system lesions
   (1) Arteriosclerosis, thrombosis, arteritis (syphilitic), or embolus of fine vessels to midbrain

7. Apparent paralysis of elevation of both eyes
   A. Physiologic in older individuals

B. Parinaud's syndrome—paralysis of vertical gaze due to lesion of superior colliculus, such as pineal gland tumor

C. Nuclear aplasia

D. Progressive supranuclear palsy

8. Paralysis of downward gaze
    A. Reverse Parinaud's syndrome
    B. Associated with choreo-athetotic syndromes
    C. Parkinsonoid syndromes
    D. Miscellaneous

Cogan, D. G.: Neurology of the Ocular Muscles, 2nd ed. Springfield, Ill., Charles C Thomas, 1969, pp. 134–135.

Cogan, D. G.: Paralysis of Down Gaze. Arch. Ophthal. *91*:192–199, 1974.

Jampel, R. S., and Fells, P.: Monocular Elevation Paresis Caused by a Central Nervous System Lesion. Arch. Ophthal. *80:45*, 1968.

Lessell, S., et al.: Brain Stem Arteriovenous Malformations. Arch. Ophthal. *86*:255–259, 1971.

Parks, M. M.: Isolated Cyclovertical Muscle Palsy. Arch. Ophthal. *60*:1027–1035, 1958.

Pfaffenbach, D. D., Layton, D. D., and Kearns, T. P.: Ocular Manifestations in Progressive Supranuclear Palsy. Amer. J. Ophthal. *74*: 1179–1189, 1972.

Vaughan, D., Cook, R., and Asbury, T.: General Ophthalmology. Los Altos, Lange Medical Publications, 1971.

Von Noorden, G. K., and Maumenee, A. E.: Atlas of Strabismus, 2nd ed. St. Louis, C. V. Mosby Co., 1973, pp. 154–160.

Walsh, F. B., and Hoyt, W. F.: Clinical Neuro-ophthalmology, 3rd ed. Baltimore, Williams & Wilkins Co., 1969.

Brown's Superior Oblique Tendon Sheath Syndrome (limitation of elevation in adduction that resembles an underaction of inferior oblique muscle)

1. Shortening of the tendon of the superior oblique so that the thickened superior oblique muscle is closer to the trochlea and acts as a ball and socket, being unable to pass through the trochlea

2. Thickening of the tendon resulting in impaired slippage through the trochlea

3. Anomalous insertion of the superior oblique muscle

4. Acquired superior oblique tendon sheath syndrome in which a tuck of the superior oblique medial to the superior rectus muscle restricts ocular movement

5. An innervational abnormality in which the inferior oblique and the superior oblique are simultaneously innervated in the field of gaze of the inferior oblique (electromyography)

Billet, E.: Superior Fascial Syndrome. J. Pediat. Ophthal. 4:47–51, 1967.

Brown, W. H.: Superior Oblique Tendon Sheath Syndrome. Strabismus Ophthalmic Symposium. St. Louis, C. V. Mosby Co., 1950, p. 219.

Goldstein, J. H.: Intermittent Superior Oblique Tendon Sheath Syndrome. Amer. J. Ophthal. 67:960–962, 1969.

Sanford-Smith, J. H.: Intermittent Superior Oblique Tendon Sheath Syndrome: A Case Report. Brit. J. Ophthal. 53:412–417, 1969.

Monocular Limitation of Elevation of the Adducted Eye with Forced Duction Test (in elevation and adduction)

Restricted	Unrestricted
A. Brown's syndrome of superior oblique tendon sheath: congenitally short superior oblique tendon sheath	A. Paresis of inferior oblique muscle such as impaired innervation (nuclear or infranuclear) or contractility of inferior oblique
B. Simulated Brown's syndrome	B. Pseudoparesis of inferior oblique muscle

Restricted

A. Brown's syndrome of superior oblique tendon sheath: congenitally short superior oblique tendon sheath
B. Simulated Brown's syndrome
   1. Congenital anomalous insertion of the superior oblique tendon
   2. Congenital anomalous check ligament from lateral orbit to insertion of inferior oblique
   3. Swelling of the superior oblique tendon restricting passage through the trochlea
   4. Infection in the region of the trochlea
   5. Shortening of the superior oblique tendon by a tuck procedure
   6. Scar produced by superior nasal quadrant operation
   7. Congenital or acquired restrictions affecting inferior orbital tissues, such as blow-out fracture

Unrestricted

A. Paresis of inferior oblique muscle such as impaired innervation (nuclear or infranuclear) or contractility of inferior oblique
B. Pseudoparesis of inferior oblique muscle
   1. Subtle mechanical restriction affecting superior oblique tendon or sheath, or affecting inferior orbital tissues
   2. Supranuclear innervation defect

Zipf, R. F., and Trokel, S. L.: Simulated Superior Oblique Tendon Sheath Syndrome Following Orbital Floor Fracture. Amer. J. Ophthal. 75:700–705, 1973.

Strabismus with Restricted Motility

1. Congenital
   A. Retraction such as in Duane's retraction syndrome
   B. Adherence such as in Johnson's adherence syndrome
   C. Sheath syndromes such as Brown's superior oblique tendon sheath syndrome
   D. Strabismus fixus
   E. Neurogenic paralysis with or without secondary contracture of antagonist muscle

2. Acquired
   A. Strabismus complicated by adhesions
   B. Orbital fracture
   C. Retinal detachment operation
   D. Excessive recession or resection of muscle
   E. Clipped muscle

Dunlap, E. A.: Use of Plastic Implants in the Management of Restricted Motility Resulting from Adhesions. *In* Manley, D. R. (Ed.): Symposium on Horizontal Ocular Deviations. St. Louis, C. V. Mosby Co., 1971, pp. 111–116.

Cyclic Strabismus (regularly recurring manifest strabismus that follows a rhythmic pattern, often appearing on alternate days)

1. Oculomotor paralysis

2. Esotropia
   A. Non-comitant
   B. Comitant

Levy, M. R.: Cyclic Oculomotor Paralysis with Optic Atrophy. Amer. J. Ophthal. 65:766–769, 1968.
Windsor, C. E., and Berg, E. F. : Circadian Heterotropia. Amer. J. Ophthal. 67:565–571, 1969.

Cyclic, Recurrent, Repetitive, Episodic Disorders of Extraocular Muscles

1. Myasthenia gravis

2. Alternate day esotropia (circadian heterotropia)

3. Alternate day vertical strabismus

4. Oculogyric crisis (see p. 133)

5. Diabetic nerve palsies

6. Petit mal epilepsy
   A. Upward deviation
   B. Exotropia

7. Periodic vertical nystagmus
   A. Familial
   B. Associated with potassium abnormality

8. Cyclic third nerve palsy (see pp. 134–136)

9. Twitch of lids (orbicularis)

10. Recurrent "fits" of superior oblique muscle (superior oblique myokymia)

11. Recurrent sixth nerve paralysis in children (see p. 141)

12. Spasmus nutans

Hoyt, W. F., and Keane, J. R.: Superior Oblique Myokymia. Arch. Ophthal. *84*:461–467, 1970.
Scott, A.: Ocular Motility. Stanford Course. 1972.
Windsor, C. E., and Berg, E. F.: Circadian Heterotropia. Amer. J. Ophthal. *67*:565–571, 1969.

Syndromes Associated with Strabismus*

1. Albright's hereditary osteodystrophy (pseudohypoparathyroidism): strabismus, refractory end-organ to parathyroid hormone with hypocalcemia and hyperphosphatemia

2. Apert's syndrome (acrocephalosyndactylic syndrome): strabismus, nystagmus, exophthalmos, slant fissure, field defect, keratitis, optic atrophy—syndactylia

3. Bloch-Sulzberger disease (incontinentia pigmenti): strabismus, nystagmus, cataract, optic nerve involvement—bullous skin eruptions and pigmentations

4. Crouzon's disease (craniofacial dysostosis): nystagmus, strabismus, exophthalmos, visual loss, anterior segment involvement—prognathism, maxillar atrophy, deformity of anterior fontanel

5. Cytomegalic inclusion disease, congenital: strabismus, failure to thrive, mental retardation, microcephaly, chorioretinitis, and seizures

6. Down's disease (mongolism, trisomy 21): strabismus, epicanthal folds, oblique palpebral fissures, protruding tongue, open mouth, mental retardation, muscular hypotonia

7. Ehlers-Danlos disease (fibrodysplasia elastica generalisata): hypotony of extraocular muscles, strabismus, ptosis, hyperelastic skin, thin sclera and cornea, keratoconus, subluxated lens, retinopathy—cutaneous hyperelasticity, atrophic skin, excessive articular laxity

8. Ellis-van Crefeld syndrome (chondroectodermal dysplasia): internal strabismus, congenital cataract, iris coloboma—polydactylia, skeletal and genital anomalies, congenital heart defects (50%)

9. Erb-Goldflam disease (myasthenia gravis): strabismus, ptosis, diplopia—myasthenia gravis, muscle weakness

*This section from Geeraets (pp. 234–235), with modifications.

10. Hallermann-Streiff syndrome (oculomandibulodyscephaly): nystagmus, strabismus, cataract, microphthalmia—malformations of skeleton, teeth anomalies, mental retardation

11. Hemifacial microsomia (otomandibular dysostosis): strabismus, microphthalmos, iris and choroidal colobomas—microtia, macrostomia, failure of development of mandibular ramus and condyle

12. Hurler's disease (mucopolysaccharidosis [MPS] type I): strabismus, ptosis, corneal opacity, optic nerve and retinal involvement—retarded development, dorsolumbar kyphosis, head deformities

13. Hydrocephalus, congenital: strabismus, increased head size, protruding eyes with deficiency in upward gaze, poor motor development, neurologic abnormalities, and mental retardation

14. Laurence-Moon-Bardet-Biedl syndrome: nystagmus, strabismus, ophthalmoplegia, visual field defect, optic nerve and retinal involvement—obesity, hypogenitalism, polydactylia, mental deficiency

15. Marfan's syndrome (dystrophia mesodermalis congenita): nystagmus, strabismus, anterior segment and lens involvement—arachnodactylia, congenital heart defect, relaxed ligaments

16. Millard-Gubler syndrome; paralysis of sixth nerve, diplopia, strabismus—hemiplegia of arm and leg

17. Naegeli's syndrome (melanophoric nevus syndrome): nystagmus, strabismus, papillitis, pseudoglioma—keratosis, pigmentary skin changes

18. Nevoid basal cell carcinoma syndrome: strabismus, nevoid basal cell carcinomas, jaw cysts, cataracts, glaucoma, coloboma, chalazions

19. Parry-Romberg disease (progressive facial hemiatrophy): strabismus, enophthalmos, Horner's syndrome, ptosis, miosis —facial hemiatrophy (loss of subcutaneous tissue)

20. Pierre Robin syndrome: strabismus, micrognathia, glossoptosis, cleft palate, respiratory distress

21. Prader-Willi syndrome (hypotonia-obesity syndrome): strabismus, obesity, hypogonadism, short stature, hypotonia, mental retardation, diabetes mellitus

22. Pseudohypoparathyroidism (Seabright-Bantam syndrome): strabismus—obesity, short stature, tetany, mental retardation

23. Ring chromosome 18: strabismus, ptosis, mental retardation, microcephaly, low-set ears, deafness

24. Rubella, congenital: strabismus, congenital heart disease, deafness, microphthalmos, cataracts, glaucoma, mental/motor retardation

25. Rubinstein-Taybi syndrome: strabismus, antimongoloid slant of lid fissure, epicanthus, high-arched brows, refractive error—broad thumbs and toes, abnormal facial features, motor and mental retardation

26. Smith-Lemli-Opitz syndrome: strabismus, ptosis, mental retardation, skeletal and genital abnormalities, epicanthal folds

27. Supravalvular aortic stenosis syndrome (infantile hypercalcemia with mental retardation): strabismus, infantile hypercalcemia, supravalvular aortic stenosis, mental retardation, "elfin-like" facies

28. Turner's syndrome (gonadal dysgenesis): strabismus, short stature, webbing and/or shortening of neck, absence of secondary sexual characteristics, broad bridge of nose, epicanthal folds, low-set ears

29. GML—Gangliosidosis: esotropia, nystagmus, optic atrophy, large head, coarse features, hypotonia, peripheral edema

30. Francois' dyscephalic syndrome: dyscephaly with bird-like head, dental anomalies, proportional dwarfism, microphthalmos, congenital cataracts, nystagmus

31. Seckel's bird-headed dwarfism: microcephaly; narrow, beaked nose; narrow face; mental retardation

32. De Lange's syndrome: synophrys and telecanthus, blue sclera, strabismus, nystagmus, myopia, ptosis

33. Leigh's disease (subacute necrotizing encephalomyelopathy)

34. Chromosome 18 short arm deletion: webbed neck, ptosis, cataracts, hypertelorism, strabismus

35. Noonan's syndrome (male Turner's syndrome): antimongoloid slant, hypertelorism, epicanthal folds, exophthalmos, high myopia, keratoconus, posterior embryotoxon

36. Chromosome 18 partial short arm deletion syndrome (Wolf's syndrome): iris and/or retinal coloboma, hypertelorism, epicanthus, strabismus, microcephaly, hydrocephalus, seizures

37. Nevus sebaceous of Jadassohn: antimongoloid lid; dermoid limbus; coloboma of iris-choroid; nystagmus; external oculomotor palsy, unilateral; thickening of bones of orbit; coloboma of lids

38. Craniocarpotarsal dysplasia (Freeman-Sheldon syndrome; whistling face syndrome): antimongoloid lid fissures, esotropia, mild ptosis, high-arched skull, protruding lips as in whistling, receding chin, high-arched palate

39. Cri du chat syndrome (crying cat syndrome): short arm deletion of chromosome 5, strabismus, decreased tearing, hypertelorism, tortuosity of retinal vessels

40. Maple syrup urine disease: nystagmus, cataracts, epicanthal folds, strabismus

Emery, J. M., et al.: GML—Gangliosidosis: Ocular and Pathological Manifestations. Arch. Ophthal. 85:177–187, 1971.

Francois, J., and Pierard, J.: The Francois Dyscephalic Syndrome and Skin Manifestations. Amer. J. Ophthal. 71:1241–1250, 1971.

Geeraets, W. J.: Ocular Syndromes. Philadelphia, Lea & Febiger, 1969, pp. 234–235.

Gellis, S. S., and Feingold, M.: Atlas of Mental Retardation. Washington, D.C., U.S. Government Printing Office, 1968.

Goodman, R. M., and Gorlin, R. J.: The Face in Genetic Disorders. St. Louis, C. V. Mosby Co., 1970, pp. 38, 46, 146.

Haslam, R. H., and Wirtschafter, J. D.: Unilateral External Oculomotor Nerve Palsy and Nevus Sebaceous of Jadassohn. Arch. Ophthal. 87:293–300, 1972.

Howard, R. O.: Ocular Abnormalities in the Cri du Chat Syndrome. Amer. J. Ophthal. 73:949–954, 1973.

Howard, R. O., and Albert, D. H.: Ocular Manifestations of Subacute Necrotizing Encephalomyelopathy (Leigh's Disease). Arch. Ophthal. *86*:386–393, 1972.

Johnson, R. V., and Kennedy, W. R.: Progressive Facial Hemiatrophy (Parry-Romberg Syndrome). Amer. J. Ophthal. *67*:561, 1969.

Levenson, J. E., Crandall, B. F., and Sparkes, R. S.: Partial Deletion Syndromes of Chromosome 18. Ann. Ophthal. *3*:756–760, 1971.

Milot, J., and Denoy, F.: Ocular Anomalies in De Lange Syndrome. Arch. Ophthal. *74*:394–399, 1972.

Roy, F. H., Dungan, T., and Inlaw, C.: Infantile Hypercalcemia and Supravalvular Stenosis. J. Pediat. Ophthal. *8*:188–194, 1971.

Roy, F. H., and Kelly, M. L.: Maple Syrup Urine Disease. J. Pediat. Ophthal. *10*:70–73, 1973.

Schwartz, D. E.: Noonan's Syndrome Associated with Ocular Abnormalities. Amer. J. Ophthal. *73*:955–960, 1972.

Horizontal Gaze Palsy (inability to look horizontally in a given direction. Analysis includes optically induced movement, voluntary or command movement, pursuit movement, or vestibular movement.)

1. Horizontal palsy of voluntary and command movement—frontal lobe gaze center (second frontal gyrus, Brodmann's area 8) or in the corresponding internal capsule gaze palsy of side opposite lesion. May be associated with facial palsy as well as hemiparesis or hemiplegia toward the side of the gaze palsy

2. Horizontal palsy of command and pursuit movements, optically induced movements, and vestibular movements—pons and posterior longitudinal bundle. The gaze palsy is toward the side of the lesion.

Huber, A.: Eye Symptoms in Brain Tumors, 2nd ed. St. Louis, C. V. Mosby Co., 1971, pp. 44–47.

Oscillations of the Eyes (involuntary, rapid, to-and-fro movement of the eyes having no rhythm or regularity)

1. *Ocular dysmetria*—"overshooting" of the eyes with attempted fixation; horizontal ocular dysmetria is associated with lesions of the cerebellum or its pathways as in limb ataxia

2. *Ocular flutter*—flutter-like oscillations, which are intermittent, rapid, to-and-fro motions, or motions of equal amplitude, interrupt maintained fixation; horizontal ocular flutter is associated with lesions of the cerebellum or its pathways as in limb ataxia, multiple sclerosis, poliomyelitis, neoplasms, or vascular accident

3. *Opsoclonia*—irregular, hyperkinetic, multidirectional spontaneous eye movement
   A. Associated with body tremulousness, and with benign encephalitis
   B. Associated with occult tumor such as neuroblastoma, bronchogenic carcinoma, or breast malignancy
   C. Sign of "myoclonic encephalopathy of infancy"
   D. Associated with severe brain stem involvement, such as that occurring with vascular accident or with severe encephalitis; continuous vertical or horizontal opsoclonia often is noted in unconscious patients
   E. Vertebrobasilar insufficiency
   F. Associated with multiple sclerosis or Friedreich's ataxia

4. *Lightning eye movements* (ocular myoclonus)—rapid, to-and-fro movements of small conjugate saccades; probably due to bilateral abnormality of pontine paramedial zone and pretectal lesions, such as vascular, inflammatory, neoplastic, demyelinating, or traumatic, of tegmentum

Atkins, A., and Bender, M. B.: "Lightning Eye Movements" (Ocular Myoclonus). J. Neurol. Sci. *1*:2–12, 1964.
Bricket, B., et al.: EMG Study of Opsoclonus Occurring in Vertebrobasilar Insufficiency. Electroenceph. Clin. Neurophysiol. *29*: 534, 1970.

5

Blenfang, D. C.: Opsoclonus in Infancy. Arch. Ophthal. *91*:203–205, 1974.

Cogan, D. G.: Ocular Dysmetria, Flutter-like Oscillations of the Eyes, and Opsoclonus. Arch. Ophthal. *51*:318–335, 1954.

Cogan, D. G.: Opsoclonus, Body Tremulousness and Benign Encephalitis. Arch. Ophthal. *79*:545, 1968.

Duke-Elder, S., and Scott, G. I.: System of Ophthalmology, Vol. XII. St. Louis, C. V. Mosby Co., 1971, pp. 851 and 858.

Kinsbourne, M.: Myoclonic Encephalopathy of Infants. J. Neurol. Neurosurg. Psychiat. *25*:271–276, 1959.

Lesser, R. L., et al.: Vertical Ocular Dysmetria. Amer. J. Ophthal. *76*:208–211, 1973.

Sandok, B. A., and Kranz, H.: Opsoclonus as the Initial Manifestation of Occult Neuroblastoma. Arch. Ophthal. *86*:235–236, 1971.

Cogwheel Eye Movements (jerky inaccurate pursuit movements)

1. Basal ganglia disease
   A. Idiopathic
   B. Drug intoxications
   C. Exposure to manganese
   D. Carbon monoxide poisoning
   E. Carbon disulfide poisoning
   F. Anoxia
   G. Trauma
   H. Parkinsonism

2. Cerebellar tumors
   A. Astrocytomas
   B. Medulloblastomas
   C. Hemangioblastomas

3. With homonymous hemianopia, indicates parietal or occipital lobe involvement

Huber, A.: Eye Symptoms in Brain Tumors, 2nd ed. St. Louis, C. V. Mosby Co., 1971, p. 49.

Walsh, F. B., and Hoyt, W. F.: Clinical Neuro-ophthalmology, 3rd ed. Baltimore, Williams & Wilkins Co., 1969, pp. 212–213, 1005–1006, 2207–2213.

Pendular Nystagmus (oscillations that are approximately equal in rate in two directions—may be horizontal or vertical)

1. Bilateral chorioretinal lesions involving the macula in early infancy
2. Albinism in which the macula does not develop
3. Aniridia
4. Total color blindness (monochromatism)
5. High myopia of early life
6. Congenital cataracts
7. Corneal scars
8. Work in poor illumination (e.g., mining)
9. Laurence-Moon-Biedl syndrome—optic nerve and retinal involvement, obesity, hypogenitalism, polydactylia, mental deficiency
10. Congenital—cause unknown, may be inherited as autosomal dominant or sex-linked recessive trait; not infrequently associated with astigmatism and convergent strabismus

Cogan, D. G.: Neurology of the Ocular Muscles, 4th ed. Springfield, Ill., Charles C Thomas, 1969, pp. 191–193, 225.
Walsh, F. B., and Hoyt, W. F.: Clinical Neuro-ophthalmology, 3rd ed. Baltimore, Williams & Wilkins Co., 1969, p. 898.

Horizontal Nystagmus (horizontal oscillatory movement of eyes)

1. Cerebellar disease, acute or chronic; fast component to side of lesion
2. Lesions of labyrinth (e.g., Meniere's syndrome) or when one labyrinth has been removed

3. Vestibular nuclei involvement as in persons with multiple sclerosis

4. Chediak-Higashi syndrome

Cogan, D. G.: Neurology of the Ocular Muscles, 4th ed. Springfield, Ill., Charles C. Thomas, 1969, pp. 154, 219.
Spaeth, G. L.: Ocular Manifestations of the Lipidoses. *In* Tasman, W. C. (Ed.): Retinal Disease in Children. New York, Harper & Row, 1971, pp. 187–188.

Vertical Nystagmus (spontaneous vertical oscillations of the eyes)

1. Up-beat nystagmus—nystagmus in which the fast component is upward and usually most marked when the gaze is directed upward; probably due to a lesion in the posterior fossa
   A. Cerebellar disease—acute or chronic, especially in the vermis
   B. Labyrinth disease—rare; has no lateralizing value
   C. Brain stem lesion, such as that of the vestibular nuclei
   D. Drugs—barbiturates and Dilantin
   E. Alcoholism
   F. Encephalitis
   G. Multiple sclerosis
   H. Idiopathic

2. Down-beat nystagmus—nystagmus in which the fast component is downward and usually most marked when the gaze is directed downward; probably due to a lesion in the lower end of the brain stem or cerebellum
   A. Platybasia (cerebellomedullary malformation syndrome)
   B. Arnold-Chiari malformation—herniation of cerebellar tonsils and part of medulla through foramen Magnum

C. Cerebellar atrophy
D. Degenerative encephalopathy
E. Multiple sclerosis
F. Alcoholic cerebellar disease
G. Arachnoidal adhesions
H. Morphine poisoning
I. Neurogenic muscular atrophy
J. Deformities of cervical spine
K. Klippel-Feil anomaly—upward displacement of odontoid process into foramen Magnum
L. Meningioma extending into pontine cistern
M. Insufficiency of basilar artery
N. Aneurysm of the supraclinoid part of left carotid siphon
O. Ependymoma of posterior part of the fourth ventricle
P. Diabetes mellitus
Q. Idiopathic

Cogan, D. G.: Down-Beat Nystagmus. Arch. Ophthal. *80*:757–768, 1968.
Cogan, D. G.: Neurology of the Ocular Muscles, 4th ed. Springfield, Ill., Charles C Thomas, 1969, pp. 154–155, 218, 223.
Duke-Elder, S., and Scott, G. I.: System of Ophthalmology, Vol. XII. St. Louis, C. V. Mosby Co., 1971, pp. 876–880.

Rotary Nystagmus (rotary oscillatory movement of eyes)

1. Cerebellar disease—acute or chronic

2. Lesion of vestibular nuclei in floor of fourth ventricle associated with multiple sclerosis, syringobulbia, or thrombosis of postero-inferior cerebellar artery or its branches

3. Vestibular involvement (e.g., labyrinthitis, Meniere's syndrome)

4. Encephalitis

5. Superior oblique myokymia—benign, intermittent, uniocular

6. Benign paroxysmal positional nystagmus—fast component toward lower ear

7. Cerebrotendinous xanthomatosis

Cogan, D. G.: Neurology of the Ocular Muscles, 4th ed. Springfield, Ill., Charles C Thomas, 1969, pp. 128, 154.

Harbert, F.: Benign Paroxysmal Positional Nystagmus. Arch. Ophthal. *84*:298–302, 1970.

Hoyt, W. F., and Keane, J. R.: Superior Oblique Myokymia. Arch. Ophthal. *84*:461–467, 1970.

Schimschack, J. R., Alvard, E. C., and Swanson, P. D.: Cerebrotendinous Xanthomatosis. Arch. Neurol. *18*:687–698, 1968.

See-Saw Nystagmus (one eye moves up as the other eye moves down; in addition there is torsion of the eyes—the eye moving up intorts, and the eye moving down extorts)

This nystagmus probably is due to lesions located in mesodiencephalic region, hypothalamus, and thalamus. It may be associated with bitemporal hemianopsia and reduced vertical optokinetic nystagmus.

1. Associated with chiasmal glioma

2. Associated with chromophobe adenoma of the pituitary gland, involving the optic chiasm and third ventricle

3. Associated with craniopharyngioma, involving the optic chiasm and hypothalamus

4. Due to brain stem vascular disease, including vertebrobasilar thrombosis

5. Due to suprasellar epidermoid tumor involving optic chiasm and hypothalamus

6. Due to toxoplasmosis of the brain stem

7. Due to oligodendroglioma involving the pons and third ventricle

8. Congenital

9. Head injury with fracture of frontal bone

10. Associated with syringomyelia and syringobulbia

11. Multiple sclerosis

12. Idiopathic

Daroff, R. B.: See-Saw Nystagmus. Neurology 15:874–877, 1965.
Druckman, R., Ellis, P., Kleinfeld, J., and Waldman, M.: See-Saw Nystagmus. Arch. Ophthal. 76:668, 1966.
Duke-Elder, S., and Scott, G. I.: System of Ophthalmology, Vol. XII. St. Louis, C. V. Mosby Co., 1971, pp. 883–886.
Fein, J. M., and Williams, R. D. B.: See-Saw Nystagmus. J. Neurol. Neurosurg. Psychiat. 32:202–207, 1969.
Walsh, F. B., and Hoyt, W. F.: Clinical Neuro-ophthalmology, 3rd ed. Baltimore, Williams & Wilkins Co., 1969, pp. 282, 2092, 2142, 2159.

Retraction Nystagmus (spasmodic retraction of the eyes when an attempt is made to move them in any direction; caused by lesions of midbrain, especially lesions in the vicinity of the aqueduct of Sylvius)

1. Koerber-Salus-Elschnig syndrome (sylvian aqueduct syndrome)—nystagmus, lid retraction, muscle palsies; headaches, hypertension, hemiparesis, ataxia

2. Parinaud's syndrome (paralysis of vertical movement)—nystagmus, ptosis, diplopia, mydriatic pupils, papilledema, vertigo, such as with pineal tumor

3. Cysticercus cyst

4. Ependymoma

5. Arteriovenous aneurysm

6. Vascular lesions

7. Brucellosis

Duke-Elder, S., and Scott, G. I.: System of Ophthalmology, Vol. XII. St. Louis, C. V. Mosby Co., 1971, pp. 886–887.

Huber, A.: Eye Symptoms in Brain Tumors, 2nd ed. St. Louis, C. V. Mosby Co., 1971, p. 48.

Smith, J. L., Zieper, I., Gay, A. J., and Cogan, D. G.: Nystagmus Retractions. Arch. Ophthal. 62:864, 1959.

Uniocular Vertical Nystagmus

1. Spasmus nutans

2. Multiple sclerosis

3. Unilateral amblyopia

4. Sleep

5. Myokymia of lower eyelid

Reinecke, R. D.: Translated Myokymia of the Lower Eyelid Causing Uniocular Vertical Pseudonystagmus. Amer. J. Ophthal. 75:150–151, 1973.

Monocular Nystagmus

1. Unilateral amblyopia

2. Unilateral opacity of the ocular media

3. Unilateral astigmatism or high refractive error

4. Nervous system disease, such as multiple sclerosis, epidemic meningitis, and congenital syphilis

5. Superior oblique myokymia—benign, intermittent, uniocular

6. Spasmus nutans—most common cause in children

7. Tumors of brain stem

8. Lesions of optic nerve, chiasm, midbrain, or brain stem

9. Congenital syphilis

Donin, J. F.: Acquired Monocular Nystagmus in Children. Canad. J. Ophthal. 2:212–215, 1967.
Duke-Elder, S., and Scott, G. I.: System of Ophthalmology, Vol. XII. St. Louis, C. V. Mosby Co., 1971, p. 882.
Hoyt, W. F., and Keane, J. R.: Superior Oblique Myokymia. Arch. Ophthal. 84:461–467, 1970.

Periodic Alternating Nystagmus (central vestibular nystagmus with rhythmic jerk type of nystagmus that undergoes phasic or cyclic changes in amplitude and direction)

1. Syringobulbia

2. Multiple sclerosis

3. Mesencephalic brain stem and cerebellar disease

4. Syphilitic optic atrophy

5. Diabetes mellitus

6. Chiasmal lesion such as craniopharyngioma

7. Friedreich's hereditary ataxia

8. Encephalitis

9. Chronic otitis media

10. Cerebral trauma or fractured skull

11. Vertebrobasilar artery insufficiency

12. Tumor of the corpus callosum

13. Congenital

14. von Recklinghausen's disease

15. Meningioma of tentorium cerebelli, cerebellar glioma, and cholesteatoma of the cerebellopontine angle

Davis, D. G., and Smith, J. L.: Periodic Alternating Nystagmus. Amer. J. Ophthal. *72*:757–762, 1971.

Duke-Elder, S., and Scott, G. I.: System of Ophthalmology, Vol. XII. St. Louis, C. V. Mosby Co., 1971, pp. 881–882.

Walsh, F. B., and Hoyt, W. F.: Clinical Neuro-ophthalmology, 3rd ed. Baltimore, Williams & Wilkins Co., 1969, pp. 284, 285, 921.

Positional Nystagmus (nystagmus that appears or changes in form or intensity after certain positional changes of the head indicates vestibular stimulation)

1. Normal individuals

2. Anxiety

3. Drugs
   A. Barbiturates
   B. Quinine
   C. Aspirin
   D. Alcohol
   E. Carbon monoxide poisoning

4. After head injury

5. After general anesthesia

6. After prolonged illness

7. Inner ear pathologic changes, including hemorrhage, inflammation, thrombosis, emboli, circulatory and secretory conditions

8. Neuritis, meningitis, tumors, vascular anomalies, degeneration, atrophy, increased intraocular pressure, syphilis, arteriosclerosis, hypertonia, vasomotor disturbance, allergic and toxic conditions, cranial trauma, hemorrhage, emboli, or thrombosis

Nylan, C. O.: Positional Nystagmus: A Review and Future Prospects. J. Laryng. *64*:295–318, 1950.

Solmon, S. D.: Positional Nystagmus. Arch. Otolaryng. *90*:58–63, 1969.

Optokinetic Nystagmus (physiologic nystagmus obtained by watching moving targets; slow component in direction targets are moving, and fast component in opposite direction)

1. Normal patient—optokinetic response present and symmetrical to each side

2. Lesions of optic tract, geniculate body, temporal and occipital lobes show no asymmetry of horizontal optokinetic responses

3. Lesions of parietal lobe give asymmetrical horizontal optokinetic responses

4. Occipital lobe involvement with homonymous hemianopia and asymmetrical horizontal optokinetic responses suggests a mass lesion extending into parietal lobe rather than a vascular lesion

5. Test for malingering in "blind" eye or eyes with obtained optokinetic responses

6. Parkinsonism—vertical optokinetic nystagmus may be reduced either upward or downward

7. See-saw nystagmus—vertical optokinetic nystagmus may be reduced either upward or downward (see p. 122)

8. Parinaud's syndrome—vertical optokinetic nystagmus with targets moving downward suppressed

9. Aberrant regeneration of third nerve—absent vertical optokinetic nystagmus, normal horizontal optokinetic nystagmus

10. Internuclear palsies—horizontal targets bring out dissociation of ocular response movements

Smith, J. L.: Optokinetic Nystagmus; Its Use in Topical Neuro-Ophthalmologic Diagnosis. Springfield, Ill., Charles C Thomas, 1963.
Walsh, F. B., and Hoyt, W. F.: Clinical Neuro-ophthalmology, 3rd ed. Baltimore, Williams & Wilkins Co., 1969, pp. 285–287.

Syndromes Associated with Nystagmus*

1. Apert's syndrome (acrocephalosyndactylia): strabismus, nystagmus, exophthalmos, slant fissure, field defect, keratitis, optic atrophy—syndactylia

2. Arnold-Chiari syndrome (platybasia syndrome): nystagmus, diplopia, hemianopia, papilledema—pyramidal tract signs, vertebral malformations

3. Babinski-Nageotte syndrome (medullary tegmental paralysis): nystagmus, enophthalmos, ptosis, miosis—cerebellar hemiataxia, hemiparesis

*This section from Geeraets (pp. 234–235), with modifications.

4. Behr's disease: nystagmus, partial optic atrophy—abortive hereditary ataxia, mental deficiency

5. Bielschowsky-Lutz-Cogan syndrome (internuclear ophthalmoplegia): dissociated nystagmus, unilateral or bilateral external ocular muscle palsies

6. Bloch-Sulzberger disease (incontinentia pigmenti): nystagmus, strabismus, cataract, optic nerve involvement—bullous skin eruptions and pigmentations

7. Cestan-Chenais syndrome: nystagmus, ptosis, enophthalmos, miosis—flaccid paralysis of soft palate and vocal cord, ataxia, contralateral hemiplegia

8. Charcot-Marie-Tooth disease (progressive peroneal muscular atrophy): nystagmus, visual loss, optic atrophy—progressive muscular atrophy

9. Chromosome 18, partial deletion of the long arm (deletion 18): nystagmus, mental retardation, microcephaly, mid-face retraction, prominent anthelix and antitragus, and acromial dimpling

10. Crouzon's disease (craniofacial dysostosis): nystagmus, strabismus, exophthalmos, visual loss, anterior segment involvement—prognathism, maxillar atrophy, deformity of anterior fontanel

11. Cytomegalic inclusion disease, congenital: failure to thrive, mental retardation, microcephaly, chorioretinitis, and seizures

12. De Lange's syndrome: severe mental retardation; bushy, confluent eyebrows; upturned nose; wide upper lip; hirsutism; pallor of optic disc; ptosis; and nystagmus

13. Diencephalic syndrome: profound emaciation, marked loss of subcutaneous tissue, euphoria—secondary to a tumor in the region of the diencephalon; culminates in death during the second or third year of life

14. Down's disease (mongolism, trisomy 21): nystagmus, myopia, slanted eyelid fissures, lens opacities, epicanthus—mental retardation, skeletal and heart anomalies

15. Hallermann-Streiff syndrome (oculomandibulodyscephaly): nystagmus, strabismus, cataract, microphthalmia—malformations of skeleton, teeth anomalies, mental retardation

16. Hennebert's syndrome (luetic-otitic-nystagmus syndrome): otitic nystagmus, interstitial keratitis—vertigo

17. Kernicterus: high levels of bilirubin in the blood, jaundice, brain damage, mental retardation, nystagmus

18. Koerber-Salus-Elschnig syndrome (sylvian aqueduct syndrome): nystagmus, muscle palsies, lid retraction—headaches, hypertension, hemiparesis, ataxia

19. Laurence-Moon-Bardet-Biedl syndrome: nystagmus, strabismus, ophthalmoplegia, visual field defect, optic nerve and retinal involvement—obesity, hypogenitalism, polydactylia, mental deficiency

20. Lenoble-Aubineau syndrome: nystagmus—head and limb tremor, myoclonia

21. Louis-Bar syndrome (ataxia-telangiectasia): pseudo-ophthalmoplegia, fixation nystagmus, conjunctival telangiectasia—ataxia, scanning speech, hypotonia, cutaneous telangiectasis

22. Lowe's disease (oculocerebrorenal syndrome): nystagmus, congenital glaucoma, anterior segment involvement, mental retardation, acidosis, osteomalacia

23. Marfan's syndrome (dystrophia mesodermalis congenita): nystagmus, strabismus, anterior segment and lens involvement—arachnodactylia, congenital heart defect, relaxed ligaments

24. Marinesco-Sjögren syndrome (oligophrenia with cerebellar ataxia and cataracts): nystagmus, cerebellar ataxia, bilateral congenital cataracts, mental retardation, and short stature

25. Meniere's syndrome: nystagmus—vertigo, tinnitus, progressive deafness

26. Naegeli's syndrome (melanophoric nevus syndrome): nystagmus, strabismus, papillitis, pseudoglioma—keratosis, pigmentary skin changes

27. Parkinson's disease (paralysis agitans): nystagmus, diplopia, blepharospasm, sluggish or absent pupil reaction—rhythmical tremor, cogwheel rigidity of arms, loss of facial expression

28. Pelizaeus-Merzbacher disease (aplasia axialis extracorticalis congenita): nystagmus, retinitis pigmentosa, optic atrophy—retarded development, athetosis, abnormal reflexes, spastic paralysis, hearing and speech disturbances

29. Pyle's disease (familial metaphyseal dysplasia): nystagmus, macrocephaly, hypertelorism, bony prominence of the glabella and prognathism

30. Rubella, congenital: nystagmus, congenital heart disease, deafness, microphthalmos, cataracts, glaucoma, mental/motor retardation

31. Schilder's disease (encephalitis periaxialis diffusa): nystagmus, extraocular palsy, visual loss, visual field defect, optic nerve involvement—spastic paralysis, hearing and speech disturbances

32. Sebaceous nevi, linear: nystagmus, convulsions, mental retardation, linear sebaceous nevi of face

33. Sylvian syndrome: central nystagmus, muscle palsy, pupillary disturbances, tonic convergence spasm, clonic convergence movements

34. Tay-Sachs disease (familial amaurotic idiocy): nystagmus, strabismus, optic atrophy, macular cherry-red spot and retinal pigmentary changes, visual loss—mental retardation, convulsions, flaccid muscles becoming spastic with progression

35. Vermis syndrome: nystagmus, papilledema—vomiting, enlarged head, incoordination

36. Wallenberg's syndrome (lateral bulbar syndrome): nystagmus, diplopia, enophthalmos, ptosis, miosis—nausea, difficulty in speaking and swallowing

37. Dawson's disease (subacute sclerosing panencephalitis): chorioretinitis, nystagmus, papilledema, cortical blindness, optic atrophy

38. Hypothyroidism (cretinism)

39. GML—Gangliosidosis: esotropia, nystagmus, optic atrophy, large head, coarse features, hypotonia, peripheral edema

40. Francois' dyscephalic syndrome: dyscephaly with bird-like head, dental anomalies, proportional dwarfism, microphthalmos, congenital cataracts, strabismus

41. Nevus sebaceous of Jadassohn: antimongoloid lid; dermoid limbus; coloboma of iris-choroid; esotropia; external oculomotor palsy, unilateral; thickening of bones of orbit; coloboma of lids

42. Leigh's disease (subacute necrotizing encephalomyelopathy)

43. Maple syrup urine disease: nystagmus, cataracts, epicanthal folds, strabismus

Emery, J. M., et al.: GML—Gangliosidosis: Ocular and Pathological Manifestations. Arch. Ophthal. *85*:177–187, 1971.

Francois, J., and Pierard, J.: The Francois Dyscephalic Syndrome and Skin Manifestations. Amer. J. Ophthal. *71*:1241–1250, 1971.

Geeraets, W. L.: Ocular Syndromes, 2nd ed. Philadelphia, Lea & Febiger, 1969, pp. 234–235.

Gellis, S. S., and Feingold, M.: Atlas of Mental Retardation. Washington, D.C., U.S. Government Printing Office, 1968.

Haslam, R. H., and Wirtschafter, J. D.: Unilateral External Oculomotor Nerve Palsy and Nevus Sebaceous of Jadassohn. Arch. Ophthal. *87*:293–300, 1972.

Howard, R. O., and Albert, D. H.: Ocular Manifestations of Subacute Necrotizing Encephalomyelopathy (Leigh's Disease). Arch. Ophthal. *86*:386–393, 1972.

Robb, R. M., and Watters, G. V.: Ophthalmic Manifestations of Subacute Sclerosing Panencephalitis. Arch. Ophthal. *83*:426–435, 1970.

Roy, F. H., and Kelly, M. L.: Maple Syrup Urine Disease. J. Pediat. Ophthal. *10*:70–73, 1973.

Shulman, J. D., and Crawford, J. D.: Congenital Nystagmus and Hypothyroidism. New Eng. J. Med. *280*:708–710, 1969.

Oculogyric Crisis (spasmodic and involuntary deviation of the eyes, usually upward, lasting from a few minutes to several hours)

1. Parkinsonism

2. Late manifestation of encephalitis

3. Neurosyphilis

4. Trauma

5. Cerebellar disease

6. Drugs, such as chlorpromazine (Thorazine) and perphenazine (Trilafon)

7. Lesions of fourth ventricle and cerebellum, especially lesions of the flocculus

8. Multiple sclerosis

Cogan, D. G.: Neurology of the Ocular Muscles, 4th ed. Springfield, Ill., Charles C Thomas, 1969, pp. 111, 122, 155.

Duke-Elder, S., and Scott, G. I.: System of Ophthalmology, Vol. XII. St. Louis, C. V. Mosby, 1971, pp. 855–857.

Walsh, F. B., and Hoyt, W. F.: Clinical Neuro-ophthalmology, 3rd ed. Baltimore, Williams & Wilkins Co., 1969, pp. 1006, 1321, 2636.

Ocular Bobbing (both globes move synchronously in the vertical plane by spontaneously and intermittently dipping downward through an arc of a few millimeters and then return to the primary position)

Ocular bobbing differs from vertical nystagmus by virtue of the absence of a fast and a slow component in the movements. It is due to advanced pontine disease.

1. Thrombosis of basilar, middle cerebral, or vertebral arteries with posterior fossa infarction

2. Hypertensive pontine hemorrhage

3. Associated with palatal myoclonus

4. Leigh's encephalopathy

Fisher, C. M.: Ocular Bobbing. Arch. Neurol. *11*:543–546, 1964.

Hemeroff, S. B., Garcia-Mullin, R., and Eckholdt, J.: Ocular Bobbing. Arch. Ophthal. *82*:774–780, 1969.

Howard, R. O., and Albert, D. H.: Ocular Manifestations of Subacute Necrotizing Encephalomyelopathy (Leigh's Disease). Arch. Ophthal. *86*:386–393, 1972.

Yap, C., Mayo, C., and Barron, K.: "Ocular Bobbing" in Palatal Myoclonus. Arch. Neurol. *18*:304–310, 1968.

Paralysis of Third Nerve (Oculomotor Nerve) (ptosis; inability to rotate eye upward, downward, or inward; a dilated unreactive pupil [iridoplegia] and paralysis of accommodation [cycloplegia])

1. Intracerebral
   A. Lesion of red nucleus (Benedikt's syndrome)—homolateral oculomotor paralysis with contralateral intention tremor
   B. Syndrome of cerebral peduncle (Weber's syndrome)—homolateral oculomotor paralysis and cross hemiplegia
   C. Occlusion of basilar artery—due to emboli especially but also to hemorrhage or aneurysm
   D. Recurrent third nerve palsy secondary to vascular spasm of migraine
   E. Tumors
   F. Nuclear types—pareses of a single or a few extraocular muscles supplied by the oculomotor nerve in one or both eyes. There may or may not be pupillary disturbances (mydriasis, sluggish pupillary reaction) and

paresis of accommodation. In tumors within or near the midbrain (pinealomas), there is a combination of isolated muscle pareses with vertical gaze palsy, possibly a disturbance of convergence, and nystagmus retractorius (Parinaud's syndrome, Sylvian aqueduct syndrome, pineal syndrome).

2. Intracranial
   A. Rupture of aneurysm at base of brain—third nerve paralysis, pain about the face (fifth nerve), and headache
   B. Polyneuritis due to toxins such as alcohol, lead, arsenic, and carbon monoxide, to dinitrophenol or carbon disulfide poisoning, or to diabetes mellitus, herpes zoster, or mumps
   C. Poliomyelitis
   D. Syphilis and tuberculosis, meningitis, or encephalitis
   E. Multiple sclerosis
   F. Subdural hematoma
   G. Temporal arteritis
   H. Ophthalmic migraine
   I. Rabies
   J. Meningococcal meningitis
   K. Myasthenia gravis—worse in afternoon
   L. Diphtheria
   M. Botulism
   N. Amebic dysentery
   O. Dengue fever
   P. Smallpox vaccination
   Q. Hepatitis

3. Lesions affecting exit of third nerve from the cranial cavity
   A. Cavernous sinus syndrome—paralysis of third, fourth, and sixth nerves with proptosis
      (1) Cavernous sinus thrombosis
      (2) Pituitary adenoma—lateral extension
      (3) Aneurysm
      (4) Carotid-cavernous fistula
      (5) Extension of nasopharyngeal tumor
      (6) Extension from lateral sinus thrombosis

B. Superior orbital fissure syndrome—same as for cavernous sinus syndrome except exophthalmosis less likely to occur and optic nerve involvement and miotic pupil are more likely
   (1) Sphenoid sinus suppuration
   (2) Skull fractures or hemorrhage
   (3) Tumors, such as sphenoid ridge meningioma, nasopharyngeal tumor, and metastatic carcinoma, rhabdomyosarcoma, cordoma, sarcoma
   (4) Aneurysm
   (5) Occlusion of superior ophthalmic vein
C. Orbital apex—involvement of III, IV, VI, first division of V cranial nerves, and optic nerve—proptosis is common

4. Other
   A. Lupus erythematosus
   B. Hodgkin's disease
   C. Sarcoid
   D. Dengue fever
   E. In association with aspirin poisoning

Huber, A.: Symptoms in Brain Tumors. St. Louis, C. V. Mosby Co., 1971, pp. 38–41.

Kass, M. A., Keltner, J. L., and Gay, A. J.: Total Third Nerve Paralysis. Arch. Ophthal. 87:107–109, 1972.

Milstein, B. A., and Morretin, L. B.: Report of a Case of Sphenoid Fissure Syndrome Studied by Orbital Venography. Amer. J. Ophthal. 72:600–603, 1971.

Rucker, C. W.: The Causes of Paralysis of the Third, Fourth, and Sixth Cranial Nerves. Amer. J. Ophthal. 61:1293, 1966.

Sananman, M. L., and Weintroub, M. I.: Remitting Ophthalmoplegia Due to Rhabdomyosarcoma. Arch. Ophthal. 86:459–461, 1971.

Walsh, F. B., and Hoyt, W. F.: Clinical Neuro-ophthalmology, 3rd ed. Baltimore, Williams & Wilkins Co., 1969.

Paralysis of Fourth Nerve (Trochlear Nerve) (produces palsy of the superior oblique muscle resulting in limitation of downward movement of the eye when it is in the adducted position—frequently associated with third cranial nerve palsy)

1. Intracerebral
   A. Thrombosis of nutrient vessels, including median penetrating branch of basilar artery to fourth nucleus
   B. Hemorrhage in the roof of the midbrain
   C. Aneurysm, including direct involvement by posterior cerebral and superior cerebellar arteries
   D. Tumors
   E. Neonatal hypoxia
   F. Nuclear type—trochlear paresis combined with a homolateral oculomotor paresis, occasionally in association with vertical gaze palsies, convergence spasm or convergence palsy, and pupillary disturbances is seen in tumors of the roof of the midbrain or pinealomas (pineal syndrome)

2. Intracranial
   A. Aneurysms, such as that of the posterior communicating artery
   B. Hematomas, traumatic
   C. Tumors, including cerebellopontine angle tumor
   D. Meningitis, encephalitis, polyneuritis—diabetes mellitus, herpes zoster, multiple sclerosis, myasthenia gravis

3. Lesions affecting exit of fourth nerve from the cranial cavity
   A. Cavernous sinus syndrome (see third nerve, p. 135)
   B. Superior orbital fissure syndrome (see third nerve, p. 136)
   C. Orbital apex syndrome

4. Orbital lesions
   A. Fracture of superior orbital rim.
   B. Sinusitis

C. Operations upon the frontal sinus in which there is trochlear displacement
D. Trochlear disturbance, such as in Paget's disease or hypertrophic arthritis
E. Adherence syndrome—adhesions between the superior rectus and superior oblique muscles
F. Abnormal insertion of superior oblique muscle or abnormal fascial attachments
G. Idiopathic

Burger, L. J., Kalvin, N. H., and Smith, J. L.: Acquired Lesions of the Fourth Cranial Nerve. Brain *93*:567–574, 1970.

Huber, A.: Eye Symptoms in Brain Tumors. St. Louis, C. V. Mosby Co., 1971, pp. 38–41.

Miller, M. T., Urist, M. J., Folk, E. R., and Chapman, L. I.: Superior Oblique Palsy Presenting in Late Childhood. Amer. J. Ophthal. *70*: 212, 1970.

Rucker, C. W.: The Causes of Paralysis of the Third, Fourth, and Sixth Cranial Nerves. Amer. J. Ophthal. *61*:1293, 1966.

Walsh, F. B., and Hoyt, W. F.: Clinical Neuro-ophthalmology, 3rd ed. Baltimore, Williams & Wilkins Co., 1969, pp. 145, 248, 921, 2390.

Pseudoabducens Palsy

1. Lack of effort involved in abducting a habitually adducted eye—patch on other eye differentiates from abducens palsy

2. Unwillingness to co-operate—doll's head phenomenon (sudden passive turning of head) differentiates from abducens palsy

3. Fibrosis of medial rectus

4. Overambitious resection of medial rectus

5. Horizontal gaze palsy (bilateral)—with or without co-contraction

6. Duane's syndrome

Von Noorden, G. K., and Maumenee, A. E.: Atlas of Strabismus, 2nd ed. St. Louis, C. V. Mosby Co., 1973, pp. 116–119.

Paralysis of Sixth Nerve (Abducens Palsy) (produces palsy of lateral rectus muscle with esotropia increasing when eye is moved laterally)

The course of the sixth nerve makes it more vulnerable than other cranial nerves to injury.

1. Intracerebral
    A. Thrombosis or aneurysm of nutrient vessels to sixth nucleus—basilar artery
    B. Wernicke's encephalopathy—thiamine deficiency in alcoholics with sixth nerve palsy, paresis of horizontal conjugate gaze, nystagmus, ataxia, and Korsakoff's psychosis
    C. Millard-Gubler syndrome—pontine lesion, such as glioma, with homolateral sixth nerve palsy, contralateral hemiplegia, and homolateral peripheral facial palsy
    D. Tumors—intracranial, pontine glioma, or metastatic tumor from breast, thyroid glands, or nasopharynx
    E. Platybasia (cerebellomedullary malformation syndrome)
    F. Nuclear aplasia
    G. Foville's syndrome—homolateral sixth nerve palsy, homolateral peripheral facial palsy, homolateral horizontal gaze palsy, possibly combined with a Horner syndrome

2. Intracranial
    A. Meningitis
    B. Skull fractures
    C. Carotid artery aneurysm
    D. Gradenigo's syndrome—osteitis of petrous tip of pyramid following homolateral mastoid or middle ear infection; facial pain (fifth nerve involvement)
    E. Subdural hematoma
    F. Increased intracranial pressure
    G. Cerebellopontine angle tumor, such as acoustic neuroma, producing unilateral deafness, facial paralysis, diplopia, and papilledema

H. Neuritis due to diseases such as diabetes mellitus, herpes zoster, poliomyelitis, lead or arsenic poisoning, multiple sclerosis, syphilis, brucellosis
I. Congenital absence of sixth nerve
J. Myasthenia gravis

3. Lesions affecting exit of sixth nerve from the cranial cavity
   A. Cavernous sinus syndrome (see third nerve, p. 135)
   B. Superior orbital fissure syndrome (see third nerve, p. 136)
   C. Sphenopalatine fossa lesion—loss of tearing and paresis of second division of fifth nerve, most frequently due to malignant tumor
   D. Orbital apex lesion

4. Other
   A. Duane's syndrome—lateral rectus muscle replaced by fibrous band with adduction; eye retracts into orbit
   B. Following lumbar puncture, lumbar anesthesia, or Pantopaque injection for myelography
   C. Toxic substances, such as arsenic, carbon tetrachloride, dichloroacetylene, Dilantin, gold salts, isoniazid, nitrofuran, thalidomide, trichloroethylene, furaltadone (Altafur)

Cogan, D. G.: Neurology of the Ocular Muscles, 4th ed. Springfield, Ill., Charles C Thomas, 1969, pp. 77–83.

Ernest, J. T., and Costenbader, F. D.: Lateral Rectus Muscle Palsy. Amer. J. Ophthal. 65:721–726, 1968.

Huber, A.: Eye Symptoms in Brain Tumors. St. Louis, C. V. Mosby Co., 1971, pp. 38–41.

Rucker, C. W.: The Causes of Paralysis of the Third, Fourth, and Sixth Cranial Nerves. Amer. J. Ophthal. 61:1293, 1966.

Schrader, E. C., and Schlezinger, N. S.: Neuro-ophthalmologic Evaluation of Abducens Paralysis. Arch. Ophthal. 63:84–91, 1960.

Smith, J. L., and Creighton, J.: Sixth Nerve Palsy Due to Furaltadone (Altafur). Arch. Ophthal. 65:61–62, 1961.

Walsh, F. B., and Hoyt, W. F.: Clinical Neuro-ophthalmology, 3rd ed. Baltimore, Williams & Wilkins Co., 1969.

Weintraub, M. I., and Sananman, M. L.: Giant Intracavernous Aneurysm and Sixth Nerve Palsy. Canad. J. Ophthal. 6:223–226, 1971.

Acquired Isolated Sixth Nerve Paresis in Children

1. Tumors—may be present with history of trauma or symptoms of infectious process
    A. Primary
        (1) Gliomas, such as astrocytomas, ependymomas, and medulloblastomas
        (2) Other primary tumors, including meningiomas, pinealomas, craniopharyngiomas, and hemangiomas
    B. Metastatic lesions, such as those from the nasopharynx, rhabdomyosarcomas, and neuroblastomas

2. Trauma—usually severe crush injury

3. Inflammatory lesions, such as meningoencephalitis, Gradenigo's syndrome (including fifth nerve), cerebellitis, and abscess

4. Vascular lesions, such as congenital aneurysm and arteriovenous anomalies

5. Other
    A. Hydrocephalus
    B. Pseudotumor cerebri
    C. Leukemia
    D. Gaucher's disease
    E. Lateral ventricular cyst
    F. Spontaneous subdural hematoma
    G. Transient in newborns

Jampel, R. S. B., and Titone, C.: Congenital Paradoxical Gustatory Lacrimal Reflex and Lateral Rectus Paralysis. Arch. Ophthal. 67: 123–126, 1962.

Lignell, K. W., and Davis, C. J.: Abducens Nerve Palsy and Optic Disc Hypoplasia in Cretinism. J. Pediat. Ophthal. 8:105–106, 1971.

Reisner, S. H., et al.: Transient Lateral Rectus Muscle Paresis in the Newborn Infant. J. Pediat. 78:461–465, 1971.

Robertson, D. M., Hines, J. D., and Rucker, C. W.: Acquired Sixth Nerve Paresis in Children. Arch. Ophthal. 83:574–579, 1970.

Acute Ophthalmoplegia (acute onset of extraocular muscle palsy)

1. Infranuclear
   A. Aneurysm of internal carotid artery or circle of Willis
   B. Trauma
      (1) Orbital fracture
      (2) Orbital hematoma
   C. Orbital cellulitis secondary to acute paranasal sinusitis
   D. Ophthalmoplegic migraine
   E. Myasthenia gravis

2. Nuclear*
   A. Acute and subacute infections
      (1) Infectious encephalitis
         a. Viral encephalitis
            1) Encephalitis lethargica and other epidemic viral encephalitides
            2) Anterior poliomyelitis
            3) Vaccinal encephalitis
            4) Rabies
            5) Zoster
            6) Post-febrile encephalitis—varicella, variola, measles, mumps, influenza, infectious mononucleosis
         b. Organismal encephalitic infections
            1) Typhoid
            2) Scarlet fever
            3) Whooping cough
            4) Gas gangrene
            5) Septicemia
            6) Pneumonia
            7) Typhus
            8) Malaria
         c. Acute central nervous system diseases
            1) Acute demyelinating diseases—acute disseminated encephalomyelitis, acute multiple sclerosis

*A through F of this section (2. Nuclear) from Duke-Elder, S., and Scott, G. I.: System of Ophthalmology, Vol. XII. London, Henry Kimpton, 1971, p. 747, with modifications.

    (2) Neuritic infections
        a. Polyradiculoneuritis
        b. Epidemic paralyzing vertigo
        c. Acute infectious (rheumatic) polyneuritis
        d. Interstitial neuritis—meningitis, cranial sinusitis, petrositis, nasal sinusitis, orbital periostitis, orbital abscess
    (3) Widespread infections
        a. Meningovascular syphilis
        b. Tuberculosis
        c. Torula and cryptococcosis
    (4) Toxic conditions
        a. Diphtheria
        b. Tetanus
        c. Botulism
    (5) Allergic conditions
        a. Sarcoidosis
        b. Recurrent multiple cranial nerve palsies

B. Metabolic diseases
    (1) Deficiency diseases
        a. Thiamine deficiency
            1) Wernicke's encephalopathy
            2) Beriberi
        b. Nicotinic acid deficiency—pellagra
        c. Ascorbic acid deficiency—scurvy
    (2) Diabetes
    (3) Anemias
        a. Primary anemia—leukemia
        b. Secondary anemia (loss of blood)
    (4) Exophthalmic ophthalmoplegia
    (5) Porphyria

C. Intoxication from exogenous poisons
    (1) Metallic—lead
    (2) Organic
        a. Carbon monoxide
        b. Sulfuric acid, ergot, phosphorus, triorthocresylphosphate, dichloroacetylene
        c. Snake poison, wasp stings
        d. Alcohol

(3) Drugs

(4) Spinal anesthetics

D. Vascular lesions

    (1) Arteriosclerosis, hemorrhage and thrombosis in the midbrain, subarachnoid hemorrhage, aneurysms, congenitally dilated arteries, giant-cell arteritis

E. Neoplasms and cysts

F. Trauma affecting the midbrain, base of the skull, and orbit

G. Idiopathic—etiologic basis undetermined

Abrahamson, I. A., and Horwitz, I. D.: Acute Ophthalmologia. Amer. J. Ophthal. *38*:781, 1954.

Duke-Elder, S., and Scott, G. I.: System of Ophthalmology, Vol. XII. St. Louis, C. V. Mosby Co., 1971, pp. 745–780.

Gonyea, E. F., and Heilman, K. M.: Neuro-Ophthalmic Aspects of Central Nervous System Cryptococcosis. Arch. Ophthal. *87*:164–168, 1972.

Chronic Ophthalmoplegias (slow onset of extraocular muscle palsy)

1. Infective conditions

    A. Tabes and general paralysis

    B. Disseminated sclerosis

    C. Diffuse sclerosis

2. Degenerative conditions

    A. Chronic progressive external ophthalmoplegia

    B. Amyotrophic lateral sclerosis—progressive bulbar palsy

    C. Hereditary ataxias—Friedreich's ataxia, Sanger-Brown's ataxia

    D. Syringomyelia (syringobulbia)

Duke-Elder, S., and Scott, G. I.: System of Ophthalmology, Vol. XII. St. Louis, C. V. Mosby Co., 1971, pp. 747, 780–782.

Bilateral Complete Ophthalmoplegia (bilateral palsy of ocular muscles, ptosis, with pupil and accommodation involvement)

1. Encephalitis
2. Syphilis
3. Wernicke's encephalopathies
4. Tumors of midbrain
5. Tumors of cerebellopontine angle
6. Arteriosclerotic softening
7. Multiple sclerosis
8. Trauma
9. Arteriosclerotic hemorrhage and occlusion

Collins, R. D.: Bilateral Nuclear Ophthalmoplegia. Amer. J. Ophthal. *51*:152, 1961.

External Ophthalmoplegia (paralysis of ocular muscles including ptosis with sparing of pupil and accommodation)

1. Familial and congenital
2. Abiotrophy—specific for one particular tissue, bilateral, symmetrical
3. Thyrotoxicosis
4. Myasthenia gravis

5. Diabetes mellitus

6. Aneurysm of internal carotid artery

7. Amyloidosis

8. Chronic progressive external ophthalmoplegia

9. Bee sting

10. Diphtheria

11. Epidemic encephalitis

12. Mumps

13. Pernicious anemia

14. Scleroderma

15. Tick paralysis

16. Wernicke's encephalopathies

17. Olivopontocerebellar atrophy

18. Polyradiculoneuronitis (Guillain-Barré and Fisher's syndromes)

19. Progressive facial hemiatrophy (Parry-Romberg syndrome)

20. Vincristine—may have fifth and seventh nerve and peripheral neuropathies

21. Friedreich's ataxia

22. Kearns-Sayre syndrome—ptosis, retinitis pigmentosa, heart block

23. Myotonic dystrophy

24. Nevus sebaceous of Jadassohn—antimongoloid lid, dermoid limbus, coloboma of iris-choroid, nystagmus, esotropia, thickening of bones of orbit, coloboma of lids

Albert, D. M., Wong, V. G., and Henderson, E. S.: Ocular Complications of Vincristine Therapy. Arch. Ophthal. 78:709–713, 1967.
DiFiare, J. A.: Diabetes Oculomotor Neuropathy. Amer. J. Ophthal. 50:808, 1960.

Haslam, R. H., and Wirtschafter, J. D.: Unilateral External Oculomotor Nerve Palsy and Nevus Sebaceous of Jadassohn. Arch.
Ophthal. *87*:293–300, 1972.

Johnson, R. V., and Kennedy, W. R.: Progressive Facial Hemiatrophy (Parry-Romberg Syndrome). Amer. J. Ophthal. *67*:561, 1969.

Kearns, T. P., and Sayre, G. P.: Retinitis Pigmentosa, External Ophthalmoplegia and Complete Heart Block: Unusual Syndrome with
Histologic Study in One of Two Cases. Arch. Ophthal. *60*:280–
289, 1958.

Kiloh, L. G., and Nevin, S.: Progressive Dystrophy of the External
Ocular Muscles (Ocular Myopathy). Brain *74*:115, 1951.

Koerner, F., and Schlote, W.: Chronic Progressive External Ophthalmoplegia. Arch. Ophthal. *88*:155–166, 1972.

Lessell, S., Coppeto, J., and Samet, S.: Ophthalmoplegia in Myotonic Dystrophy. Amer. J. Ophthal. *71*:1231–1235, 1971.

Macoul, K. L., and Winter, F. C.: External Ophthalmoplegia. Arch.
Ophthal. *79*:182, 1968.

Schultz, R. O., Hamilton, H. E., and Braley, A. E.: Ocular Changes
Related to Endocrine Dysfunction. Amer. J. Ophthal. *59*:26, 1960.

Walsh, F. B., and Hoyt, W. F.: Clinical Neuro-ophthalmology, 3rd
ed. Baltimore, Williams & Wilkins Co., 1969.

Internuclear Ophthalmoplegia (paralysis of medial rectus muscles on attempted conjugate lateral gaze without
other evidence of third nerve paralysis due to involvement of medial longitudinal fasciculus. Jerk nystagmus
of the abducting eye and vertical nystagmus, usually on
upward gaze, may be present.)

* = Most important

1. Bilateral
   *A. Multiple sclerosis
    B. Inflammation, such as upper respiratory infection
    C. Neoplasms—usually medulloblastomas or infiltrative
       gliomas
    D. Myasthenia gravis
    E. Occlusive vascular disease
    F. Syphilis

147

G. Arnold-Chiari malformation

H. Pontine hematoma

2. Unilateral

   *A. Vascular lesion—infarct of small branch of basilar artery

   B. Tumors of the brain stem

   C. Multiple sclerosis

   D. Myasthenia gravis

   E. Cryptococcosis

Cogan, D. G.: Internuclear Ophthalmoplegia. Typical and Atypical. Arch. Ophthal. *84*:583–589, 1970.

Cogan, D. G., Kubik, C. S., and Smith, W. L.: Unilateral Internuclear Ophthalmoplegia. Arch. Ophthal. *44*:783, 1950.

Glaser, J. S.: Myasthenic Pseudo-internuclear Ophthalmoplegia. Arch. Ophthal. *75*:363, 1966.

Gonyea, E. F., and Heilman, K. M.: Neuro-Ophthalmic Aspects of Central Nervous System Cryptococcosis. Arch. Ophthal. *87*:164–168, 1972.

Koos, W. T., Sunder-Plassmonn, M., and Salak, S.: Successful Removal of a Large Intrapontine Hematoma. J. Neurosurg. *31*:690–694, 1969.

Swick, H. M.: Pseudointernuclear Ophthalmoplegia in Acute Idiopathic Polyneuritis (Fisher's Syndrome). Amer. J. Ophthal. *77*:725–728, 1974.

Painful Ophthalmoplegia (palsy of ocular muscles with pain)

1. Diabetic ophthalmoplegia

2. Intracavernous carotid aneurysm

3. Nasopharyngeal tumor

4. Tolosa-Hunt syndrome—inflammation of cavernous sinus

5. Pseudotumor of orbit

6. **Ophthalmoplegic migraine**

7. Orbital myositis

8. Orbital periostitis

9. Alternating exophthalmos with painful ophthalmoplegia

10. Adenocarcinoma metastatic to the orbit

11. Superior orbital fissuritis (see p. 136)

12. Orbital abscess

13. Collier's sphenoidal palsy

14. Postherpetic neuralgia

15. Atypical facial neuralgia

16. Tic douloureux of the first trigeminal division

17. Sphenoidal fissure syndrome (Rochon-Duvigneaud syndrome)

18. Osteoperiostitis, anterior (orbital)

19. Osteoperiostitis, posterior (orbital)

20. Orbital apex syndrome

21. Cavernous sinus syndrome (see p. 135)

Hedges, T. R.: Alternating Exophthalmos with Painful Ophthalmoplegia. Arch. Ophthal. 74:625–627, 1965.
Lessor, R., and Jampol, L. M.: Tolosa-Hunt Syndrome and Antinuclear Factor. Amer. J. Ophthal. 77:732–734, 1974.
Milstein, B. A., and Morretin, L. B.: Report of a Case of Sphenoid Fissure Syndrome Studied by Orbital Venography. Amer. J. Ophthal. 72:600–603, 1971.
Sacks, J. G., and O'Grady, R. B.: Painful Ophthalmoplegia and Enophthalmos Due to Metastatic Carcinoma. Trans. Amer. Acad. Ophthal. Otolaryng. 75:351–354, 1970.
Sananman, M. L., and Weintroub, M. I.: Remitting Ophthalmoplegia Due to Rhabdomyosarcoma. Arch. Ophthal. 86:459–461, 1971.
Smith, J. L.: Letter to Editor. Amer. J. Ophthal. 63:1815, 1967.
Smith, J. L., and Taxda, D. S. R.: Painful Ophthalmoplegia, the Tolosa-Hunt Syndrome. Amer. J. Ophthal. 61:1466, 1966.

Transient Ophthalmoplegia (extraocular muscle paralysis of short duration)

1. Multiple sclerosis—usually the lateral rectus
2. Tabes
3. Lethargic encephalitis
4. Cerebral syphilis
5. Recurrent oculomotor palsy

O'Brien, C. S.: Ophthalmology, Notes for Students. Iowa City, Athens Press, 1930, p. 334.

Painful Ocular Movements (pain with movement of the eyes)

1. Retrobulbar neuritis
2. Influenza
3. Orbital cellulitis
4. Orbital periostitis
5. Myositis
   A. "Collagen diseases"
   B. Infectious myositis
   C. Trichinosis
6. Bone-break fever (dengue fever)

Jampel, R. S., and Fells, P.: Monocular Elevation Paresis Caused by a Central Nervous System Lesion. Arch. Ophthal. *80*:45, 1968.
O'Brien, C. S.: Ophthalmology, Notes for Students. Iowa City, Athens Press, 1930, p. 333.

Poor Convergence (inability of both eyes to fixate simultaneously on a near object)

1. Functional
   A. Convergence insufficiency
   B. Hysteria
   C. Poor attention span of patient
   D. Exophoria
   E. Exotropia

2. Organic
   A. Third nerve paralysis (see p. 134)
   B. Exophthalmic goiter—Möbius' sign
   C. Exophthalmos
   D. Encephalitis
   E. Multiple sclerosis
   F. Syphilis and tabes
   G. Brain lesion, to include bilateral occipital lobe lesions, superior colliculi, and anterior internuclear ophthalmoplegia, such as in hemorrhage, trauma, or tumors
   H. Postencephalitis
   I. Narcolepsy
   J. Myotonic dystrophy
   K. Poor visual acuity in one or both eyes
   L. Whiplash injury

Cogan, D. G.: Neurology of the Ocular Muscles, 4th ed. Springfield, Ill., Charles C Thomas, 1969.
Duke-Elder, S., and Scott, G. I.: System of Ophthalmology, Vol. XII. St. Louis, C. V. Mosby Co., 1971, pp. 829–832.
Roca, P. D.: Ocular Manifestations of Whiplash Injuries. Ann. Ophthal. *4*:63–73, 1972.
Walsh, F. B., and Hoyt, W. F.: Clinical Neuro-ophthalmology, 3rd ed. Baltimore, Williams & Wilkins Co., 1969.

Spasm of Convergence (occurs with spasm of accommodation and miosis, i.e., spasm of the near reflex)

1. Encephalitis—accompanied with nystagmus
2. Tabes dorsalis
3. Labyrinthine fistulas
4. Trauma
5. Hysteria—may be confused with lateral rectus palsy
6. Paralysis of horizontal gaze with compensatory spasm of near reflex
7. Parinaud's syndrome
8. Wernicke's encephalopathy
9. Oculogyric crisis in myasthenia

Cogan, D. G.: Neurology of the Ocular Muscles, 4th ed. Springfield, Ill., Charles C Thomas, 1969.
Thompson, R. A., and Zynde, R. H.: Convergence Spasm Associated with Wernicke's Encephalopathy. Neurology *19*:711–712, 1969.

Divergence Paralysis (supranuclear cause with sudden onset of comitant esotropia and uncrossed diplopia at distance, fusion at near [usually 1 to 2 meters], normal ductions and versions, and gross impairment of fusional amplitudes of divergence)

1. Epidemic encephalitis
2. Syphilis

152

3. Multiple sclerosis

4. Head injuries

5. Vascular disease
   A. Occlusion of subclavian artery with reversal of flow in vertebral artery
   B. Hypertension
   C. Vertebral basilar insufficiency
   D. Diabetes mellitus

6. Increased intracranial pressure

7. Cerebral hemorrhage

8. Diphtheria

9. Poliomyelitis

10. Influenza

11. Lead poisoning

12. Brain stem lesions
    A. Hemangioma
    B. Cerebellar cyst
    C. Tumors, such as cerebellar and acoustic neuromas

13. Functional

14. Unknown

Chamlin, M., and Davidoff, L.: Divergence Paralysis with Increased Intracranial Pressure. Arch. Ophthal. 46:145, 1951.
Cunningham, R. D.: Divergence Paralysis. Amer. J. Ophthal. 74: 630–633, 1972.
Duke-Elder, S., and Scott, G. I.: System of Ophthalmology, Vol. XII. St. Louis, C. V. Mosby Co., 1971, pp. 833–835.
Rutkowski, P. C., and Burian, H. M.: Divergence Paralysis Following Head Trauma. Amer. J. Ophthal. 73:660–662, 1972.
Walsh, F. B., and Hoyt, W. F.: Clinical Neuro-ophthalmology, 3rd ed. Baltimore, Williams & Wilkins Co., 1969.

Oculocardiac Reflex (bradycardia, nausea and faintness dependent upon trigeminal sensory stimulation evoked by pressure upon or within the eyeball or from sensory impulses by stretching of ocular muscles)

1. Intraocular injections

2. Acute glaucoma

3. Orbital hematoma

4. Traction on extraocular muscles including levator palpebrae superioris

5. Retinal detachment operation

6. Severe injury to eye or orbit

7. Pressure on globe

8. Intermittent exophthalmos due to congenital venous malformations of the orbit

9. Exaggerated in epidemic encephalitis

Walsh, F. B., and Hoyt, W. F.: Clinical Neuro-ophthalmology, 3rd ed. Baltimore, Williams & Wilkins Co., 1969, pp. 379–380, 1318, 1696.

Retraction of the Globe (on horizontal conjugate gaze)

1. Medial wall fracture with incarceration of orbital contents —retraction of globe with attempted abduction

2. Retraction of convergent non-fixating eye associated with loss of conjugate lateral gaze and occurrence of the near reflex on attempted lateral gaze

3. Duane's syndrome—retraction of globe with attempted adduction
    A. Fibrotic lateral rectus
    B. Co-contraction of horizontal rectus muscles, lateral rectus, and both vertical muscles, or medial and inferior rectus muscles

Holtz, S. J.: Congenital Ocular Anomalies Associated with Duane's Retraction Syndrome, the Nevus of Ota, and Axial Anisometropia. Amer. J. Ophthal. 77:729–731, 1974.
Miller, G. R., and Glaser, J. S.: The Retraction Syndrome and Trauma. Arch. Ophthal. 76:662, 1966.
Zauberman, H., Magora, A., and Chaco, J.: An Electromyographic Evaluation of the Retraction Syndrome. Amer. J. Ophthal. 64: 1103, 1967.
Zweifach, P. H., Walton, D. S., and Brown, R. H.: Isolated Congenital Horizontal Gaze Paralysis. Arch. Ophthal. 81:345, 1969.

Forced Duction Test (the eyeball is moved away from the muscle being tested by grasping with a forceps the conjunctiva and episclera close to the limbus)

1. Supraduction–Infraduction
    A. Resistance
        (1) Orbital floor fracture
        (2) Thyroid myopathy of inferior rectus muscle
        (3) Abnormal fascial or muscle attachments
    B. Unrestricted
        (1) Elevator paresis
        (2) Paresis of inferior rectus muscle

2. Supraduction in adduction
    A. Brown's superior oblique tendon sheath syndrome—resistance
    B. Paresis of inferior oblique muscle—unrestricted

3. Adduction
    A. Resistance
        (1) Tight lateral rectus following excessive resection operation

155

    (2) Duane's retraction syndrome due to fibrosis of
      lateral rectus muscle
    (3) Abnormal fascial or muscle attachments
  B. Unrestricted
    (1) Extensive medial rectus recession
    (2) Duane's retraction syndrome due to central or
      peripheral co-contraction of medial and lateral
      rectus on attempted adduction

 4. Abduction
  A. Resistance
    (1) Tight medial rectus following excessive resection
      operation
    (2) Abnormal fascial or muscle attachments includ-
      ing strabismus fixus
  B. Unrestricted
    (1) Extensive lateral rectus recession
    (2) Paralysis of lateral rectus muscle

Von Noorden, G. K., and Maumenee, A. E.: Atlas of Strabismus,
2nd ed. St. Louis, C. V. Mosby Co., 1973, pp. 112–115.

CONJUNCTIVA

Contents

Cellular Responses

1. Basophilic reaction—significant only when seen in large numbers; allergic inflammation, especially vernal conjunctivitis

2. Eosinophilic reaction
   A. Vernal conjunctivitis—characteristic with fragmentation of eosinophil
   B. Hay fever conjunctivitis—rarely fragmentation of eosinophil
   C. Allergic conjunctivitis due to various drugs, cosmetics, and other antigens
   D. Atropine sensitivity—not present when Eserine or pilocarpine is employed

3. Mononuclear reaction
   A. Viral disease—100% without secondary infection; usually lymphocytic
      (1) Epidemic keratoconjunctivitis—adenovirus type 8
      (2) Pharyngoconjunctival fever—adenovirus type 3
      (3) Herpetic keratoconjunctivitis
      (4) Acute follicular conjunctivitis of Beal
   B. Chronic ocular infections

4. Neutrophilic reaction
   A. All bacteria but two—*Neisseria catarrhalis* and *Haemophilus duplex* (Morax-Axenfeld diplobacillus)
   B. Viruses of the family Chlamydiaceae (Tric agent)
      (1) Trachoma
      (2) Inclusion conjunctivitis
      (3) Lymphogranuloma venereum
   C. Fungal diseases
      (1) Streptothrix conjunctivitis secondary to canaliculitis
      (2) Nocardial corneal ulcers
      (3) Monilial corneal ulcers

D. Unknown cause
    (1) Erythema multiforme
    (2) Conjunctivitis of Reiter's disease
E. Vernal conjunctivitis—eosinophilic and neutrophilic reaction
F. Epidemic keratoconjunctivitis and herpetic keratoconjunctivitis have a shift from mononuclear to polymorphonuclear reaction when a membrane is formed

5. Plasma-cell reaction
Trachoma—especially with spontaneous rupturing of follicles

6. Epithelial changes
  A. Keratinization of conjunctival epithelial cells
    (1) Vitamin A deficiency
    (2) Exposure
    (3) Cicatrization
    (4) Keratoconjunctivitis sicca—partially keratinized epithelial cells, specific
    (5) Epithelial plaque
  B. Large, multipointed epithelial cells
    (1) Characteristic of viral infection
    (2) Most often found in herpetic keratitis
  C. Intracellular granules
    (1) Pseudoinclusion bodies—extension of nuclear material into cytoplasm
    (2) Intracellular free green pigment in cytoplasm—present in individuals with dark complexion
    (3) Intracellular free blue granules—present in cytoplasm in about 12% of normal individuals
    (4) Sex chromatin—present in nuclei only of females

7. Cellular inclusions
  A. Trachoma and inclusion conjunctivitis have identical inclusions—basophilic, cytoplasmic (Halberstadter-Prowazek)
  B. Molluscum contagiosum—eosinophilic, cytoplasmic
  C. Lymphogranuloma venereum—eosinophilic
  D. Herpes simplex and herpes zoster—eosinophilic, internuclear (Lipschutz)

E. Measles—multinucleated giant cells with eosinophilic, internuclear inclusion bodies and cytoplasmic, eosinophilic masses

F. Chickenpox—eosinophilic, internuclear

G. Smallpox—eosinophilic, cytoplasmic

Fedukowicz, H. B.: External Infections of the Eye. New York, Appleton-Century-Crofts, Inc., 1963.

Kimura, S. J., and Thygeson, P.: The Cytology of External Ocular Disease. Amer. J. Ophthal. *39*:137–144, 1955.

Locatcher-Khorazo, D., and Seegal, B. C.: Microbiology of the Eye. St. Louis, C. V. Mosby Co., 1972, pp. 44–51.

Purulent Conjunctivitis (violent acute conjunctival inflammation, great swelling of the lids, copious secretion of pus, and a marked tendency to corneal involvement, and even possible loss of the eye)

1. Gram-positive group
   A. Staphylococcus
   B. Streptococcus
   C. Pneumococcus
   D. Bacillus of Doderlein (lactobacillus sp.)

2. Gram-negative group
   A. *Neisseria gonorrhoeae*
   B. *Neisseria meningitidis*
   C. *Haemophilus aegyptius* (Koch-Weeks baciilus)
   D. *Escherichia coli*
   E. *Aerobacter aerogenes*
   F. *Klebsiella pneumoniae*
   G. *Serratia marcescens*

3. Vaccinia virus

4. Fungus
   A. Actinomyces
   B. Nocardia

Atlee, W. E., Burns, R. P., and Oden, M.: Serratia marcescens Kerato-conjunctivitis. Amer. J. Ophthal. 70:31–33, 1970.

Duke-Elder, S.: Diseases of the Outer Eye. System of Ophthalmology, Vol. VIII, Part 1. St. Louis, C. V. Mosby Co., 1965, pp. 82–89.

Fedukowicz, H. B.: External Infections of the Eye. New York, Appleton-Century-Crofts, Inc., 1963.

Harbin, T., and Curran, R. E.: Gonococcal Conjunctivitis. Ann. Ophthal. 6:221–228, 1974.

Thygeson, P.: Historical Review of Oculogenital Disease. Amer. J. Ophthal. 71:975–985, 1971.

Acute Mucopurulent Conjunctivitis (epidemic pink eye—marked hyperemia and a mucopurulent discharge, which tends toward spontaneous recovery)

1. Gram-positive group
    A. Staphylococcus—eyelid lesions and punctate staining of the lower cornea may occur
    B. Pneumococcus

2. Gram-negative group
    A. *Haemophilus aegyptius* (Koch-Weeks bacillus)
    B. *Haemophilus influenzae*

3. Associated with exanthems and viral infections to include
    A. Measles
    B. German measles
    C. Scarlet fever
    D. Mumps

4. Fungus
    A. Leptothrix
    B. *Candida albicans*

5. Lyell's disease—toxic epidermal necrolysis or scalded skin syndrome

6. Etiology obscure in many cases

Fedukowicz, H. B.: External Infections of the Eye. New York, Appleton-Century-Crofts, Inc., 1963.

Givner, I.: Catarrhal Conjunctivitis. Infectious Diseases of the Conjunctiva and Cornea. Symposium of the New Orleans Academy of Ophthalmology. St. Louis, C. V. Mosby Co., 1963, p. 57.

Okumoto, M., and Smolin, G.: Pneumococcal Infections of the Eye. Amer. J. Ophthal. 77:346–352, 1974.

Ostler, H. B., Conant, M. A., and Groundwater, J.: Lyell's Disease, the Stevens-Johnson Syndrome and Exfoliative Dermatitis. Trans. Amer. Acad. Ophthal. Otolaryng. 74:1254–1265, 1970.

Chronic Mucopurulent Conjunctivitis (mucopurulent discharge, moderate hyperemia with a chronic course)

1. Infective element—lids or lacrimal apparatus
   A. Staphylococcus
   B. Morax-Axenfeld diplobacillus (angular conjunctivitis)
   C. *Streptothrix foersteri*
   D. Pneumococcus
   E. Monilia
   F. Pubic lice

2. Allergic—cosmetic

3. Irritative
   A. Overtreatment by drugs—antibiotics, miotics, mydriatics
   B. Direct irritants—foreign body, mascara, dust, wind, smog, insecticides, chlorinated water, and many others
   C. Associated infection or irritation of lids, lacrimal apparatus, nose, or skin
   D. Metabolic conditions—gout, alcoholism—or prolonged digestive disturbances
   E. Deficiency of lacrimal secretions
   F. Exposure—ectropion, facial paralysis, exophthalmos, and many others
   G. Eyestrain

Duke-Elder, S.: Diseases of the Outer Eye. System of Ophthalmology, Vol. VIII, Part 1. St. Louis, C. V. Mosby Co., 1965, pp. 74–80.

Okumoto, M., and Smolin, G.: Pneumococcal Infections of the Eye. Amer. J. Ophthal. 77:346–352, 1974.

Membranous Conjunctivitis (exudate permeates the epithelium to such an extent that removal of the membrane is difficult and a raw bleeding surface results)

Membranous conjunctivitis may lead to symblepharon, ankyloblepharon, and entropion with trichiasis.

1. *Corynebacterium diphtheriae*

2. Streptococcus

3. Pneumococcus

4. Ligneous conjunctivitis—chronic, cause unknown

5. Uncommon—Actinomyces, glandular fever, measles, *Neisseria catarrhalis,* variola, *Pseudomonas aeruginosa,* herpes simplex, Leptothrix, and epidemic keratoconjunctivitis (type 8 adenovirus)

6. Chemical irritants
   A. Acids, such as acetic or lactic
   B. Alkalis, such as ammonia or lime
   C. Metallic salts, such as silver nitrate or copper sulfate

Duke-Elder, S.: Diseases of the Outer Eye. System of Ophthalmology, Vol. VIII, Part 1. St. Louis, C. V. Mosby Co., 1965, pp. 89–95.
Fedukowicz, H. B.: External Infections of the Eye. New York, Appleton-Century-Crofts, Inc., 1963.

Pseudomembranous Conjunctivitis (fibrin network, which can be easily peeled off leaving the conjunctiva intact, forms on the conjunctiva)

1. Bacterial
   A. *Corynebacterium diphtheriae*
   B. Streptococcus
   C. Staphylococcus

D. Pneumococcus

E. Meningococcus

F. Gonococcus

G. Uncommon—*Haemophilus aegyptius, Haemophilus influenzae, Neisseria catarrhalis, Pseudomonas aeruginosa, Escherichia coli, Bacillus subtilis, Shigella, Bacillus faecalis alcaligenes, Salmonella paratyphi B, Mycrobacterium tuberculosis,* and *Treponema pallidum*

2. Viral

   A. Herpes simplex

   B. Vaccinia

   C. Epidemic keratoconjunctivitis (type 8 adenovirus)

3. Fungal—*Candida albicans*

4. Allergic—vernal conjunctivitis

5. Toxic

   A. Erythema multiforme

   B. Benign mucous membrane pemphigoid

   C. Lyell's disease—toxic epidermal necrolysis or scalded skin syndrome

6. Chemical irritants

   A. Acids, such as acetic or lactic

   B. Alkalis, such as ammonia or lime

   C. Metallic salts, such as silver nitrate or copper sulfate

   D. Vegetable and animal irritants

7. Traumatic or operative healing of wounds

8. Ligneous conjunctivitis—chronic, cause unknown

9. Superior limbic keratoconjunctivitis

Duke-Elder, S.: Diseases of the Outer Eye. System of Ophthalmology, Vol. VIII, Part 1. St. Louis, C. V. Mosby Co., 1965, pp. 89–98.

Givner, I.: Purulent, Membranous, and Pseudomembranous Conjunctivitis—Infectious Diseases of the Conjunctiva and Cornea. Symposium of the New Orleans Academy of Ophthalmology. St. Louis, C. V. Mosby Co., 1963, p. 67.

Ostler, H. B., Conant, M. A., and Groundwater, J.: Lyell's Disease, the Stevens-Johnson Syndrome and Exfoliative Dermatitis. Trans. Amer. Acad. Ophthal. Otolaryng. *74*:1254–1265, 1970.

Theodore, F. H., and Ferry, A. P.: Superior Limbic Keratoconjunctivitis. Arch. Ophthal. *84*:481–484, 1970.

Ophthalmia Neonatorum (conjunctivitis occurring in newborns)

1. Staphylococcus

2. Pneumococcus

3. Streptococcus

4. Inclusion blennorrhea

5. *Haemophilus influenzae*

6. *Neisseria gonorrhoeae* and *N. catarrhalis*

7. *Haemophilus aegyptius* (Koch-Weeks bacillus)

8. *Corynebacterium diphtheriae*

9. Meningococcus

10. Chemical conjunctivitis, such as from silver nitrate instillation

11. Listeriosis (*Listeria monocytogenes*)

12. Coliform bacillus, such as *Escherichia coli*

13. Tric virus

14. *Pseudomonas pyocyanea*

15. Moraxella

16. Herpes simplex

17. Mima polymorpha—gram negative

18. Candida

19. Mycoplasma

20. *Trichomonas vaginalis*

21. *Serratia marcescens*

Burdin, J. C., et al.: Human Listeriosis of the Eye. Presse Med. *73*: 1461–1464, 1965.

Duke-Elder, S.: Diseases of the Outer Eye. System of Ophthalmology, Vol. VIII, Part 1. St. Louis, C. V. Mosby Co., 1965, pp. 115–125.

Lazachek, G. W., et al.: Serratia marcescens, an Ocular Pathogen. Arch. Ophthal. *86*:599–603, 1971.

Sood, N. N., and Madhaven, H. N.: Ophthalmia Neonatorum Caused by Mima Polymorpha. J. Pediat. Ophthal. *5*:242, 1968.

Thygeson, P.: Historical Review of Oculogenital Disease. Amer. J. Ophthal. *71*:975–985, 1971.

Parinaud's Oculoglandular Conjunctivitis (conjunctivitis of acute onset—usually of uniocular incidence and complicated by regional lymphadenopathy)

1. Leptothricosis including cat-scratch fever

2. Tuberculosis

3. Tularemia

4. Lymphogranuloma venereum

5. Syphilis

6. Sporotrichum

7. Boeck's sarcoid

8. Trachoma

9. *Corynebacterium diphtheriae*

10. Conjunctival vaccinia

11. Coccidioidomycosis

12. Listeriosis (*Listeria monocytogenes*)

13. Marseilles fever (rickettsial)

14. Pasteurellosis (*Pasteurella pseudotuberculosis* and *P. septica*)

Bedrossian, E. H.: The Eye. Springfield, Ill., Charles C Thomas, 1958, pp. 178–181.

Duke-Elder, S.: Diseases of the Outer Eye. System of Ophthalmology, Vol. VIII, Part 1. St. Louis, C. V. Mosby Co., 1965, pp. 106–113.

Margileth, A. M.: Cat Scratch Disease: Nonbacterial Regional Lymphoadenitis. Pediatrics *42*:803, 1968.

Wood, T. R.: Ocular Coccidioidomycosis. Amer. J. Ophthal. *64*:587, 1967.

Acute Follicular Conjunctivitis (lymphoid follicles [cobblestoning] of conjunctiva with rapid onset)

1. Inclusion conjunctivitis—rare except in newborn infants or in adults who have derived their infection from inclusion urethritis in the male or inclusion cervicitis in the female

2. Adenovirus conjunctivitis
   A. Pharyngoconjunctival fever—usually due to type 3 adenovirus; common in swimming-pool epidemics in summer and fall
   B. Epidemic keratoconjunctivitis—due to adenovirus type 8 (rarely occurs in children)

3. Primary herpetic keratoconjunctivitis—conjunctival reaction may be follicular or pseudomembranous

4. Newcastle disease conjunctivitis—usually seen in poultry handlers, veterinarians, etc.

5. Influenza virus A

6. Herpes zoster

7. Cat-scratch fever

8. Trachoma (sometimes)

9. Bacterial (rare)—streptococcus, moraxella, and treponema

10. Mesantoin use

168

11. Unknown types—a case that resists etiologic classification is encountered occasionally; it is probable that other viruses can occasionally produce acute follicular conjunctivitis

12. Associated with regional adenitis
    A. Syndrome of Beal—transient unilateral disease, usually bilateral later, without purulent discharge, resolving within two weeks
    B. Inclusion conjunctivitis in adults—acute mucopurulent follicular inflammation, persisting as long as several months, sometimes with scarring
    C. Syndrome of Parinaud—acute follicular inflammation becoming chronic after general illness (see p. 167)

13. Chlamydia epizootic (feline pneumonitis)

Duke-Elder, S.: Diseases of the Outer Eye. System of Ophthalmology, Vol. VIII, Part 1. St. Louis, C. V. Mosby Co., 1965, pp. 103–108.
Ostler, H. B., Schacter, J., and Dawson, C. R.: Acute Follicular Conjunctivitis of Epizootic Origin. Arch. Ophthal. 82:587, 1969.
Thygeson, P.: Follicular Conjunctivitis. Infectious Diseases of the Conjunctiva and Cornea. Symposium of the New Orleans Academy of Ophthalmology. St. Louis, C. V. Mosby Co., 1963, p. 103.
Thygeson, P., and Dawson, C. R.: Trachoma and Follicular Conjunctivitis in Children. Arch. Ophthal. 75:3, 1966.

Chronic Follicular Conjunctivitis (lymphoid follicles [cobblestoning] of conjunctiva with long-term course)

1. Chronic follicular conjunctivitis—Axenfeld's type (orphan's) frequently found in institutionalized children; almost asymptomatic; long duration (twelve to twenty-four months or longer): no keratitis; cause unknown

2. Chronic follicular conjunctivitis, toxic type
    A. Miotics, such as Eserine, pilocarpine, and diisopropyl fluorophosphate (DFP)

B. Cycloplegics, such as atropine

C. Bacterial origin, such as that due to a diplobacillus or other microorganism

3. Molluscum contagiosum conjunctivitis—due to desquamation into the conjunctival sac of toxic products from a nodule of the lid margin; often resembles trachoma, exhibiting keratitis and upper tarsal follicles; heals rapidly after removal of the viral nodule

4. Chronic follicular conjunctivitis with epithelial keratitis; differentiated from Axenfeld's type by shorter duration (four to five months) and by epithelial keratitis involving upper third of cornea; epidemic in schools; can be transmitted by mascara pencil; cause unknown

5. Folliculosis—associated general lymphoid hypertrophy

6. Trachoma—stages 1, 2, and 3

7. With generalized lymphadenopathy

8. Neurocutaneous syndrome (ectodermal dysgenesis)

Benjamin, S. N., and Allen, H. F.: Classification for Limbal Dermoid Choristomas and Brachial Arch Anomalies. Arch. Ophthal. 87: 305–314, 1972.

Fedukowicz, H. B.: External Infections of the Eye. New York, Appleton-Century-Crofts, Inc., 1963.

Thygeson, P., and Dawson, C. R.: Trachoma and Follicular Conjunctivitis in Children. Arch. Ophthal. 75:3, 1966.

Cicatricial Conjunctivitis (scarring of the conjunctiva)

1. General: an infectious type of membranous conjunctivitis such as beta streptococcal infection, ocular diphtheria, or primary herpetic keratoconjunctivitis

2. Upper lid: trachoma

170

3. Lower lid:
   A. Erythema multiforme (Stevens-Johnson disease)
   B. Reiter's syndrome
   C. Ocular pemphigoid
   D. Chemical (especially alkali)
   E. Radium burns
   F. Vaccinia
   G. Dermatitis herpetiformis
   H. Epidermolysis bullosa
   I. Sjögren's syndrome
   J. Chronic cicatricial conjunctivitis—occurs in the elderly; has a chronic course; may have concurrent skin and mucous membrane lesions
   K. Erythroderma ichthyosiforme
   L. Exfoliative dermatitis
   M. Acne rosacea
   N. Epidemic keratoconjunctivitis
   O. Staphylococcal granuloma
   P. Hydroa vacciniforme
   Q. Congenital syphilis
   R. Chlamydia (psittacosis-lymphogranuloma group)

Chalkley, T. H. F.: Chronic Cicatricial Conjunctivitis. Amer. J. Ophthal. 67:526, 1969.

Duke-Elder, S.: Diseases of the Outer Eye. System of Ophthalmology, Vol. VIII. St. Louis, C. V. Mosby Co., 1965, p. 500.

Mordhorst, C. H., and Dawson, C.: Sequelae of Neonatal Inclusion Conjunctivitis and Associated Disease in Parents. Amer. J. Ophthal. 71:861–867, 1971.

Newell, F. W.: Ophthalmology, Principles and Concepts. St. Louis, C. V. Mosby Co., 1969, p. 171.

Taylor, R.: Modern Treatment of Severe "Shrinkage of the Conjunctiva." Brit. J. Ophthal. 51:31–43, 1967.

Conjunctival Disorders Associated with Dermatologic Disorders

1. Mucocutaneous eruptions
    A. Pemphigus—vulgaris, vegetans, foliaceus
    B. Benign mucous membrane pemphigoid
    C. Hydroa vacciniforme (recurrent summer eruption)
    D. Dermatitis herpetiformis (Duhring-Brocq disease)
    E. Erythema multiforme (Stevens-Johnson disease)
    F. Epidermolysis bullosa
    G. Reiter's disease
    H. Behcet's disease
    I. Pyostomatitis vegetans

2. Dermatoses
    A. Acne rosacea
    B. Atopic eczema dermatitis
    C. Seborrhea
    D. Erythroderma exfoliativa (Wilson-Brocq disease)
    E. Ichthyosis
    F. Acanthosis nigricans
    G. Xeroderma pigmentosum
    H. Psoriasis vulgaris
    I. Keratosis follicularis spinulosa decalvans
    J. Lichen planus
    K. Pityriasis rubra pilaris; lichen acuminatus
    L. Keratosis follicularis
    M. Porokeratosis
    N. Acrodermatitis chronica atrophica
    O. Acrodermatitis enteropathica
    P. Diffuse cutaneous mastocytosis

Duke-Elder, S.: Diseases of the Outer Eye. System of Ophthalmology, Vol. VIII, Part 1. St. Louis, C. V. Mosby Co., 1965, pp. 498–561.

Conjunctival Disorders Associated with Genital Disorders

1. Bacteria
   A. Staphylococcus species
   B. Streptococcus species
   C. *Neisseria gonorrhoeae*
   D. *Mycobacterium tuberculosis*
   E. *Mycobacterium leprae*
   F. *Escherichia coli*
   G. Proteus species
   H. *Pseudomonas aeruginosa*
   I. *Haemophilus vaginalis*
   J. *Haemophilus ducreyi*
   K. *Calymmatobacterium granulomatis* (granuloma inguinale)
   L. Mimeae species
   M. Bacteroides species

2. Fungi
   A. Candida species
   B. Other

3. Viruses
   A. Herpesvirus hominis 2
   B. Cytomegalovirus
   C. Varicella zoster
   D. Verruca virus
   E. Molluscum contagiosum virus
   F. Rubella

4. Spirochetes
   A. *Treponema pallidum*

5. Chlamydiae
   A. *Chlamydia oculogenitalis*
   B. *Chlamydia lymphogranulomatis*
   C. Unclassified Chlamydia from Reiter's disease

6. Parasites
   A. *Phthirus pubis*
   B. *Trichomonas vaginalis*

C. Fly larvae
D. Beetles
E. Moths

Thygeson, P.: Historical Review of Oculogenital Disease. Amer. J. Ophthal. *71*:975–985, 1971.
Vergnani, R. J., and Smith, R. S.: Reiter Syndrome in a Child. Arch. Ophthal. *91*:165–166, 1974.

Congestion of the Conjunctiva (non-infectious hyperemia of the conjunctiva)

1. Polycythemia vera

2. Gout

3. Hypothyroidism

4. Malignant lymphoma

5. Acute lupus erythematosus

6. Irritative follicular conjunctivitis (see follicular conjunctivitis, pp. 168 and 169)
   A. Toxic conjunctivitis due to drugs, such as miotics or cycloplegics
   B. Chemical conjunctivitis, such as that due to lime, Zephiran, indelible pencil, or turpentine
   C. Topical drugs that are hypotonic, hypertonic or in which the pH is above or below 6.9, or a drug degradation causing chemical irritation
   D. Vegetable irritants, e.g., caster bean

7. Allergic conjunctivitis, such as that due to contact with drugs, plastic, or cosmetics

8. Conjunctivitis caused by air pollution (smog, dust, and/or smoke)

9. Photosensitive conjunctivitis

10. Alcoholism

11. Hormone deficiency (estrogenic)

12. Avitaminosis

13. Sjögren's syndrome

14. Vascular changes
    A. Hereditary hemorrhagic telangiectasis (Rendu-Osler-Weber disease)
    B. Petechial hemorrhage of conjunctiva (see subconjunctival hemorrhage, p. 180)
    C. Facial paralysis (see p. 63)

15. Carotid-cavernous fistula or arteriovenous aneurysm

16. Ophthalmic vein thrombosis

17. Cavernous sinus thrombosis

18. Carcinoid syndrome

Boniuk, M.: The Ocular Manifestations of Ophthalmic Vein and Aseptic Cavernous Sinus Thrombosis. Trans. Amer. Acad. Ophthal. Otolaryng. 76:1519–1534, 1972.

Givner, I.: Noninfectious Conjunctival Congestion. Infectious Diseases of the Conjunctiva and Cornea. Symposium of the New Orleans Academy of Ophthalmology. St. Louis, C. V. Mosby Co., 1963, p. 48.

Wong, V. G., and Melmon, K. L.: Ophthalmic Manifestations of the Carcinoid Flush. New Eng. J. Med. 277:406–409, 1967.

Ciliary Flush (circumcorneal congestion) (congestion of the ciliary vessels immediately surrounding the cornea. The individual vessels are not seen, the color is violaceous, the redness fades toward the fornices, and the vessels do not move with the conjunctiva.)

1. Iritis

2. Iridocyclitis

3. Glaucoma, especially acute glaucoma

4. Iris irritation, such as with corneal foreign bodies

5. Corneal disease, such as with inflammations and erosions

Vaughan, D., Asbury, T., and Cook, R.: General Ophthalmology, 6th ed. Los Altos, Calif., Lange Medical Publishers, 1971.

Conjunctival Aneurysms, Varicosities, Tortuosities, and Telangiectasis

1. Local causes
   A. Acne rosacea
   B. Long-standing ocular inflammation
   C. Irradiation of the eye
   D. Delayed mustard-gas keratitis

2. Systemic causes
   A. Arteriosclerosis
   B. Hypertension
   C. Diabetes
   D. Syphilis
   E. Rheumatic fever or rheumatic heart disease
   F. Scleroderma
   G. Varicose veins—generalized
   H. Hereditary hemorrhagic telangiectasia (Rendu-Osler-Weber disease)
   I. Ataxic telangiectasia (Louis-Bar syndrome)
   J. Degos' syndrome (malignant atrophic papulosis)
   K. Renal failure
   L. Fabry's disease
   M. Normal individuals

Berlyne, G. M., and Shae, A. B.: Red Eyes in Renal Failure. Lancet 1:4–7, 1967.

Duke-Elder, S.: Diseases of the Outer Eye. System of Ophthalmology, Vol. VIII, Part 1. St. Louis, C. V. Mosby Co., 1965, pp. 24–33.

Grace, E.: Diffuse Angiokeratosis (Fabry's Disease). Amer. J. Ophthal. 62:139–145, 1966.

Howard, R. O., Klaus, S. N., Savin, R. C., and Fenton, R.: Malignant Atrophic Papulosis. Arch. Ophthal. 79:262, 1968.

Hyams, S. W., Reisner, S. H., and Newmann, E.: The Eye Signs in Ataxia-Telangiectasia. Amer. J. Ophthal. 62:118, 1966.

Conjunctival Sludging and Segmentation

1. Local
   A. Vasodilator drugs that are applied locally
   B. Hypothermia
   C. Sympathetic irritation
   D. Old age

2. Systemic or hyperviscosity with increase in serum proteins— erythrocyte sedimentation rate is usually above 30 mm in first hour
   A. Hypertension
   B. Multiple myeloma
   C. Macroglobulinemia
   D. Cryoglobulinemia
   E. Sickle-cell disease
   F. Hyperglobinemia

Duke-Elder, S.: Diseases of the Outer Eye. System of Ophthalmology, Vol. VIII. Part 1. St. Louis, C. V. Mosby Co., 1965, pp. 21–24.

Luxenberg, M. N., and Mansoff, F. A.: Retinal Circulation in Hyperviscosity Syndrome. Amer. J. Ophthal. 70:588–598, 1970.

Conjunctival Edema (chemosis)

1. Local inflammatory conditions
   A. Eye—viral conjunctivitis, corneal ulcer, fulminating iritis, or panophthalmitis
   B. Lids—styes, vaccinia, acute meibomitis, insect bites, or vaccinal pocks
   C. Orbit—cellulitis, periostitis, dacryoadenitis, tenonitis
   D. Lacrimal passages—dacryocystitis
   E. Nasal cavity—sinusitis
   F. Cerebral cavity—acute meningitis

2. Local or systemic irritants—drugs, such as iodides, sanguinarine, and Dionin; glandular fever

3. Hypersensitivity—local topical allergies

4 Vasomotor instability—angioneurotic edema or premenstrual phase of water retention

5. Venous congestion—local obstruction of orbital apex, carotid-cavernous fistula, thrombosis of cavernous sinus, or right-sided heart failure

6. Reduced plasma protein level—nephrotic state

7. Acquired blockage of orbital lymphatics following orbital surgery (lateral orbitotomy) or due to erysipelas or lymphogranuloma venereum

8. Myxedema—infiltration with mucopolysaccharides

9. Increased bulk of orbital contents—orbital tumors, cysts, or endocrine exophthalmos

10. Chronic hereditary lymphedema (Nonne-Milroy-Meige disease)

Duke-Elder, S.: Diseases of the Outer Eye. System of Ophthalmology, Vol. VIII, Part 1. St. Louis, C. V. Mosby Co., 1965, pp. 42–46.
Tabbara, K. F., and Baghdassarian, S. A.: Chronic Hereditary Lymphedema of the Legs with Congenital Conjunctival Lymphedema. Amer. J. Ophthal. 73:531–532, 1972.

Conjunctival Xerosis (dryness of the conjunctiva)

1. Vitamin A deficiency
   A. Dietary deficiencies, including malnutrition and cystic fibrosis
   B. Pregnancy
   C. Liver disease, such as chronic cirrhosis
   D. Thyroid gland disorder, such as hyperthyroidism
   E. Digestive tract disorders
      (1) In stomach—achlorhydria, chronic gastritis or diarrhea, peptic ulcer
      (2) In pancreas—chronic pancreatitis
      (3) Colitis and enteritis
   F. Skin disorders, such as pityriasis rubra pilaris
   G. Pulmonary tuberculosis
   H. Malaria

2. Following cicatricial conjunctivitis (see p. 170)

3. Result of exposure of conjunctiva to air
   A. Excessive proptosis, such as in exophthalmic goiter or orbital tumor
   B. Deficient closure of lids, such as with paralysis of orbicularis, as part of facial palsy, spasm of the levator, or ectropion

4. Absence of blinking

5. Lack of closure of lids in sleep

6. Illness or coma

Duke-Elder, S., and Leigh, A. G.: System of Ophthalmology, Vol. III. St. Louis, C. V. Mosby Co., 1965, pp. 128, 593, 803.

Joyle, G. E., Ourgand, A. G., Baisinger, L. F., and Holmes, W. J.: Night Vision. Springfield, Ill., Charles C Thomas, 1959, pp. 174–300.

Newell, F. W.: Ophthalmology, Principles and Concepts. St. Louis, C. V. Mosby Co., 1969, p. 171

Sullivan, W. R., McCulley, J. P., and Dohlman, C. H.: Return of Goblet Cells after Vitamin A Therapy in Xerosis of the Conjunctiva. Amer. J. Ophthal. 75:720–725, 1973.

Subconjunctival Hemorrhage (blood under the conjunctiva)

1. Local trauma, including surgical trauma

2. Injury to orbital or adjacent structures, such as sinus; basal skull fracture; subarachnoid hemorrhage

3. Remote injury associated with fractured bones and fat emboli causing "splinter" subconjunctival hemorrhage

4. Local acute inflammation, including acute pneumococcal conjunctivitis, leptospirosis ictero-hemorrhagica, epidemic typhus, and scrub typhus

5. Spontaneous rupture of telangiectasis, varicosities, aneurysm, or angiomatous tumor (see p. 176)

6. Sudden severe venous congestion of head, including that due to coughing, vomiting, an epileptic fit, strangulation, or an orbital tumor (neuroblastoma)

7. Fragility of vessel walls due to systemic vascular disease
   A. Age
   B. Arteriosclerosis
   C. Hypertension
   D. Nephritis
   E. Diabetes

8. Blood dyscrasias
   A. Thrombocytopenia purpura
   B. Associated with thrombocytopenia
      (1) Leukemia
      (2) Anemias, especially aplastic anemia
      (3) Splenic disorders, such as Banti's or Gaucher's disease, Felty's syndrome, and hemolytic icterus
      (4) Septicemias
      (5) Systemic lupus erythematosus
      (6) Drugs, including pyrimethamine, sulfonamides, Butazolidin, chloramphenicol, tolbutamide, and propylthiouracil

C. Scurvy

D. Secondary, such as that due to nephritic, cardiac, or hepatic disease

E. Hemochromatosis

F. Ehlers-Danlos syndrome (fibrodysplasia elastica generalisata)

G. Schomberg's disease

9. Acute febrile systemic infections

A. Parasites, such as plasmodia (malaria)

B. Bacteria, such as those responsible for meningococcal septicemia, subacute bacterial endocarditis, scarlet fever, diphtheria, typhoid fever, or cholera

C. Rickettsia, such as those causing typhus fever

D. Viruses, such as those responsible for influenza, smallpox, measles, yellow fever, or sandfly fever

E. Unknown infective agents, such as those causing glandular fever

10. Spontaneous during menstruation

11. Following angiography

12. Bacterial endocarditis

13. Following open heart operation

14. Without apparent cause—most common

Duke-Elder, S.: Diseases of the Outer Eye. System of Ophthalmology, Vol. VIII, Part 1. St. Louis, C. V. Mosby Co., 1965, pp. 33–39.

Givner, I.: Noninfectious Conjunctival Congestion. Infectious Diseases of the Conjunctiva and Cornea. Symposium of the New Orleans Academy of Ophthalmology. St. Louis, C. V. Mosby Co., 1963, p. 48.

Russo, C. E., and Ruiz, R. S.: Silicone Sponge Rejection. Arch. Ophthal. 85:647–650, 1971.

Willerson, J. T., et al.: Conjunctival Petechiae after Open Heart Surgery. New Eng. J. Med. 284:539, 1971.

7

Bitot's Spots (small gray or white sharply outlined areas, cheese-like or foamy, occurring on either side of the limbus but especially in the temporal area)

1. Vitamin A deficiency—(see night blindness, p. 545)

2. Pellagra or other poor nutritional states

3. Congenital anomaly

4. Associated with coloboma of lid (see p. 80)

5. Exposure (drying)

6. Idiopathic

Duke-Elder, S., and Leigh, A. G.: Diseases of the Outer Eye. System of Ophthalmology, Vol. VIII, Part 2. St. Louis, C. V. Mosby Co., 1965, pp. 1117–1125.

Levine, R. A., and Raab, M. F.: Bitot's Spot Overlying a Pinquecula. Arch. Ophthal. 86:525–528, 1971.

Snood, N. N., and Rotnaraj, A.: Bitot's Spots. Orient. Arch. Ophthal. 5:223, 1967.

Tumors of the Conjunctiva

1. Epithelial tumors
    A. Kerato-acanthoma
    B. Dyskeratosis
        (1) Epithelial plaques—leukoplakia, hereditary benign intraepithelial dyskeratosis
        (2) Intraepithelial epithelioma (Bowen's disease)
    C. Papilloma
    D. Epithelioma
    E. Adenoma

      (1) Papillary cystadenoma lymphomatosum (Warthin's tumor)

      (2) Oncocytoma (oxyphil-cell adenoma)

      (3) Pleomorphic adenoma of Krause's glands

2. Mesoblastic tumors
   A. Inflammatory hyperplasias
      (1) Granuloma
      (2) Plasmoma
   B. Connective tissue tumors
      (1) Fibroma
      (2) Lipoma
      (3) Myxoma

3. The reticuloses
   A. Lymphoma
   B. Lymphosarcoma
   C. Mycosis fungoides

4. Vascular tumors—angiomas
   A. Polymorphous hemangioma, telangiectatic granuloma, granuloma pyogenicum
   B. Lymphangioma
   C. Angiosarcoma—monomorphous angioma, Kaposi's (hemorrhagic) sarcoma

5. Pigmented tumors
   A. Nevus
   B. Malignant melanoma
   C. Intraepithelial melanoma—precancerous melanosis

6. Peripheral nerve tumors
   A. Neurofibroma
      (1) Neurilemmoma (neurinoma, schwannoma)
      (2) Malignant schwannoma (neurogenic sarcoma; neurofibrosarcoma)
      (3) Plexiform neurofibromatosis
   B. Tuberous sclerosis (Bourneville's disease)
   C. Intrascleral nerve loops

Doughman, D. J., and Wenk, R. E.: Epibulbar Myxoma. Amer. J. Ophthal. *69*:483–485, 1970.

Duke-Elder, S.: System of Ophthalmology, Vol. VIII, Part 2. St. Louis, C. V. Mosby Co., 1965, p. 1144–1242.

Wilson, F. M., and Ostler, H. B.: Conjunctival Papillomas in Siblings. Amer. J. Ophthal. *77*:103–107, 1974.

Conjunctival Cysts

1. Congenital corneoscleral cysts (rare)

2. Epibulbar dermoids with cystic form

3. Traumatic cyst (epithelial implantation), such as that following operation for correction of strabismus

4. Limbal wounds with iris prolapse

5. Parasitic cyst, such as filarial cyst

6. Epithelial cyst
   A. Glandular retention—involvement of Krause's glands in chronic inflammatory conditions, including trachoma and pemphigus
   B. Downgrowth of epithelium—chronic inflammatory conditions, such as that following inflammation of the pterygium
   C. Apposition of folds of conjunctival mucosa (common)
   D. Pigmented cyst appearing after prolonged topical use of cocaine or epinephrine

7. Lymphatic cyst

Duke-Elder, S., and Leigh, A. G.: Diseases of the Outer Eye. System of Ophthalmology, Vol. VIII, Part 2. St. Louis, C. V. Mosby Co., 1965, pp. 1137–1143.
Jampol, L. M., Albert, D. M., and Taylor, M.: Multiple Retention Cysts of Conjunctiva. Arch. Ophthal. 91:60, 1974.

Limbal Mass

1. Pterygia

2. Papillomas

3. Nevi

4. Granulomas

5. Lymphomas

6. Sarcomas

7. Dermoids

8. Allergic reaction
   A. Phlyctenules (see p. 187)
   B. Vernal limbal lesions

9. Epithelial hyperplasia

10. Malignant melanomas

11. Intraepithelial epitheliomas (Bowen's)

12. Ectopic lacrimal gland tissue

13. Benign nodular fascitis

14. Squamous cell carcinoma

15. Hemangioma

16. Amyloid-perilimbal

17. Associated with skin disease
    A. Acne rosacea
    B. Pityriasis rubra pilaris
    C. Psoriasis
    D. Hereditary benign intraepithelial dyskeratosis
    E. Reticulum cell sarcoma—raised, pink, smooth lesions
    F. Hodgkin's disease
    G. Limbal squamous carcinoma in xeroderma pigmentosa

Boockvar, W., Wessely, Z., and Ballen, P.: Recurrent Granuloma Pyogenicum of Limbus. Arch. Ophthal. *91*:42–44, 1974.
Grayson, M., and Keates, R. H.: Manual of Diseases of the Cornea. Boston, Little, Brown & Co., 1969.

Large, Flat, Fleshy Lesions of Palpebral Conjunctiva

1. Granuloma pyogenicum

2. Ligneous conjunctivitis

3. Papillary hyperplasia of vernal conjunctivitis

4. Embryonal rhabdomyosarcoma of children

Friedman, A. H., and Henkind, P.: Granuloma Pyogenicum of the Palpebral Conjunctiva. Amer. J. Ophthal. *71*:868–872, 1971.

Chronic or Recurrent Ulcers of the Conjunctiva

1. Mucous membrane pemphigoid

2. Tuberculosis

3. Syphilis

4. Soft chancre

5. Fungi

6. Herpes simplex

Nauheim, J. S.: Recurrent Herpes Simplex Conjunctival Ulceration. Arch. Ophthal. *81*:592–595, 1969.

Phlyctenular Keratoconjunctivitis (localized conjunctival, limbal, or corneal nodule about 1 to 3 mm in size)

1. Delayed hypersensitivity to bacterial protein, particularly tuberculoprotein and staphylococci; lymphopathia venereum and coccidioidomycosis may also be allergens

2. Systemic infection

3. Malnutrition

4. Secondary infection of the conjunctiva, especially from *Staphylococcus aureus,* pneumococcus, and Koch-Weeks bacillus

Bedrossian, E. H.: The Eye. Springfield, Ill., Charles C Thomas, 1958, p. 176.

Davis, P. L., and Watson, J. I.: Experimental Conjunctival Phlyctenulosis. Canad. J. Ophthal. *4*:183–190, 1969.

Newell, F. W.: Ophthalmology, Principles and Concepts. St. Louis, C. V. Mosby Co., 1969, p. 177.

Pigmentation of the Conjunctiva (see pigment spots of sclera and episclera, p. 212)

1. Blood pigment
   A. After subconjunctival hemorrhage—fine brown spots (see p. 180)
   B. Yellow tinge of malaria, blackwater fever, or yellow fever
   C. Pigmentary limbal ring associated with senile, traumatic, or diseased conditions

2. Bile pigments (yellow)—obstructive or hemorrhagic jaundice

3. Melanin pigmentation
   A. Addison's disease
   B. Endogenous ochronosis
   C. Keratomalacia
   D. Trachoma—near the limbus
   E. Vernal conjunctivitis
   F. Acanthosis nigricans
   G. Xeroderma pigmentosum
   H. Vitiligo (leukoderma)—increased conjunctival pigmentation
   I. Use of epinephrine, or epinephrine bitartrate, borate, and hydrochloride
   J. Chlorpromazine (Thorazine)

4. Foreign substances
   A. Silver (argyrosis)
   B. Iron (siderosis)
   C. Copper (chalcosis)
   D. Arsenic (arsenic melanosis)
   E. Gold (chrysiasis)
   F. Epinephrine bitartrate, borate, and hydrochloride
   G. Other—including quinones, aniline dyes, and eye cosmetics containing carbon black

5. Benign melanosis—overactivity of melanocytes
   A. Epithelial—congenital or acquired, e.g., following radiation or use of chemicals (arsenic); in Addison's disease; due to chronic conjunctivitis (trachoma, vernal conjunctivitis, onchocerciasis, keratomalacia)
   B. Subepithelial—congenital or in association with melanosis oculi or nevus of Ota

6. Neoplasms
   A. Nevus—most common in children, localized, stationary, elevated, cystic, may or may not have pigmentation
   B. Malignant melanoma arising from pre-existing nevus, apparently normal conjunctiva, or from an area of acquired pigmentation (intraepithelial melanoma), middle age, diffuse, flat, pigmentation, progressive, no cysts

7. Secondary melanotic tumors

8. Incidentally pigmented tumors, such as a melanocarcinoma

Bernstein, H. N.: Some Iatrogenic Ocular Diseases from Systemically Administered Drugs. *In* Symposium on Ocular Pharmacology and Therapeutics. Transactions of New Orleans Academy of Ophthalmology. St. Louis, C. V. Mosby, 1970, pp. 143–163.

Duke-Elder, S., and Leigh, A. G.: Diseases of the Outer Eye. System of Ophthalmology, Vol. VIII, Part 2. St. Louis, C. V. Mosby Co., 1965, pp. 595–598, 1210–1231.

Reinecke, R. D., and Kuwabara, T.: Corneal Deposits Secondary to Topical Epinephrine. Arch. Ophthal. *70*:170–172, 1963.

Sugar, H. S., and Koberwick, S.: Subconjunctival Pigmentation Associated with the Use of Eye Cosmetics Containing Carbon Black. Amer. J. Ophthal. *62*:146, 1966.

Verdaguea, J., Valenzuela, H., and Strozzi, L.: Melanocytoma of the Conjunctiva. Arch. Ophthal. *91*:363–366, 1974.

Symblepharon (fusing of eyelid to opposing surface, such as eyelid and bulbar conjunctiva)

1. Physical trauma with denuded epithelium, including purulent, membranous, bullous, or ulcerative conjunctivitis and trauma

2. Chemical burns especially lime or caustic burns

3. Longstanding acute inflammation
   A. Pemphigus
   B. Stevens-Johnson disease
   C. Erythema multiforme exudativum

4. Congenital

Duke-Elder, S.: System of Ophthalmology. Vol. III, Part 1. St. Louis, C. V. Mosby Co., 1965, pp. 6–7.

Fox, S. A.: Ophthalmic Plastic Surgery, 4th ed. New York, Grune & Stratton, 1970, p. 234.

GLOBE

Contents

Microphthalmia (small globe)

1. Hallerman-Streiff malformation (dyscephalia mandibulo-oculofacialis)—beaked nose, small mouth, cataracts, hypotrichosis

2. Oculodentodigital dysplasia—hypoplastic enamel, syndactylia of fourth and fifth fingers and thin nose

3. Pierre Robin syndrome—micrognathia, glossoptosis, and respiratory distress

4. Congenital rubella—congenital heart disease, deafness, cataracts, glaucoma, mental-motor retardation

5. Congenital toxoplasmosis—hydrocephalus, chorioretinitis, intracranial calcifications, mental retardation

6. Cytomegalic inclusion disease—chorioretinitis

7. Treacher Collins syndrome (mandibulofacial dysostosis, Franceschetti-Klein syndrome)—malformed ears, micrognathia, beaked nose, colobomas, conduction deafness, sloping forehead, depressed nasal bridge, malformed or low-set ears, cleft lip

8. Trisomy 13-15

9. Microphthalmia associated with
   A. Coloboma—dominant and sex-linked inheritance
   B. Cataract—dominant inheritance
   C. Retinitis pigmentosa and glaucoma—dominant inheritance
   D. Ectopic pupils—dominant inheritance
   E. High hypermetropia—?recessive inheritance
   F. Glaucoma—?recessive inheritance
   G. Oligophrenia—sex-linked recessive
   H. Congenital spastic diplegia (Little's disease)—sex-linked recessive
   I. Malformation of hands and feet—autosomal recessive
   J. Polydactyly—autosomal recessive
   K. Harelip and cleft palate—autosomal recessive

10. Maternal vitamin A deficiency—colobomas and microphthalmia

11. Maternal thalidomide ingestion

12. Chromosome 18 deletion

13. Oculovertebral dysplasia (Weyers and Thier)—unilateral maxillary dysplasia, macrostomia, dental malocclusion

14. Oculoauriculovertebral syndrome (Goldenhar)—frontal bossing, epibulbar cyst, microtia, hypoplastic nostrils

15. Dyscraniopygophalangea (Ullrich's syndrome)

16. Focal dermal hypoplasia syndrome (Goltz's syndrome)— papillomas of the lips, strabismus, uveal colobomas, microphthalmus, and usually female

17. Meckel's syndrome—autosomal recessive with developmental abnormalities incompatible with life, and anophthalmos or microphthalmia

18. Ring chromosome in the D group (13-15)—microphthalmus, epicanthus, blepharophimosis, cataracts

19. Myotonic dystrophy

20. Francois' dyscephalic syndrome—dyscephaly with bird-like head, dental anomalies, proportional dwarfism, hypotrichiasis, skin atrophy, congenital cataracts, nystagmus

21. Conradi's syndrome (chondrodystrophia calcificans congenita syndrome)

22. Idiopathic

Bilchik, R. C., et al.: Anomalies with Ring D Chromosome. Amer. J. Ophthal. 73:83–89, 1972.

Duke-Elder, S.: System of Ophthalmology, Vol. III, Part 2. St. Louis, C. V. Mosby Co., 1964, pp. 493–494.

Francois, J., and Pierard, J.: The Francois Dyscephalic Syndrome and Skin Manifestations. Amer. J. Ophthal. 71:1241–1250, 1971.

Gellis, S. S., and Feingold, M.: Atlas of Mental Retardation. Washington, D.C., U.S. Government Printing Office, 1968.

Goldberg, M. F., and McKusick, V. A.: X-Linked Colobomatous Microphthalmus and Other Congenital Anomalies. Amer. J. Ophthal. 71:1128–1133, 1971.

Goodman, R. M., and Gorlin, R. J.: The Face in Genetic Disorders. St. Louis, C. V. Mosby Co., 1970, p. 70.

Ide, C. H., Miller, G. W., and Wollschlaeger, P. B.: Familial Facial Dysplasia. Arch. Ophthal. *84*:427–432, 1970.

Ide, C. H., Wollschlaeger, P. B., and Wollschlaeger, G.: Oculovertebral Syndrome Associated with Cardiovascular Abnormalities. Ann. Ophthal. *4*:836–841, 1972.

Lessell, S., Coppeto, J., and Samet, S.: Ophthalmoplegia in Myotonic Dystrophy. Amer. J. Ophthal. *71*:1231–1235, 1971.

MacRae, D. W., et al.: Ocular Manifestations of the Meckel Syndrome. Arch. Ophthal. *88*:106–113, 1972.

Rains, D. E., McCoy, D. A., and Nelson, E. J.: Bilateral Microphthalmus in Monozygous Twins. Ann. Ophthal. *4*:646–652, 1972.

Sorsby, A.: Ophthalmic Genetics, 2nd ed. New York, Appleton-Century-Crofts, Inc., 1970.

Yanoff, M., Rorke, L. B., and Niederer, B. S.: Ocular and Cerebral Abnormalities in Chromosome 18 Deletion Defect. Amer. J. Ophthal. *70*:391–402, 1970.

Zimmerman, L. E., and Font, R. L.: Congenital Malformations of the Eye; Some Recent Advances in Knowledge of the Pathogenesis and Histopathological Characteristics. J.A.M.A. *196*:684–692, 1966.

Buphthalmos (large globe)

This is usually associated with corneal abnormalities such as opacities and rupture of Descemet's membrane. Transition from cornea to sclera is unclear and a thin bluish sclera may be present.

1. Congenital glaucoma (see p. 266)

2. Autosomal recessive inheritance

3. Sporadic occurrence

4. Associated with anterior chamber cleavage syndrome

5. Lowe's syndrome (oculocerebrorenal syndrome)

6. Neurofibromatosis (von Recklinghausen's disease)

7. Sturge-Weber syndrome

8. Cerebrohepatorenal syndrome

9. Chondrodystrophia calcificans congenita (Conradi's syndrome)

10. Oculodentodigital dysplasia

11. Rieger's syndrome (hypodentia and iris dysgenesis)

12. Congenital rubella

Gellis, S. S., and Feingold, M.: Atlas of Mental Retardation. Washington, D.C., U.S. Government Printing Office, 1968.
Sorsby, A.: Ophthalmic Genetics, 2nd ed. New York, Appleton-Century-Crofts, Inc., 1970.

Pseudo-endophthalmitis (conditions that simulate endophthalmitis)

1. Severe postoperative iridocyclitis

2. Chemical reactions from irritating chemicals introduced into the anterior chamber

3. Retained lenticular material

4. Metastatic carcinoma

Levine, R. A., and Williamson, D. E.: Metastatic Carcinoma Simulating a Post-operative Endophthalmitis. Arch. Ophthal. *83*:59–60, 1970.
Theodore, F. H.: Complications after Cataract Surgery: Part I. Int. Ophthal. Clin., *4*:853–885, 1964.

Endophthalmitis (intraocular infection)

1. Bacterial
    A. Responsible bacteria
        (1) Gram positive
            a. *Staphylococcus aureus*
            b. *Staphylococcus albus*
            c. *Diplococcus pneumoniae* (*Pneumococcus*)
            d. Hemolytic streptococcus
            e. *Streptococcus viridans*
            f. *Bacillus subtilis*
            g. *Bacillus megatherium*
            h. *Clostridium perfringens* (*B. welchii*)
        (2) Gram negative
            a. *Pseudomonas aeruginosa* (*B. pyocyaneus*)
            b. *Proteus vulgaris* (*B. proteus*)
            c. *Klebsiella pneumoniae* (*Friedländer's bacillus*)
            d. *Escherichia coli*
            e. *Aerobacter aerogenes*
            f. *Serratia marcescens*
            g. *Neisseria catarrhalis*
            h. Other coliform bacteria
    B. Clinical picture
        (1) Pain, of an intensity much more severe than usually experienced following operation
        (2) Marked tenderness on removing the dressing or touching any of the area adjacent to the eye
        (3) Marked swelling of the upper lid, with redness as well as edema
        (4) Marked inability to open the eyelids
        (5) Extreme redness and chemosis of the bulbar conjunctiva
        (6) Haziness of the cornea with or without microscopic corneal epithelial edema
        (7) A cloudy and turbid anterior chamber, which is usually well reformed
        (8) Hypopyon

2. Fungal
   A. Responsible fungi
      (1) *Cephalosporium* sp.
      (2) *Volutella* sp.
      (3) *Neurospora sitophila*
      (4) *Hormodendrum*
      (5) *Hyalosporus*
      (6) *Cephalosporium* or *Penicillium*
      (7) *Cephalosporium* or *Hyphas*
      (8) *Hyalopus bogolepofi*
      (9) *Actinomyces* sp.
      (10) *Sporotrichum schenkii*
      (11) *Candida* sp.
      (12) *Nocardiosis*
   B. Clinical picture
      (1) Delayed onset—eight to fourteen days or more
      (2) Pain and redness
      (3) Localized gray-white area in anterior vitreous adjacent to pupillary border
      (4) Transient hypopyon
      (5) Gradual extension of membrane on face of vitreous
      (6) Appearance of additional satellite lesions in anterior vitreous at other locations in pupillary zone
      (7) Occasional, less atypical, explosive massive exudative process in anterior vitreous bulging into anterior chamber
      (8) Good light-perception

Allen, H. F., and Mangiaracine, A. B.: Bacterial Endophthalmitis after Cataract Extraction. Arch. Ophthal. *91*:3–7, 1974.

Aronson, S. B.: Starch Endophthalmitis. Amer. J. Ophthal. *73*:570–579, 1972.

Bigger, J. F., et al.: Serratia marcescens Endophthalmitis. Amer. J. Ophthal. *72*:1102–1105, 1971.

Greene, W. H., and Wiesnik, P. H.: Candida Endophthalmitis. Successful Treatment in a Patient with Acute Leukemia. Amer. J. Ophthal. *74*:1100–1102, 1972.

Griffin, R. J., et al.: Blood-borne Candida Endophthalmitis. Arch. Ophthal. *89*:450–456, 1973.

Hattenhauer, J. H., and Lipsich, M. P.: Late Endophthalmitis after Filtering Surgery. Amer. J. Ophthal. *72*:1097–1101, 1971.

Meyer, S. L., Font, R. L., and Shaver, R. P.: Intraocular Nocardiosis. Arch. Ophthal. *83*:536–541, 1970.

Salceda, S. R., Lapuy, J., and Vizconde, R.: Serratia marcescens Endophthalmitis. Arch. Ophthal. *89*:163–166, 1973.

Theodore, F. H.: Complications after Cataract Surgery: Part I. Int. Ophthal. Clin. *4*:839–882, 1964.

Valenton, M. J., Brubaker, R. F., and Allen, H. F.: Staphylococcus epidermidis (albus) Endophthalmitis. Arch. Ophthal. *89*:94–96, 1973.

Wassermann, H. E.: Avian Tuberculosis Endophthalmitis. Arch. Ophthal. *89*:321–323, 1973.

Intraocular Cartilage

1. Persistent hyperplastic primary vitreous

2. Trisomy 13-15 (globe less than 10 mm in diameter)

3. Embryonal medulloepitheliomas (diktyomas)

4. Incidental finding in microphthalmic eye, microphthalmus with cyst, microphthalmic eye from a cyclopic orbit, in eyes with coloboma of the choroid and retina or ciliary body

5. Angiomatosis of the retina

6. Chromosome 18 deletion

7. Incontinenta pigmenti (Bloch-Sulzberger disease)

8. Retinal dysplasia

9. Chronic inflammation

Anderson, S. R.: Medulloepithelioma of the Retina. Int. Ophthal. Clin. *2*:483–506, 1962.

Cogan, D. G., and Kuwabara, T.: Ocular Pathology of the 13-15 Trisomy Syndrome. Arch. Ophthal. *72*:246–253, 1964.

Duke-Elder, S.: System of Ophthalmology, Vol. III, Part 2. St. Louis, C. V. Mosby Co., 1964, pp. 456–488, 542.

Reese, A. B., and Payne, F.: Persistence and Hyperplasia of the Primary Vitreous. Amer. J. Ophthal. *29*:1–19, 1964.

Riley, F. C.: Intraocular Cartilage. Arch. Ophthal. *85*:256, 1971.

Yanoff, M., and Font, R. L.: Intraocular Cartilage in a Microphthalmic Eye of an Otherwise Healthy Girl. Arch. Ophthal. *81*:238–240, 1969.

Yanoff, M., Rorke, L. B., and Niederer, B. S.: Ocular and Cerebral Abnormalities in Chromosome 18 Deletion Defect. Amer. J. Ophthal. *70*:391–402, 1970.

Intraocular Calcifications

1. Retinoblastoma

2. Retrolental fibroplasia

3. Intraocular sarcoma

4. Sites of intraocular calcification
   A. Posterior pole to ora serrata in region of choroid and pigment epithelium
   B. Cyclitic membrane
   C. Peripapillary choroid
   D. Lens
   E. Retina
   F. Vitreous
   G. Calcific emboli of retinal and ciliary arteries

5. Intraocular calcifications following:
   A. Trauma (perforating, non-perforating, or surgical)
   B. Congenital deformity
   C. Recurrent iritis and keratitis
   D. Retinal detachment

Baghdassarian, S. A., Crawford, J. B., and Rathbun, J. E.: Calcific Emboli of the Retinal and Ciliary Arteries. Amer. J. Ophthal. *69*:372–375, 1970.

Finkelstein, E. M., and Boniuk, M.: Intraocular Ossification and Hematopoiesis. Amer. J. Ophthal. *68*:683, 1969.

Hartman, E., and Gilles, E.: Roentgenologic Diagnosis in Ophthalmology. Philadelphia, J. B. Lippincott Co., 1958, pp. 126–127.

Intraocular Adipose Tissue

1. Missile passing through orbit carrying orbital fat into the eye
2. Embolic phenomenon secondary to crush wounds of the thorax and abdomen or fracture of long bones of the extremities
3. Congenital malformations
   A. Dermoid or dermolipoma extending from the cornea or limbus into the globe
   B. Persistent hyperplastic vitreous and other related ocular malformations, such as microphthalmia, persistent hyloid vessels, cataract, and abnormal differentiation of the angle of the anterior chamber
   C. Malformed optic nerve
4. Formation of fatty tissue within the marrow spaces of metaplastic bone

Font, R. L., Yanoff, M., and Zimmerman, L. E.: Intraocular Adipose Tissue and Persistent Hyperplastic Primary Vitreous. Arch. Ophthal. *82*:43–59, 1969.

Hogan, M. J., and Zimmerman, L. E. (Eds.): Ophthalmic Pathology, an Atlas and Textbook, ed. 2. Philadelphia, W. B. Saunders Company, 1962, Fig. 81, p. 131; and Fig. 83, p. 134.

Willis, R., et al.: Heterotropic Adipose Tissue and Smooth Muscle in the Optic Disc: Association with Isolated Colobomas. Arch. Ophthal. *86*:139–146, 1972.

Soft Globe (decreased intraocular pressure)

1. Fistula from intraocular source, including penetrating intraocular trauma or surgery and ruptured wall of the globe
2. Phthisis bulbi (see p. 202)

3. Choroidal detachment (see p. 456)

4. Injury to the cervical sympathetic nerve

5. Serous detachment of the retina

6. Myotonic dystrophy

7. Systemic disturbances
   A. Diabetic coma
   B. Uremic coma
   C. Cardiac edema
   D. Extreme or rapid dehydration due to malnutrition, cholera, or diarrhea
   E. Severe abdominal disturbances, such as intestinal perforation or obstruction
   F. Profound anemias
   G. Giant-cell arteritis
   H. Fall in ocular blood pressure due to hypotension, ligation of the carotid artery, carotid occlusion, or pulseless disease (aortic arch syndrome; Takayasu's syndrome)
   I. Postencephalitic syndrome following severe cerebral trauma, barbiturate poisoning, in deep anesthesia, following leukotomy, or on the paralyzed side in cases of cerebral hemiplegia

8. Drugs, such as Eserine, pilocarpine, epinephrine bitartrate, Diamox, and ouabain

9. Detachment of the ciliary body, planned or inadvertent

10. Hyperosmotic agents, such as mannitol or urea

11. Iritis or iridocyclitis

12. After central retinal vein occlusion

13. Myopia—low scleral rigidity may give false low readings with schiotz but normal readings with applanation

14. Parkinson's disease

15. Herpes zoster

16. Following irradiation by x rays or beta rays

17. Congenital lesions, including microphthalmus, aniridia, and coloboma

18. Concussion trauma

19. Necrosis of anterior segment of the eye

20. Leprosy

21. Idiopathic, including normal variation

Cherry, P. M. H.: Rupture of the Globe. Arch. Ophthal. *88*:498–507, 1972.

Chandler, P. A., and Maumenee, A. E.: A Major Cause of Hypotony. Amer. J. Ophthal. *52*:609, 1961.

Duke-Elder, S.: System of Ophthalmology, Vol. XI. St. Louis, C. V. Mosby Co., 1969, pp. 726–746.

Lessell, S., Coppeto, J., and Samet, S.: Ophthalmoplegia in Myotonic Dystrophy. Amer. J. Ophthal. *71*:1231–1235, 1971.

Pradham, J. S., Shukla, B. R., and Ahuja, O. P.: Shallow Anterior Chamber after Cataract Extraction. Eye Ear Nose Throat Monthly *47*:53, 1968.

Slem, G.: Clinical Studies of Ocular Leprosy. Amer. J. Ophthal. *71*: 431–434, 1971.

Vannas, S., and Raitta, C.: Intraocular Hypotony vs Hypotony after Central Retinal Vein Occlusion. Ann. Ophthal. *2*:213–217, 1970.

Walsh, F. B., and Hoyt, W. F.: Clinical Neuro-ophthalmology, 3rd ed. Baltimore, Williams & Wilkins Co., 1969, pp. 1850–1853.

Phthisis Bulbi (degenerative shrinkage of the eyeball with hypotony)

1. Panophthalmitis

2. Endophthalmitis

3. Sympathetic ophthalmia

4. Severe ocular injury with loss of tissue

5. Tumor, such as retinoblastoma or malignant melanoma

6. Severe uveitis

7. Following cataract surgery, especially with rubella syndrome

Boniuk, J., and Boniuk, M.: The Incidence of Phthisis Bulbi as a Complication of Cataract Surgery in the Congenital Rubella Syndrome. Trans. Amer. Acad. Ophthal. Otolaryng. *74*:360–369, 1970.

Duke-Elder, S., and Perkins, E. S.: Diseases of the Uveal Tract. System of Ophthalmology, Vol. IX. St. Louis, C. V. Mosby Co., 1966.

Hogan, M. J., and Zimmerman, L. E.: Ophthalmic Pathology, 2nd ed. Philadelphia, W. B. Saunders Co., 1962.

Newell, F. W.: Ophthalmology, Principles and Concepts, 2nd ed. St. Louis, C. V. Mosby Co., 1969.

Clinical Anophthalmos (apparent absence of globe)

1. Idiopathic

2. Oculovertebral dysplasia (Weyers and Thier)—unilateral maxillary dysplasia, macrostomia, dental malocclusion

3. Gross midline facial defects

4. Trisomy 13-15—frontal bossing, acentric pupils, cleft palate, hypoplastic mandible, low-set and malformed ears

5. Otocephaly—transverse facial cleft, anophthalmos, ear remnants meeting near mid-line

6. Anencephaly—exposed cerebrum, midbrain, flat nose, puffy eyelids, short neck

7. Dyscraniopygophalangea—microphthalmia, sunken nose, cleft palate, macrostomia or microstomia, polydactyly

8. Hallermann-Strieff syndrome (oculomandibulodyscephaly)—microbrachycephaly, cataract, small face, high-arched palate, dental anomalies

203

9. Goldenhar's syndrome (oculoauriculovertebral syndrome) —frontal bossing, epibulbar cyst, microtia, hypoplastic nostrils

10. Meckel's syndrome—autosomal recessive with developmental abnormalities incompatible with life, and anophthalmos or microphthalmia

11. Kleinfelter's syndrome—XXY chromosome

Aita, J. A.: Congenital Facial Anomalies with Neurologic Defects. Springfield, Ill., Charles C Thomas, 1969, pp. 5, 57, 73, 80, 92, 161, 184, 261.

Ide, C. H., Wollschlaeger, P. B., and Wollschlaeger, G.: Oculovertebral Syndrome Associated with Cardiovascular Abnormalities. Ann. Ophthal. *4*:836–841, 1972.

MacRae, D. W., et al.: Ocular Manifestations of the Meckel Syndrome. Arch. Ophthal. *88*:106–113, 1972.

Welter, D. A., et al.: Kleinfelter's Syndrome with Anophthalmos. Amer. J. Ophthal. *77*:895–898, 1974.

Oculodigital Stimulation (patient presses on globe through lids with index finger or hand; poor visual acuity)

1. Leber's amaurosis congenita or other congenital retinal degeneration

2. Congenital rubella syndrome

3. Congenital glaucoma

4. Bilateral congenital cataracts

5. Total corneal leukomas

6. Combined retinal detachment and congenital cataract

7. Norrie's disease

Fradkin, A. H.: Norrie's Disease. Amer. J. Ophthal. *72*:947–948, 1971.

Roy, F. H.: Ocular Autostimulation. Amer. J. Ophthal. *63*:1776–1777, 1967.

SCLERA

Contents

Pseudoepiscleritis (lesions resembling episcleritis)

1. Lids
    A. Ingrowing lash
    B. Lash in punctum

2. Conjunctiva
    A. Inflamed pinguecula
    B. Phlyctenular conjunctivitis
    C. Conjunctivitis

3. Cornea
    A. Punctate keratitis, such as that due to viral kerato-conjunctivitis, Sjögren's disease, or psoriasis (p. 235)
    B. Sclerosing keratitis due to scleritis
    C. Rosacea keratitis associated with sector nebulae

4. Sclera, such as scleritis with thinning

5. Tumor, such as malignant melanoma

Lyne, A. J., and Pitkeathley, D. A.: Episcleritis and Scleritis. Arch. Ophthal. *80*:171, 1968.

Episcleritis (inflammation of the episcleral tissues causing discomfort rather than pain, not affecting visual acuity, and resolving spontaneously)

Episcleritis may be nodular or diffuse.

1. Single, short episode that does not recur—idiopathic

2. Recurrent attacks over years that do not produce scleritis
    A. Episcleral foreign body
    B. Associated with skin diseases, such as psoriasis, lichen planus, and erythema elevantum diutinum

C. Collagen disorders, such as rheumatoid arthritis and polyarteritis nodosa
D. Arteritis and systemic vasculitis
E. Weber-Christian disease
F. Inflammatory pseudotumor
G. Insect bite granuloma

Ferry, P. A.: The Histopathology of Rheumatoid Episcleral Nodules. Arch. Ophthal. *82*:77, 1969.
Friedman, A. H., and Henkind, P.: Unusual Causes of Episcleritis. Trans. Amer. Acad. Ophthal. Otolaryng. In press.
Horwitz, J. A., and Worthen, D. M.: Episcleral Nodule in Systemic Vasculitis. Ann. Ophthal. *4*:482–483, 1972.
Lyne, A. J., and Pitkeathley, D. A.: Episcleritis and Scleritis. Arch. Ophthal. *80*:171, 1968.

Scleritis (inflammation of the scleral coat of the eye)

Scleritis may cause severe pain, scleral thinning, and even perforation. It may be nodular (localized) or brawny (generalized).

1. Exogenous infections—by ulceration or injury, infection penetrates through the conjunctiva
   A. Bacterial
   B. Viral
   C. Fungal
   D. Chemical, animal, or vegetable irritants

2. Secondary infections that spread directly from:
   A. Conjunctiva
   B. Cornea
   C. Uvea
   D. Periorbital tissues, such as those of the nose or sinuses
   E. Associated with skin disease

3. Endogenous infections
   A. Acute suppurative metastatic lesions

B. Granulomatous lesions of tuberculosis, syphilis, and leprosy

C. Viral infections, such as herpes simplex, herpes zoster, and mumps

4. Allergic or toxic—imprecise etiologic background
   A. Erythema nodosum
   B. Felty's syndrome (rheumatoid arthritis with hypersplenism)
   C. Wegener's granuloma

5. Systemic diseases
   A. Collagen diseases, such as rheumatoid arthritis
   B. Metabolic disease, such as gout

Lyne, A. J., and Pitkeathley, D. A.: Episcleritis and Scleritis. Arch. Ophthal. *80*:171–176, 1968.

Ostriker, P. J., Ostriker, M., and Lasky, M. A.: Keratitis and Scleritis Associated with Felty's Syndrome. Arch. Ophthal. *54*:858, 1955.

Staphyloma of the Sclera (stretching and thinning of the sclera with incarceration of uveal tissue)

1. Scleritis, such as that secondary to rheumatoid arthritis (see scleritis, p. 207)

2. Syphiloma

3. Tuberculoma

4. Uveitis (see pp. 329–335)

5. Endarteritis

6. Trauma

7. Herpes zoster (rare)

8. Corneoscleral ectasia

9. Myopia with increased anteroposterior diameter

10. Buphthalmos (see p. 194)

11. Marfan's syndrome associated with myopia

12. Retinal detachment associated with meridonal staphyloma

13. Wegener's granuloma

14. Beta radiation

Ferry, A. P., and Leopold, I. H.: Marginal (Ring) Corneal Ulcer as Presenting Manifestation of Wegener's Granuloma. Trans. Amer. Acad. Ophthal. Otolaryng. 74:1276–1282, 1970.

Goldberg, M. F., and Ryan, S. J.: Intercalary Staphyloma in Marfan's Syndrome. Amer. J. Ophthal. 67:329, 1969.

Vail, F.: The Scleral-Resection (Eyeball Shortening) Operation: The DeSchweintz Lecture. Amer. J. Ophthal. 29:785, 1946.

Young, C. A.: Equatorial Scleral Staphyloma. Amer. J. Ophthal. 40:12, 1955.

Zagora, E.: Eye Injuries. Springfield, Ill., Charles C Thomas, 1970, p. 480.

Differential Diagnosis of Scleromalacia Perforans

	Scleromalacia Perforans	Scleromalacia Perforans with Porphyria	Necrotizing Nodular Scleritis	Spontaneous Intercalary Perforation	Hyaline Plaques	Episcleritis; Scleritis
Age	50–75	over 40	50–75	25–50	60–75	Variable
Sex	Females	Males	Either	Either	Either	Either
Rheumatoid arthritis	Constant	Unrelated	50%	Unrelated	Unrelated	Variable
Binocularity	Bilateral	Bilateral	Either	Either	Bilateral	Variable
Distribution	Multiple	Single	Random	Single	Symmetrical	Variable
Inflammation	Nil	Nil	Marked	Nil	Nil	Marked
Pathology	Necrosis	Necrosis	Inflammation and necrosis	Unknown (? atrophy)	Degeneration	Inflammation
Pain	Nil	Nil	Marked	Nil	Nil	Marked
Evolution	Progressive	Slowly progressive	Sometimes resolution	Stationary	Stationary	Often resolution
Prognosis	Bad	Poor	Poor	Good	Good	Usually good

Duke-Elder, S.: System of Ophthalmology, Vol. VIII, Part 2. London, Henry Kimpton, 1965, p. 1055.

Blue Sclera (localized or generalized blue coloration of the sclera due to thinness and loss of water content allowing the underlying dark choroid to be seen)

1. Osteogenesis imperfecta (van der Hoeve's syndrome)—deafness and brittle bones

2. Hereditary anomaly characterized by defective mesodermal structures including brittle corneas

3. Corneal encroachment into sclera

4. Crouzon's disease (craniofacial dysostosis)

5. Ehlers-Danlos syndrome (fibrodysplasia elastica generalisata)

6. Staphyloma (see staphyloma, p. 208)

7. Marfan's syndrome (dystrophia mesodermalis congenita)

8. Hypophosphatasia

9. Albright's hereditary osteodystrophy (pseudohypoparathyroidism)—refractory end-organ to parathyroid hormone with hypocalcemia and hyperphosphatemia

10. Hallerman-Streiff syndrome (dyscephalia mandibulo-oculo-facialis)—dwarfism associated with thin, beaked nose; small mouth; bilateral microphthalmia; cataracts; atrophied skin; and hypotrichosis

11. Pycnodysostosis—short stature, persistent cranial sutures, frontal bossing, hypoplastic facial bones, dental abnormalities

12. Turner's syndrome (gonadal dysgenesis)—short stature, webbing and/or shortening of neck, absence of secondary sexual characteristics, broad bridge of nose, epicanthal folds, low-set ears

13. De Lange's syndrome—synophrys and telecanthus, blue sclera, strabismus, nystagmus, myopia, ptosis

14. Werner's syndrome—dwarfism, premature balding and graying, skin atrophy, beaked nose

Brenner, R. L., Smith, J. L., Cleveland, W. W., Bejar, R. L., and Lockhart, W. S., Jr.: Eye Signs of Hypophosphatasia. Arch. Ophthal. *81*:614, 1969.

Bullock, J. D., and Howard, R. O.: Werner Syndrome. Arch. Ophthal. *90*:53–56, 1973.

Duke-Elder, S.: Normal and Abnormal Development. System of Ophthalmology, Vol. III, Part 2. St. Louis, C. V. Mosby Co., 1964, pp. 539–542.

Duke-Elder, S., and Leigh, A. G.: Diseases of the Outer Eye. System of Ophthalmology, Vol. VIII, Part 2. St. Louis, C. V. Mosby Co., 1965, pp. 998–1003.

Geeraets, W. J.: Ocular Syndromes, 2nd ed. Philadelphia, Lea & Febiger, 1969, p. 224.

Gellis, S. S., and Feingold, M.: Atlas of Mental Retardation. Washington, D.C., U.S. Government Printing Office, 1968.

Milot, J., and DeMay, F.: Ocular Anomalies in DeLange Syndrome. Amer. J. Ophthal. *74*:394–399, 1972.

Stein, R., Lazar, M., and Adam, A.: Brittle Cornea, a Familial Trait Associated with Blue Sclera. Amer. J. Ophthal. *66*:67, 1968.

Wilson, F. M., Grayson, M., and Pieroni, D.: Corneal Changes in Ectodermal Dysplasia: Case Report, Histopathology and Differential Diagnosis. Amer. J. Ophthal. *75*:17–27, 1973.

Pigment Spots of Sclera and Episclera (see pigmentation of conjunctiva, p. 187)

1. Uveal melanocytes carried by the scleral emissaria into the episclera—most often in eyes with dark irides in superior, inferior, temporal, and nasal quadrants in descending frequency. Conjunctiva freely movable over them

2. Intrascleral nerve loops with uveal pigment—painful to touch

3. Nevi

4. Cysts

5. Extension of adjacent or underlying malignant melanoma

6. Ochronosis with melanin deposition

7. Transscleral migration of pigment following cryotherapy of intraocular tumor or trauma

8. Resolving hemorrhage

9. Staphyloma

10. Acquired melanosis

11. Topically applied epinephrine

12. Foreign body

Boniuk, M., and Hawkins, W. R.: Transscleral Migration of Pigment Following Cryotherapy of Intraocular Glioma. Trans. Amer. Acad. Ophthal. Otolaryng. 75:60–69, 1971.

Shields, J. A., Green, W. R., and McDonald, P. R.: Uveal Pseudo-melanoma Due to Post-traumatic Pigmentary Migration. Arch. Ophthal. 89:519–522, 1973.

Yanoff, M.: Pigment Spots of the Sclera. Arch. Ophthal. 81:151, 1969.

Dilated Episcleral Vessels

1. Glaucoma, untreated

2. Uveal neoplasm with localized engorgement

3. Occlusion of orbital veins of the apex of the orbit
   A. Endocrine exophthalmos of rapid development
   B. Inflammatory lesions
   C. Orbital thrombophlebitis
   D. Neoplasm (rare)

4. Carotico-cavernous fistula

5. Right-sided heart failure due to bronchitis, emphysema, bronchiectasis, or other type of chronic respiratory difficulty

8

6. Increased viscosity of circulating blood
   A. Polycythemia vera
   B. Leukemia (early)

7. Ophthalmic vein thrombosis

8. Cavernous sinus thrombosis

Boniuk, M.: The Ocular Manifestations of Ophthalmic Vein and Aseptic Cavernous Sinus Thrombosis. Trans. Amer. Acad. Ophthal. Otolaryng. *76*:1519–1534, 1972.

Duke-Elder, S.: Diseases of the Outer Eye. System of Ophthalmology, Vol. VIII, Part 1. St. Louis, C. V. Mosby Co., 1965, pp. 17–20.

Minas, T. F., and Podos, S. M.: Familial Glaucoma Associated with Elevated Episcleral Venous Pressure. Arch. Ophthal. *80*:202–213, 1968.

Weekers, R., and Delmarcelle, Y.: Pathogenesis of Intraocular Hypertension in Cases of Arteriovenous Aneurysm. Arch. Ophthal. *48*: 338–343, 1952.

Scleral Rigidity

1. Age—increase, decrease, or stay the same

2. Myopia—increase or decrease

3. Increased intraocular pressure—increase, decrease, or stay the same

4. Thyrotropic exophthalmos—decrease

5. Following intraocular procedures—increase or decrease

6. Diabetes mellitus—increase

7. Use of strong miotics, such as phospholine iodide—decrease

8. Drinking of water—decrease

Kolker, A. E., and Hetherington, J.: Becker-Shaffer's Diagnosis and Therapy of the Glaucomas, 3rd ed. St. Louis, C. V. Mosby Co., 1970, pp. 460–471.

Vucicevic, Z. M., and Ralston, J.: Influences of the Volume and Hydration Changes on Scleral Rigidity. Ann. Ophthal. *4*:715–732, 1972.

CORNEA

Contents

216

Crystals of the Cornea (deposition of crystalline substances in the cornea)

1. Cystinosis
   A. Congenital
   B. Benign adult

2. Crystalline dystrophy of Schnyder

3. Dysproteinemia
   A. Cryoglobulinemia
   B. Multiple myeloma

4. Bietti's marginal crystalline dystrophy

5. Uremia

6. Gout

7. Elevated bilirubin with crystalline dystrophy

8. Drugs, such as indomethacin (Indocin), chloroquine, and Mellaril

9. Hyperparathyroidism

10. Cholesterol crystals—primary or secondary with vascularization

11. Fine multicolored glittering crystals following successful transplant that later underwent graft rejection and was treated with steroids

12. Calcium oxalate—diffenbachia and other plants

Burns, C. A.: Indomethacin, Reduced Retinal Sensitivity, and Corneal Deposits. Amer. J. Ophthal, 66:825, 1968.

Burns, R. P.: Quantitative Biology of the Conjunctiva in Symposium on Ocular Pharmacology and Therapeutics. Transactions of the New Orleans Academy of Ophthalmology. St. Louis, C. V. Mosby Co., 1970, pp. 83–93.

Cogan, D. G.: Ocular Correlates of Inborn Metabolic Defects. Canad. Med. Assoc. J. 95:1055, 1966.

Duke-Elder, S., and Leigh, A. G.: Diseases of the Outer Eye. System of Ophthalmology, Vol. VIII, Part 2. St. Louis, C. V. Mosby Co., 1965, pp. 946, 1062, 1093.

Ellis, W., Barfort, P., and Mastman, G. J.: Keratoconjunctivitis with Corneal Crystals Caused by the Diffenbachia Plant. Amer. J. Ophthal. 76:143–147, 1973.

Grayson, M., and Keates, R. H.: Manual of Diseases of the Cornea. Boston, Little, Brown & Co., 1969, p. 296.

Sanderson, P. O., et al.: Cystinosis. Arch. Ophthal. 91:270–274, 1974.

Anesthesia of the Cornea (hypesthesia or diminished corneal sensation)

1. Herpes simplex

2. Congestive glaucoma

3. Recent burn

4. Neuroparalytic keratitis

5. Exposure keratitis

6. Leprosy and malaria

7. Postoperative cataract extraction

8. Constant wearing of contact lens

9. Corneal dystrophy—lattice, granular, and macular

10. Within corneal transplant

11. After electrocautery of Bowman's membrane

12. In young diabetic patients—becoming more marked with age

13. Following operation for detached retina—from an encircling band or, less frequently, a circumscribed buckle

14. Riley-Day syndrome (congenital familial dysautonomia), Barré-Liéou syndrome (posterior cervical sympathetic syndrome), Gradenigo's syndrome (temporal syndrome), Rochon-Duvigneaud syndrome (superior orbital fissure syndrome)

15. Radiation keratitis

16. Herpes zoster ophthalmicus

17. Interruption of trigeminal nerve or gasserian ganglion, including cerebellopontine angle tumor or other space-occupying lesion in the region of the superior orbital fissure

18. Oculoauriculovertebral dysplasia—unilateral or bilateral congenital failure of the trigeminal nerve

19. Psoriasis (lower portion)

20. Hydroa vacciniforme (lower portion)

21. Corneal edema

22. Carbon disulfide

23. Congenital

24. Hydrogen sulfide

25. Scholz's subacute cerebral sclerosis

26. Stelazine and Steladex

27. Hereditary fleck dystrophy of the cornea

Birndorf, L. A., and Ginsberg, S. P.: Hereditary Fleck Dystrophy Associated with Decreased Corneal Sensitivity. Amer. J. Ophthal. 73:670–672, 1972.
DeVoe, A. G.: Electrocautery of Bowman's Membrane. Arch. Ophthal. 76:768, 1966.
Geeraets, W. J.: Ocular Syndromes, 2nd ed. Philadelphia, Lea & Febiger, 1969, pp. 220–222.
Grayson, M., and Keates, R .H.: Manual of Disease of the Cornea. Boston, Little, Brown & Co., 1969, p. 294.
Pannarole, M. R., and Pannarole, C.: Research into Corneal Sensitivity in Cases Operated on for Retinal Detachment. Boll. Oculist. 44:929–943, 1965.
Petursson, G. J.: Corneal Sensitivity in Lattice Dystrophy. Amer. J. Ophthal. 64:880, 1967.
Schwartz, D. E.: Corneal Sensitivity in Diabetics. Arch. Ophthal. 91:174–178, 1974.
Stewart, H. L., Wind, C. A., and Kaufman, H. E.: Unilateral Congenital Corneal Anesthesia. Amer. J. Ophthal. 74:334–335, 1972.
van Bijsterveld, O. P.: Unilateral Corneal Anesthesia in Oculo-auriculo-vertebral Dysplasia. Arch. Ophthal. 82:189, 1969.

Hyperplastic Corneal Nerves (overgrowth of corneal nerves up to twenty times the normal number)

This nonspecific change may occur in association with the following:

1. Neurofibromatosis
2. Phthisis bulbi
3. Ocular pemphigus
4. Opaque corneal grafts
5. Neuroparalytic keratitis
6. Normal eyes at advanced age

Wolter, J. R.: Corneal Involvement in Choroidal Neurofibromatosis. J. Pediat. Ophthal. 3:19–24, 1966.

Increased Visibility of Corneal Nerves

1. Fuch's dystrophy
2. Keratoconus
3. Ichthyosis
4. Neurofibromatosis
5. Neurofibromatosis associated with pheochromocytoma and thyroid carcinoma
6. Refsum's syndrome—night blindness, retinal degeneration, ataxia, ichthyosis, deafness, polyneuritis
7. Leprosy

8. Siemen's disease (keratosis follicularis spinulosa decalvans) —circumferential pannus with diffuse superficial farinaceous corneal opacities, small hyperkeratotic spines at openings of hair follicles (gooseflesh)

9. Primary amyloidosis

10. "Colloidin" skin syndrome

11. Idiopathic

Baum, J. L., and Adler, M. E.: Pheochromocytoma, Medullary Thyroid Carcinoma, Multiple Mucosal Neuroma. Arch. Ophthal. *87*: 574–584, 1972.

Grayson, M., and Keates, R. H.: Manual of Diseases of the Cornea. Boston, Little, Brown & Co., 1969, p. 296.

Knox, D. L., Payne, J. W., and Hartman, W. H.: The Thickened Corneal Nerves and Eyelids as Signs of Neurofibromatosis and Medullary Thyroid Carcinoma. Prog. Neuro-Ophthal. 1966, pp. 262–266.

Wilson, F. M., Grayson, M., and Pieroni, D.: Corneal Changes in Ectodermal Dysplasia: Case Report, Histopathology, and Differential Diagnosis. Amer. J. Ophthal. *75*:17–27, 1973.

Pigmentation of the Cornea

1. Melanin pigmentation
    A. Epithelial melanosis
        (1) Congenital
        (2) Presence of limbal malignant melanoma
        (3) Sequel to trachoma and other inflammations
        (4) Melanocytic migration in heavily pigmented individuals
    B. Stromal pigmentation such as that in ochronosis
    C. Endothelial melanosis
        (1) Congenital
        (2) Senile

(3) Degenerative, including atrophic and inflammatory conditions, such as cornea guttata, myopia, diabetes mellitus, senile cataract, chronic glaucoma, and melanoma

(4) Krukenberg's spindle, with or without pigmentary glaucoma, may be present in association with diabetes mellitus

(5) Trauma—from contusions, wounds, or intraocular operations

(6) Turk's line—fine vertical line in the lower portion of the cornea

2. Hematogenous pigmentation
   A. Blood-staining of the cornea, most often due to total hyphema associated with elevated intraocular pressure
   B. Hemorrhage into cornea—following subconjunctival hemorrhage and intracorneal hemorrhage from newly formed vessels, as in interstitial keratitis or mustard-gas keratitis
   C. Epithelial deposit associated with spherocytic anemia

3. Metallic pigmentation
   A. Copper (chalcosis)
      (1) Kayser-Fleischer ring—limbal ring associated with Wilson's disease
      (2) Copper foreign body in cornea or intraocular region
      (3) Occupational exposure or topical therapeutic use of copper-containing substance
      (4) Advanced cirrhosis of the liver, such as that associated with parasitic infestation (schistosomiasis)
   B. Silver (argyrosis)—from topical, local, or systemic use; also occupational use
   C. Gold (chrysiasis)—from topical, local, or systemic use
   D. Iron (siderosis)
      (1) Foreign body in cornea or intraocular area
      (2) Iron lines
         a. Fleischer's ring—associated with keratoconus around base of the cone
         b. Hudson-Stahli line—horizontal line at the

junction of the middle and lower one third of the cornea, believed to be related to exposure, trauma of lid closure, and chronic corneal infection

    c. Stocker's line—line running parallel with head of the pterygium

    d. Ferry's line—associated with filtering blebs, believed to result from minute, repeated, localized trauma caused by eyelid striking the elevated bleb

    e. Circular lesion associated with congenital spherocytosis

  E. Bismuth (bismuthiasis)—from therapeutic use

4. Drug pigmentation

  A. Chloroquine and related drugs, as quinacrine, amodiaquin, and hydrochloroquine, give epithelial deposits—yellowish brown

  B. Excessive vitamin D intake with calcium deposition

  C. Epinephrine bitartrate, borate, and hydrochloride

5. Other color changes

  A. White discoloration—scars, fatty degeneration or infiltration, and calcified areas

  B. Yellow discoloration—hyaline or colloid degeneration, and Tangier's disease (familial deficiency of high-density lipoprotein)

  C. Black discoloration—powder, dirt, or ink (tattooing)

  D. Yellow-brown discoloration—Kyrle's disease—hyperkeratosis follicularis et parafollicularis in cutem penetrans

Dalgleish, R.: Ring-like Corneal Deposit in a Case of Congenital Spherocytosis. Brit. J. Ophthal. *49*:40, 1965.

Duke-Elder, S.: Normal and Abnormal Development. System of Ophthalmology, Vol. III, Part 2. St. Louis, C. V. Mosby Co., 1965, pp. 978–992.

Ferry, A. P.: A "New" Iron Line of the Superficial Cornea. Arch. Ophthal. *79*:142, 1968.

Gass, J. D.: The Iron Lines of the Superficial Cornea. Arch. Ophthal. *71*:348–358, 1964.

Grant, W. M.: Toxicology of the Eye. Springfield, Ill., Charles C Thomas, 1962.

Hoffman, H. N., and Fredrickson, D. S.: Tangier Disease (Familial High Density Lipoprotein Deficiency). Amer. J. Med. *39*:582–593, 1965.

O'Brien, C. S.: Ophthalmology, Notes for Students. Iowa City, Athens Press, 1930, pp. 277–278.

Reinecke, R. D., and Kuwabara, T.: Corneal Deposits Secondary to Topical Epinephrine. Arch. Ophthal. *70*:170–172, 1963.

Tessler, H., Apple, D. J., and Goldberg, M. F.: Ophthalmologic Findings in a Kindred with Kyrle's Disease (Hyperkeratosis Follicularis et Parafollicularis in Cutem Penetrans). Invest. Ophthal. *11*:626, 1972.

Corneal Edema

1. Mechanical trauma, including stripping Descemet's membrane

2. Exposure, such as in exophthalmos (see exposure keratitis, p. 238)

3. Radiation injury, such as from UV, X rays, gamma rays

4. Anoxia of epithelium, such as from excessive wearing of contact lens (Sattler's veil).

5. Osmotic, such as irrigation of cornea or anterior chamber with distilled water

6. Chemical, such as tear gas injury

7. Associated with inflammatory conditions especially when endothelium or fresh keratitic precipitates are present

8. Degenerative conditions, such as with corneal dystrophy or neuropathic conditions

9. Glaucoma, intraocular pressure parallels edema

10. Metabolic, such as myxedema and hypercholesterolemia

11. Vitreous touch of cornea

12. Essential corneal edema—idiopathic episodes, often cyclic

13. Acute hydrops with keratoconus (see p. 253)

14. Foreign bodies in anterior chamber angle

15. Late peripheral corneal edema following cataract extraction

16. Chandler's syndrome

17. Anhidrotic ectodermal dysplasia

18. Anterior segment necrosis

Dohlman, C. H.: Corneal Edema. Int. Ophthal. Clin. 8:523–759, 1968.

Grayson, M., and Keates, R. H.: Manual of Diseases of the Cornea. Boston, Little, Brown & Co., 1969, p. 292.

Laibson, P.: Inferior Bullous Keratopathy. Arch. Ophthal. 74:191, 1965.

Simpson, G. U.: Corneal Edema. Trans. Amer. Ophthal. Soc. 47: 692–737, 1949.

Stocker, F.: The Endothelium of the Cornea and Its Clinical Implications. Trans. Amer. Ophthal. Soc. 51:669, 1953.

Taylor, D. M., and Dolburg, L. A.: Corneal Complications from Cryoextraction of Cataracts. Arch. Ophthal. 79:3–7, 1968.

Treissman, H.: Some Observations on the Causation and Elimination of Sattler's Veil. Brit. J. Ophthal. 33:555, 1949.

Worthen, D. M., and Brubaker, R. F.: An Evaluation of Cataract Cryoextraction. Arch. Ophthal. 79:8, 1968.

Ytteborg, J., and Dohlman, C.: Corneal Edema and Intraocular Pressure. I. Arch. Ophthal. 74:375, 1965; II. Arch. Ophthal. 74: 477, 1965.

Microcornea (cornea having a diameter of less than 10 mm)

1. Autosomal recessive or dominant trait

2. Ehlers-Danlos syndrome (fibrodysplasia elastica generalisata)

3. Meyer-Schwickerath-Weyers syndrome (oculodentodigital dysplasia)

4. Rieger's syndrome (hypodontia and iris dysgenesis)

5. Locally associated with hyperopia, narrow-angle glaucoma, congenital glaucoma, sclerocornea, or Axenfeld's syndrome

6. Laurence-Moon-Biedl syndrome

7. Marchesani's syndrome (mesodermal dysmorphodystrophy)

8. Rubella syndrome

9. Gansslen's syndrome

10. Hallermann-Streiff syndrome (dyscephalia mandibulooculofacialis)

11. Hemifacial microsomia syndrome

12. Trisomy 13-15 (D trisomy)

Geeraets, W. J.: Ocular Syndromes, 2nd ed. Philadelphia, Lea & Febiger, 1969, pp. 237–238.
Gellis, S. S., and Feingold, M.: Atlas of Mental Retardation Syndromes. Washington, D. C., U.S. Government Printing Office, 1969.
Scheie, H. G.: Congenital Glaucoma. Symposium on Surgical and Medical Management of Congenital Anomalies of the Eye. St. Louis, C. V. Mosby Co., 1968, p. 357.

Megalocornea (cornea having a horizontal diameter of more than 14 mm)

1. Sex-linked recessive trait

2. Autosomal dominant or recessive trait

3. Posterior embryotoxon

4. Oculocerebrorenal syndrome (Lowe's syndrome)

5. Osteogenesis imperfecta—blue sclera, deafness, brittle bones

6. Rieger's syndrome (hypodontia and iris dysgenesis)

7. Congenital glaucoma (rare)

8. Marfan's syndrome (dystrophia mesodermalis congenita)

Gellis, S. S., and Feingold, M.: Atlas of Mental Retardation. Washington, D.C., U.S. Government Printing Office, 1968.
Grayson, M., and Keates, R. H.: Manual of Diseases of the Cornea. Boston, Little, Brown & Co., 1969, p. 208.

Corneal Opacification in Infancy (see conditions simulating congenital glaucoma, p. 264)

1. Congenital malformations
   A. Anterior chamber cleavage syndromes
      (1) Congenital central anterior synechiae
      (2) Rieger's syndrome—hypoplasia of anterior iris, iridocorneal angle adhesions, posterior embryotoxon
      (3) Axenfeld's syndrome—prominent anteriorly displaced Schwalbe's line and iridocorneal angle adhesions
      (4) Peter's anomaly—central opacity with defect in corneal stroma and Descemet's membrane
      (5) Congenital anterior staphyloma—corneal protrusion lined with iris
   B. Sclerocornea
   C. Congenital glaucoma
   D. Dermoid tumors (see p. 255)
   E. Amyloidosis
   F. Xanthomas

2. Birth trauma, such as Descemet's membrane rupture

3. Corneal dystrophy
   Congenital hereditary corneal dystrophy—autosomal recessive

4. Inflammatory processes
   A. Interstitial keratitis
   B. Herpes simplex
   C. Rubella syndrome

5. Inborn errors of metabolism
   A. Mucopolysaccharidoses (MPS)
      (1) Hurler's (type I)
      (2) Morquio-Brailsford (type IV)
      (3) Scheie's (type V)
      (4) Maroteaux-Lamy (type VI)
   B. Lowe's syndrome
   C. Von Gierke's disease (glycogen disease)
   D. Corneal lipoidosis—later
   E. Mucolipidosis
      (1) Generalized gangliosidosis (GM$_1$-gangliosidosis I and II)
      (2) MLS I (lipomucopolysaccharidosis)
      (3) MLS III (pseudo-Hurler's polydystrophy)
   F. Riley-Day syndrome

6. Chromosomal aberrations
   A. Mongolism (Down's syndrome)—trisomy 21
   B. Trisomy 13-15 (Patau's syndrome)

7. Idiopathic

Becker, B., and Shaffer, R. N.: Diagnosis and Therapy of Glaucoma, 3rd ed. St. Louis, C. V. Mosby Co., 1970, pp. 263–264.

Ching, F. C.: Corneal Opacification in Infancy. Med. Coll. Va. Qtr. 8:230–240, 1972.

Emery, J. M., et al.: GM1-Gangliosidosis: Ocular and Pathological Manifestations. Arch. Ophthal. 85:1677–1787, 1971.

Fergin, R. D., and Caplan, D. B.: Corneal Opacities in Infancy and Childhood. J. Pediat. 69:383–392, 1966.

Geeraets, W. J.: Ocular Syndromes, 2nd ed. Philadelphia, Lea & Febiger, 1969, pp. 221–222.

Goldberg, M. F., Scott, C. I., and McKusick, V. A.: Hydrocephalus and Papilledema in the Maroteaux-Lamy Syndrome (Mucopolysaccharidosis Type VI). Amer. J. Ophthal. 69:969–974, 1970.

Grayson, M., and Keates, R. H.: Manual of Diseases of the Cornea. Boston, Little, Brown & Co., 1969, p. 295.

Harboyan, G., et al.: Congenital Corneal Dystrophy. Arch. Ophthal. 85:27–32, 1971.

Howard, R. O., and Abrahams, I. W.: Sclerocornea. Amer. J. Ophthal. 71:1254–1260, 1971.

Kenyon, K. R., and Sensenbrenner, J. A.: Mucolipidosis II (I-Cell Disease): Ultrastructure Observations of Conjunctiva and Skin. Invest. Ophthal. 10:555–567, 1971.

Liebman, S. D., Crocker, A. C., and Geiser, C. F.: Corneal Xanthomas in Childhood. Arch. Ophthal. 76:221–229, 1966.

McPherson, S. D., Jr., Kiffney, G. T., and Freed, C. C.: Corneal Amyloidosis. Amer. J. Ophthal. 62:1025, 1966.

Reese, A. B., and Ellsworth, R.: The Anterior Chamber Cleavage Syndrome. Arch. Ophthal. 75:307, 1966.

Rodger, F. C., and Sinclair, H. M.: Metabolic and Nutritional Eye Diseases. Springfield, Ill., Charles C Thomas, 1969, p. 104.

Rodrigues, M. M., Calhoun, J., and Weinreb, S.: Sclerocornea with an Unbalanced Translocation (17p, 10q). Amer. J. Ophthal. 78:49–53, 1974.

Band-shaped Keratopathy (corneal opacification extending horizontally over the cornea at the level of Bowman's membrane in exposed part of palpebral aperture)

1. Local degenerative diseases, including chronic uveitis, phthisis bulbi, absolute glaucoma, infantile polyarthritis (Still's disease), rheumatoid arthritis, and interstitial keratitis

2. Traumatic—chronic exposure to irritants, such as mercury fumes, calomel, calcium bichromate vapor, and hair

3. Hypercalcemia
    A. Hyperparathyroidism
    B. Excessive vitamin D as with oral intake, Boeck's sarcoid with liver involvement, and acute osteoporosis
    C. Renal failure, such as that associated with Fanconi's syndrome (cystinosis)
    D. Hypophosphatasia
    E. Milk-alkali syndrome

229

F. Paget's disease

G. Idiopathic hypercalcemia

4. Discoid lupus erythematosus

5. Gout (urate crystals)

6. Tuberous sclerosis

7. Associated with anterior mosaic dystrophy, primary type
   A. Episkopi (sex-linked recessive)
   B. Labrador keratopathy

8. Ichthyosis vulgaris—dry skin with gray-brown scales

9. Rothmund's syndrome—bilateral cataracts, skin pigmentation, telangiectasis

10. Long-term miotic therapy

11. Dysproteinemia

12. Progressive facial hemiatrophy (Parry-Romberg syndrome)

13. High levels of visible electromagnetic radiation such as xenon arc photocoagulation and laser causing acute severe anterior uveitis

14. Idiopathic or unknown cause

Cogan, D. G., Albright, F., and Bartler, F. C.: Hypercalcemia and Band Keratopathy. Arch. Ophthal. *40*:624, 1948.

Duke-Elder, S., and Leigh, A. G.: Diseases of the Outer Eye. System of Ophthalmology, Vol. VIII, Part 2. St. Louis, C. V. Mosby Co., 1965, p. 898.

Fishman, R. S., and Sunderman, F. W.: Band Keratopathy in Gout. Arch. Ophthal. *75*:367, 1966.

Grayson, M., and Keates, R. H.: Manual of the Diseases of the Cornea. Boston, Little, Brown & Co., 1969, p. 293.

Grayson, M., and Pieroni, D.: Progressive Facial Hemiatrophy with Bullous and Band-Shaped Keratopathy. Amer. J. Ophthal. *70*:42–44, 1970.

Kennedy, R. E., Roca, P. D., and Landers, P. H.: Atypical Band Keratopathy in Glaucomatous Patients. Amer. J. Ophthal. *72*:917–922, 1971.

Leibowitz, H. M., and Berkow, I. W.: Band Keratopathy after Ocular Exposure to Visible Laser Radiation. Amer. J. Ophthal. *76*:468–471, 1973.

Walsh, F. B., and Howard, J. E.: Conjunctival and Corneal Lesions in Hypercalcemia. J. Clin. Endocr. *7*:644, 1947.

Punctate Keratitis or Keratopathy

1. Diseases of the lids associated with punctate keratitis
    A. Nodules
        (1) Molluscum contagiosum
        (2) Warts
        (3) Acne rosacea
    B. Vesicles or ulcers
        (1) Herpes simplex
        (2) Herpes zoster
        (3) Vaccinia
        (4) Benign mucous membrane pemphigoid
    C. Folliculitis (blepharitis, p. 76)
        (1) Staphylococcal blepharitis
        (2) Seborrheic blepharitis
        (3) Blepharitis due to *Demodex folliculorum*
    D. Dermatitis
        (1) Seborrheic blepharitis
        (2) Psoriasis
    E. Trichiasis or entropion with traumatic keratitis (see p. 70)
    F. Ectropion (see p. 69)
        (1) Exposure keratopathy
        (2) Neuroparalytic keratopathy
    G. Lid retraction (see p. 58)
        (1) Exposure keratopathy
        (2) Endocrine exophthalmos
    H. Madarosis, such as that associated with leprosy (stiff immobile lids)

2. Diseases of the skin associated with punctate keratitis
    A. Acne rosacea
    B. Benign mucous membrane pemphigoid
    C. Erythema multiforme
    D. Leprosy
    E. Psoriasis
    F. Follicular hyperkeratosis of the palms and soles
    G. Ichthyosis

3. Conjunctival inflammation associated with punctate keratitis
   A. Follicular (see pp. 168–170)
       (1) Adenovirus
       (2) Herpes zoster
       (3) Molluscum contagiosum
       (4) Inclusion conjunctivitis
       (5) Trachoma
       (6) Herpes simplex
   B. Giant papillary, such as in vernal conjunctivitis
   C. Papillary
       (1) Sjögren's syndrome
       (2) Trachoma
   D Diffuse catarrhal (see pp. 162–163)
       (1) Bacterial conjunctivitis
       (2) Reiter's disease
       (3) Erythema multiforme
       (4) Mild adenovirus
       (5) Vaccinia
       (6) Superior limbic keratoconjunctivitis
   E. Cicatrizing (see p. 170)
       (1) Trachoma
       (2) Benign mucous membrane pemphigoid
       (3) Erythema multiforme (Stevens-Johnson)
       (4) Sjögren's keratoconjunctivitis sicca
       (5) Diphtheria
       (6) Radium burns
       (7) Chemical burns

4. Conjunctival discharge associated with punctate keratitis
   A. Mucopurulent (see pp. 162–163)
       (1) Gonococcal
       (2) Meningococcal
       (3) Reiter's disease
       (4) Erythema multiforme (Stevens-Johnson)
       (5) Vernal conjunctivitis
       (6) Trachoma (acute stage)
       (7) Inclusion conjunctivitis (acute stage)
   B. Mucoid
       (1) Sjögren's disease
       (2) Other types of keratoconjunctivitis sicca

C. Serous
    (1) Adenovirus
    (2) Herpes zoster
    (3) Molluscum contagiosum
    (4) Warts
    (5) Trachoma (later)
    (6) Inclusion conjunctivitis (later)
    (7) Herpes simplex

5. Punctate keratitis preceded by lymphadenopathy
   A. Adenovirus
   B. Herpes zoster
   C. Vaccinia
   D. Acute trachoma
   E. Inclusion conjunctivitis
   F. Herpes simplex

6. Limbal conditions associated with punctate keratitis
   A. Follicles
      (1) Trachoma
      (2) Inclusion conjunctivitis
      (3) Molluscum contagiosum
      (4) Herpes simplex
      (5) Acne rosacea
      (6) Other viral infections
   B. Focal necrotic lesions
      (1) Phlyctenular disease
      (2) Herpes simplex
      (3) Vaccinia
   C. Nodules and plaques
      (1) Limbal vernal conjunctivitis
      (2) Bowen's disease
      (3) Intra-epithelial melanoma
      (4) Avitaminosis A (Bitot's spots) (see p. 182)

7. Corneal conditions associated with punctate keratitis
   A. Vascularization (see pp. 244–247)
      (1) Trachoma
      (2) Acne rosacea
      (3) Phlyctenular disease
      (4) Sjögren's keratoconjunctivitis sicca

   (5) Molluscum contagiosum
   (6) Vaccinia
   (7) Benign mucous membrane pemphigoid
  B. Deep keratitis, disciform or irregular
   (1) Herpes simplex
   (2) Herpes zoster and other viral diseases
   (3) Lattice dystrophy
  C. Thinned facets due to previous ulcerative or other lesions
   (1) Herpes simplex
   (2) Acne rosacea
   (3) Sjögren's keratoconjunctivitis sicca
   (4) Erythema multiforme

 8. Respiratory diseases associated with punctate keratitis
  A. Adenovirus infections
  B. Myxovirus infections (influenza, Newcastle disease, mumps)
  C. Recurrent herpes complicating any fever

 9. Articular disease associated with punctate keratitis
  A. Sjögren's syndrome
  B. Psoriasis arthropathica
  C. Reiter's disease

10. Genitourinary disease associated with punctate keratitis
  A. Inclusion blennorrhea
  B. Reiter's disease
  C. Erythema multiforme
  D. Benign mucous membrane pemphigoid

11. Alimentary disorders associated with punctate keratitis
  A. Mouth
   (1) Dry mouth as in Sjögren's syndrome
   (2) Ulcers, such as primary herpes, benign mucous membrane pemphigoid, and erythema multiforme
  B. Stomach
   (1) Indigestion as in Sjögren's syndrome and acne rosacea

C. Lower alimentary tract
  (1) Ulcerative colitis as in Sjögren's disease
  (2) Mild colitis, such as that due to an adenovirus

Jones, B. R.: Differential Diagnosis of Punctate Keratitis. Int. Ophthal. Clin. 2:591–611, 1962.
Newell, F. W.: Ophthalmology, Principles and Concepts. St. Louis, C. V. Mosby Co., 1969, p. 171.

Morphologic Classification of Punctate Corneal Lesions (classification by anatomic location)

1. Punctate epithelial erosions—fine, very slightly depressed spots scarcely visible without staining with fluorescein
   A. Warts
   B. Artificial-silk keratitis
   C. Staphylococcal blepharoconjunctivitis (lower cornea)
   D. Keratoconjunctivitis sicca (interpalpebral area)
   E. Exposure keratitis (interpalpebral area)
   F. Neuroparalytic keratitis (anesthesia of cornea, p. 218)
   G. Trichiasis

2. Punctate epithelial keratitis—very small, whitish flecks on the surface of the epithelium
   A. Fine
      (1) Scattered—staphylococcal blepharitis; viral keratitis, especially trachoma and molluscum contagiosum, sometimes inclusion conjunctivitis, and not infrequently herpetic keratitis and rubeola and rubella
      (2) Confluent—keratitis sicca, exposure keratitis, vernal conjunctivitis, topical steroid-induced and early viral keratitis

B. Coarse
  - (1) Thygeson's superficial punctate keratitis (characteristic)
  - (2) Herpes zoster
  - (3) Adenovirus infection
  - (4) Early herpes simplex
  - (5) Acne rosacea (lower cornea)

C. Areolar—spots have enlarged to occupy a large area
  - (1) Herpes simplex
  - (2) Thygeson's superficial punctate keratitis
  - (3) Herpes zoster
  - (4) Vaccinia

3. Filamentary keratitis or keratopathy—formation of fine epithelial filaments that are attached at one end
  A. Keratoconjunctivitis sicca (frequent)
  B. Infectious, such as that due to adenovirus, herpes, vaccinia, and bacteria
  C. Trauma, such as wounds, abrasions, exposure to short-wave diathermy, and prolonged eye-patching
  D. Edema of cornea, such as that due to recurrent erosions or wearing of contact lens
  E. Sarcoid with infiltration of conjunctiva and lacrimal gland
  F. Heerfordt's syndrome and Mikulicz's syndrome (see p. 86)
  G. After irradiation of the lacrimal gland
  H. Keratoconus (see keratoconus, p. 253)
  I. Neuropathic keratopathy (anesthesia of cornea, p. 218)
  J. Conjunctival cicatrization, such as that associated with benign mucous membrane pemphigoid, erythema multiforme, ocular psoriasis, and advanced trachoma (see cicatrizing conjunctivitis, p. 170)
  K. Degenerative condition of corneal epithelium, such as in advanced glaucoma
  L. Superior limbic keratoconjunctivitis
  M. Hereditary hemorrhagic telangiectasis (Rendu-Osler-Weber disease)
  N. Aerosol keratitis

O. Diabetes mellitus
P. Ectodermal dysplasia
Q. Following cataract surgery
R. Idiopathic

4. Punctate subepithelial keratitis—punctate epithelial keratitis may progress to combined epithelial and subepithelial lesions followed by healing of the epithelial component, leaving a punctate subepithelial keratitis typical of viral punctate keratitis

   A. Areolar or stellate lesions—grayish-white in color
      (1) Herpes simplex (usually)
      (2) Herpes zoster
      (3) Vaccinia
   B. Fine or medium-sized lesions, typically
      (1) Adenovirus, especially types 3 and 7—grayish-white
   C. Yellowish tinge—typical of trachoma, inclusion conjunctivitis, acne rosacea, and marginal "catarrhal infiltrates" associated with staphylococcal blepharitis, Neisseria conjunctivitis, and Reiter's disease

5. Punctate opacifications of Bowman's membrane—gray, homogeneous, thickened spots, often having irregular edges
   A. Salzmann's dystrophy
   B. Punctate lesion of trachoma, measles, or phlyctenular disease

Dodds, H. T., and Laibson, P. R.: Filamentary Keratitis Following Cataract Extraction. Arch. Ophthal. 88:609–612, 1972.
Jones, B. R.: Differential Diagnosis of Punctate Keratitis. Int. Ophthal. Clin. 2:591–611, 1962.
Lemp, M. A., Chambers, R. W., and Lundy, J.: Viral Isolate in Superficial Punctate Keratitis. Arch. Ophthal. 91:8–10, 1974.
Smolin, G.: Report of a Case of Rubella Keratitis. Amer. J. Ophthal. 74:197–199, 1972.
Westkamp, C.: Parenchymatous Origin of Filamentary Keratitis. Amer. J. Ophthal. 42:115, 1956.
Winters, D. H., and Asbury, T.: Filamentary Keratitis. Amer. J. Ophthal. 51:1292, 1961.
Wolper, J., and Laibson, P. R.: Hereditary Hemorrhagic Telangiectasis (Rendu-Osler-Weber Disease). Arch. Ophthal. 81:272–277, 1969.

Sicca Keratitis (dry eye with secondary corneal changes [see p. 92])

1. Sjögren's syndrome
2. Boeck's sarcoid (Schaumann's syndrome)
3. Herpes simplex
4. Pemphigoid
5. Trachoma
6. Dermatitis herpetiformis
7. Polychondritis
8. Lye burns
9. Vitamin A deficiency (xerosis)
10. Diabetes mellitus

Grayson, M., and Keates, R. H.: Manual of Diseases of the Cornea. Boston, Little, Brown & Co., 1969, p. 292.

White Rings of the Cornea (Coats') (rings, 1 mm or less in diameter, made up of a series of tiny white dots which may coalesce at the level of Bowman's membrane or just below it)

1. Congenital
2. Trauma
    A. Foreign body
    B. Occupational—in working with limestone there may be deposition of some of the substance's components, especially calcium oxide, in the cornea

3. Intraocular disease

4. Iron deposition

Miller, E. M.: Genesis of White Rings of the Cornea. Amer. J. Ophthal. *61*:904, 1966.
Nevins, R. C., and Elliott, J. H.: White Ring of the Cornea. Arch. Ophthal. *82*:457, 1969.

Dry Spots of the Cornea (precorneal tear film drying in spot-wise fashion)

The precorneal tear film is best examined by using fluorescein and cobalt-blue filtered light. Patients may have difficulty in wearing contact lenses or have corneal pain. Normal tear films breakup time is greater than 10 seconds and averages 25 to 30 seconds.

1. Keratitis sicca

2. Congenital alacrima

3. Vitamin A deficiency

4. Stevens-Johnson syndrome

5. Ocular pemphigus

6. Associated with corneal dellen (see p. 247)

7. Chronic bacterial or viral conjunctivitis

8. Chemical burns

9. Sometimes in elderly persons without obvious pathology

10. Instillation of topical anesthetic

Baum, J. L., Mishima, S., and Boruchoff, S. A.: On the Nature of Dellen. Arch. Ophthal. *79*:657–662, 1968.

Brown, S. I.: Further Studies on the Pathophysiology of Keratitis Sicca of Rollet. Arch. Ophthal. *83*:542–547, 1970.

Brown, S. I., and Dervichian, D. G.: The Oils of the Meibomian Glands. Arch. Ophthal. *82*:537–540, 1969.

Dohlman, C. H.: The Function of the Corneal Epithelium in Health and Disease. Invest. Ophthal. *10*:376–407, 1971.

Girard, L. J., Soper, J. W., and Sampson, W. G.: Fitting of the Lens. *In:* Girard, L. J. (Ed.): Corneal Contact Lenses. St. Louis, C. V. Mosby Co., 1964.

Lemp, M. A., and Hamill, J. R.: Factors Affecting Tear Film Break-up in Normal Eyes. Arch. Ophthal. *89*:103–105, 1973.

Anterior Embryotoxon (Arcus) (white or gray substance deposited at level of Descemet's membrane and Bowman's membrane initially, then in stroma with a clear limbal interval)

1. Isolated phenomenon

2. Ocular anomaly association, such as blue sclera, megalo-cornea, or aniridia

3. Associated with corneal disease, such as interstitial keratitis

4. Long exposure to irritating dust or chemicals

5. Familial hypercholesterolemia (type II, familial beta-lipo-proteins, and type III, familial hyper-beta- and pre-beta-lipoproteins [carbohydrate-induced hyperlipemia])

6. Hereditary—autosomal dominant or autosomal recessive inheritance

7. Secondary to ocular disease, such as large corneal scars, sclerokeratitis, limbal dermoid, nevus, or epithelial cyst

8. Age—may be present normally in a Caucasian older than 40 years of age or in a Negro older than 30 years of age

9. Alport's syndrome

Chavis, R. M., and Groshong, T.: Corneal Arcus in Alport's Syndrome. Amer. J. Ophthal. 75:793–794, 1973.

Cogan, D. G., and Kuwabara, T.: Arcus Senilus, Its Pathology and Histochemistry. Arch. Ophthal. 61:553–560, 1959.

Duke-Elder, S.: System of Ophthalmology, Vol. VIII, Part 2. St. Louis, C. V. Mosby Co., 1965, pp. 874–876.

Macaraeg, P. V., Jr., Lasagna, L., and Snyder, B.: Arcus Not So Senilus. Ann. Intern. Med. 68:345–354, 1968.

Rodger, F. C., and Sinclair, H. M.: Metabolic and Nutritional Eye Diseases. Springfield, Ill., Charles C Thomas, 1969.

Spaeth, G. L.: Ocular Manifestations of the Lipidoses. In Tassman, W. (Ed.): Retinal Diseases in Children. New York, Harper & Row, 1971, pp. 127–206.

Stanbury, J. B., Wyngaarden, J. B., and Fredrickson, D. S.: The Metabolic Basis of Inherited Disease, 2nd ed. New York, McGraw-Hill Book Co., 1966, p. 434.

Bowman's Membrane Folds

1. Lowering of intraocular pressure, such as occurs in association with phthisis bulbi

2. Inflammation

3. Bullous keratopathy

4. Idiopathic

Duke-Elder, S., and Leigh, A. G.: Diseases of the Outer Eye. System of Ophthalmology, Vol. VIII, Part 2. St. Louis, C. V. Mosby Co., 1965, p. 701.

Differential Diagnosis of Anterior Corneal Abnormalities

Entity	Distinguishing Features
Vortex dystrophy	Corneal pattern, ocular and systemic findings of Fabry's disease, drug history
Meesmann's dystrophy	Corneal pattern, family history
Reis-Bücklers dystrophy	Family history, histopathology
Keratosis palmaris et plantaris	Dermatologic, systemic findings
Post-traumatic recurrent erosion	History of trauma, localized corneal pathology
Map-dot fingerprint	Corneal pattern, no family history

Trobe, J. D., and Laibson, P. R.: Dystrophic Changes in the Anterior Cornea. Arch. Ophthal. *87*:378–382, 1972. Copyright 1972, American Medical Association.

Bullous Keratopathy (terminal stages of severe or prolonged epithelial edema secondary to endothelial damage)

1. Long-standing glaucoma

2. Fuch's epithelial-endothelial dystrophy

3. Following perforating wounds, especially when the lens capsule or vitreous is adherent to the cornea

4. Chronic uveitis

5. Prolonged inflammation of corneal stroma, such as in disciform or interstitial keratitis (rare)

6. Associated with progressive facial hemiatrophy (Parry-Romberg syndrome)

Baum, J. L., and Martolo, E.: Corneal Edema and Corneal Vascularization. Amer. J. Ophthal. 65:881–884, 1968.

Duke-Elder, S., and Leigh, A. G.: Diseases of the Outer Eye. System of Ophthalmology, Vol. VIII, Part 2. St. Louis, C. V. Mosby Co., 1965, p. 671.

Grayson, M., and Pieroni, D.: Progressive Facial Hemiatrophy with Bullous and Band-Shaped Keratopathy. Amer. J. Ophthal. 70:42–44, 1970.

Nummular Keratitis (coin-shaped lesions of cornea)

1. Brucellosis
2. Infectious mononucleosis
3. Onchocerciasis

Grayson, M., and Keates, R. H.: Manual of Diseases of the Cornea. Boston, Little, Brown & Co., 1969, p. 292.

Deep Keratitis

1. Stromal herpes
2. Deep pustular keratitis
3. Behcet's disease
4. Keratitis profunda
5. Disciform keratitis
6. Vaccinia
7. Herpes zoster
8. Varicella

Grayson, M., and Keates, R. H.: Manual of Diseases of the Cornea. Boston, Little, Brown & Co., 1969, p. 291.

Interstitial Keratitis (corneal stromal inflammation, not primarily on the anterior or posterior surfaces of the stroma)

1. Syphilis—superior limbus initially

2. Tuberculosis—lower limbus initially

3. Mumps

4. Lymphogranuloma venereum

5. Trypanosomiasis

6. Cogan's syndrome—non-syphilitic interstitial keratitis associated with vestibuloauditory symptoms

7. Sarcoidosis

8. Hodgkin's disease

9. Mycosis fungoides

10. Chemical poisons, such as those due to gold and arsenic

11. Leprosy

12. Relapsing recurrent fever

13. Brucellosis

14. Filariasis

15. Vaccinia

16. Incontinentia pigmenti (Bloch-Sulzberger syndrome)

17. Disciform keratitis

18. Hydroa vacciniforme

19. Pityriasis rubra pilaris

Duke-Elder, S., and Leigh, A. G.: Diseases of the Outer Eye. System of Ophthalmology, Vol. VIII, Part 2. St. Louis, C. V. Mosby Co., 1965, pp. 811–839.

Grayson, M., and Keates, R. H.: Manual of Diseases of the Cornea. Boston, Little, Brown & Co., 1969, p. 292.

Oksala, A.: Interstitial Keratitis. Amer. J. Ophthal. *44*:217, 1957.

Wilson, F. M., Grayson, M., and Pieroni, D.: Corneal Changes in Ectodermal Dysplasia: Case Report, Histopathology, and Differential Diagnosis. Amer. J. Ophthal. *75*:17–27, 1973.

Pannus (superficial vascular invasion confined to a segment of the cornea or extending around the entire limbus)

1. Trachoma—upper limbus, associated tarsal changes, vessels between epithelium and Bowman's membrane (early) (micropannus)

2. Leprosy—may have associated interstitial keratitis, scrapings from pannus show *Mycobacterium leprae*

3. Phlyctenular—may occur anywhere on the cornea beneath Bowman's membrane following phlyctenular keratoconjunctivitis

4. Acne rosacea—associated with acne rosacea facies; pannus similar to phlyctenular pannus and may extend all around the limbus

5. Degenerative—blind degenerative eyes; often associated with bullous keratopathy

6. Molluscum contagiosum—secondary to severe long-standing conjunctivitis, lid lesion present, similar to trachoma pannus

7. Lymphopathia venereum—initially the upper cornea is involved in the superficial vascularization, punctate epithelial staining precedes

8. Ariboflavinosis keratopathy

9. Vernal conjunctivitis (micropannus)

9

10. Leishmaniasis

11. Onchocerciasis

12. Keratoconjunctivitis sicca

13. Use of contact lens

14. Inclusion conjunctivitis in infants and adults (micropannus)

15. Superior limbic keratoconjunctivitis (micropannus)

16. Allergic marginal infiltration

17. Fuch's dystrophy (degenerative pannus)

18. Glaucoma (degenerative pannus)

19. Lyell's disease (toxic epidermal necrolysis or scalded skin syndrome)

20. Siemen's disease (keratosis follicularis spinulosa decalvans) —circumferential pannus with diffuse superficial farinaceous corneal opacities, small hyperkeratotic spines at opening of hair follicles (gooseflesh)

21. Staphylococcal keratoconjunctivitis (micropannus)

22. Hypoparathyroidism

Bodion, M.: Trachoma. Arch. Ophthal. *38*:450–460, 1947.

Duke-Elder, S., and Leigh, A. G.: Diseases of the Outer Eye. System of Ophthalmology, Vol. VIII, Part 2. St. Louis, C. V. Mosby Co., 1965, pp. 680, 731.

Dixon, W. S., and Bron, A. J.: Fluorescein Angiographic Demonstration of Corneal Vascularization in Contact Lens Wearers. Amer. J. Ophthal. *75*:1010–1015, 1973.

Forster, R. K., Dawson, C. R., and Schachter, J.: Late Follow-up of Patients with Neonatal Inclusion Conjunctivitis. Amer. J. Ophthal. *69*:467–472, 1970.

Fritz, M. H., Thygeson, P., and Durham, D. G.: Phlyctenular Keratoconjunctivitis among Alaskan Natives. Amer. J. Ophthal. *34*:177–184, 1951.

Grayson, M., and Keates, R. H.: Manual of Diseases of the Cornea. Boston, Little, Brown & Co., 1969, p. 291.

Ostler, H. B., Grant, M. A., and Groundwater, J.: Lyell's Disease, the Stevens-Johnson Syndrome, and Exfoliative Dermatitis. Trans. Amer. Acad. Ophthal. Otolaryng. *74*:1254–1265, 1970.

Sysi, R.: Molluscum Contagiosum of the Cornea. Acta Ophthal. *19*:25–27, 1941.

Thygeson, P.: Corneal Changes in Tric Agent Infections. Amer. J. Ophthal. *63*:1278–1282, 1967.

Thygeson, P.: Historical Review of Oculogenital Disease. Amer. J. Ophthal. *71*:975–985, 1971.

Wilson, F. M., Grayson, M., and Pieroni, D.: Corneal Changes in Ectodermal Dysplasia: Case Report, Histopathology, and Differential Diagnosis. Amer. J. Ophthal. *75*:17–27, 1973.

Dellen (shallow corneal excavation near the limbus, usually on temporal side, with the base of the lesion hazy and dry)

1. In elderly persons—limbal vasosclerosis

2. Swelling of perilimbal tissues
    A. Episcleritis
    B. Pinguecula
    C. Limbal tumor
    D. Subconjunctival effusion or injection
    E. Allergic conjunctival edema
    F. Postoperative advancement of rectus muscle
    G. Postoperative retinal detachment

3. Lagophthalmos (see p. 61)

4. Lengthy administration of cocaine

5. Postcataract section

6. With hemeralopia (see p. 547)

7. Following the wearing of contact lens

Baum, J. L., Mishima, S., and Boruchoff, S. A.: On the Nature of Dellen. Arch. Ophthal. *79*:657–662, 1968.

Norton, E. W. D.: Complications of Retinal Detachment Surgery. Symposium on Retina and Retinal Surgery. Transactions of New Orleans Academy of Ophthalmology. St. Louis, C. V. Mosby Co., 1969, p. 230.

Rosenberg, S.: Corneal Dellen: Following Contact Lens Wear. Amer. J. Ophthal. *67*:970, 1969.

Phlyctenular Keratoconjunctivitis (localized conjunctival, limbal, or corneal nodule about 1 to 3 mm in size)

1. Delayed hypersensitivity to bacterial protein, particularly tuberculoprotein and staphylococci. Lymphopathia venereum and coccidioidomycosis may also be allergens

2. Systemic infection

3. Malnutrition

4. Secondary infection of the conjunctiva, especially from *Staphylococcus aureus,* pneumococcus, and Koch-Weeks bacillus

Bedrossian, E. H.: The Eye. Springfield, Ill., Charles C Thomas, 1958, p. 176.

Davis, P. L., and Watson, J. I.: Experimental Conjunctival Phlyctenulosis. Canad. J. Ophthal. *4*:183–190, 1969.

Newell, F. W.: Ophthalmology, Principles and Concepts. St. Louis, C. V. Mosby Co., 1969, p. 177.

Corneal Ring Lesion

1. Ring abscess—rapidly destructive purulent lesion in the deepest parts of the cornea

2. Mooren's ulcer—deeply undermined central edges and chronic course with little inflammation

3. Marginal dystrophy—degenerative chronic corneal lesion with stromal thinning and intact epithelium; occurs in individuals younger than 40 years of age

4. Marginal ulceration—secondary to massive granuloma of sclera or necrotizing nodular scleritis (see p. 207)

5. Ring ulcer—see marginal corneal ulcers (p. 256)

6. Double-ring formation—allergic keratitis

7. Associated with rheumatoid arthritis—inferior

8. Associated with Sjögren's syndrome

9. Terrien's marginal degeneration—usually begins superiorly

10. Steroid use in furrow dystrophy

11. Wegener's granuloma

Brown, S. I., and Grayson, M.: Marginal Furrows. Arch. Ophthal. 79:563, 1968.

Duke-Elder, S., and Leigh, A. G.: Diseases of the Outer Eye. System of Ophthalmology, Vol. VIII, Part 2. St. Louis, C. V. Mosby Co., 1965, pp. 775–776.

Edwards, W. C., and Reed, R. E.: Mooren's Ulcer. Arch. Ophthal. 80:361–364, 1968.

Ferry, A. P., and Leopold, I. H.: Marginal (Ring) Corneal Ulcer as Presenting Manifestation of Wegener's Granuloma. Trans. Amer. Acad. Ophthal. Otolaryng. 74:1276–1282, 1970.

Gupta, S. D., Gupta, J. S., and Singh, K. : Ring-Forming Keratitis. Amer. J. Ophthal. 63:517, 1967.

Kietzman, B.: Mooren's Ulcer in Nigeria. Amer. J. Ophthal. 65: 679–685, 1968.

Corneoscleral Keratitis

1. Boeck's sarcoid

2. Syphilis

3. Tuberculosis

4. Leprosy

5. Sarcoma

6. Gout

7. Malformations, such as in sclerocornea

8. 13-15 Trisomy (trisomy D)

Grayson, M., and Keates, R. H.: Manual of Diseases of the Cornea. Boston, Little, Brown & Co., 1969, p. 292.

Central Corneal Ulcer

1. Of bacterial origin
   A. *Diplococcus pneumoniae* (pneumococcus)—infiltrated gray-white or yellow disc-shaped central ulcer typically associated with diffuse keratitis, severe iridocyclitis, and hypopyon; follows corneal abrasion, occurs especially in the presence of chronic dacryocystitis, and is enhanced by general debility
   B. Beta-hemolytic streptococcus
   C. *Pseudomonas aeruginosa*—primary corneal involvement, rapid spread often to panophthalmitis, large hypopyon, thick, greenish pus; may be contaminant of Eserine and fluorescein
   D. *Escherichia coli*
   E. *Moraxella liquefaciens* (diplococcus of Petit)—morphologically resembles diplobacillus of Morax-Axenfeld, which is never seen in central corneal ulcers
   F. *Klebsiella pneumoniae*
   G. *Proteus vulgaris*
   H. Actinomyces
   I. Tuberculous—secondary to conjunctival or uveal infections
   J. *Serratia marcescens*—gram-negative coccobacillus
   K. Others

2. Of viral origin
   A. Herpes simplex virus
   B. Vaccinia virus
   C. Variola
   D. Herpes zoster
   E. Others

3. Of mycotic origin—follows corneal trauma, such as foreign bodies in the cornea or corneal abrasions caused by vegetable matter, or diseases, such as radiation keratitis, exposure keratitis, herpes zoster, and ocular pemphigus; chronic course; shallow crater; absent corneal vascularization; may follow treatment with antibiotics or, more likely, treatment with steroid-antibiotic combinations

   A. *Candida albicans*
   B. Nocardia
   C. Cephalosporum
   D. Aspergillus
   E. *Fusarium solani*
   F. *Blastomyces dermatitidis*
   G. Others

4. Soluble tyrosine aminotransferase (STAT) deficiency

5. Chemical—latex keratitis

Atlee, W. E., Burns, R. P., and Oden, M.: Serratia marcescens Keratoconjunctivitis. Amer. J. Ophthal. *70*:31, 1970.

Bamert, W.: Etiology and Treatment of Corneal Ulcers. Klin. Mbl. Augenheilk. *121*:271, 1952.

Burns, R. P.: Soluble Tyrosine Amino-Transferase Deficiency: An Unusual Cause of Corneal Ulcers. Amer. J. Ophthal. *73*:400–402, 1972.

Hutton, W. L., and Sexton, R. R.: Atypical Pseudomonas Corneal Ulcers in Semi-comatose Patients. Amer. J. Ophthal. *73*:37–39, 1972.

Jenes, D. B., Forster, R. K., and Rebell, G.: Fusarium solani Keratitis Treated with Natamycin (Pimaricin). Arch. Ophthal. *88*:147–154, 1972.

Kimura, S. J.: Infectious Diseases of the Conjunctiva and Cornea. Symposium of the New Orleans Academy of Ophthalmology. St. Louis, C. V. Mosby Co., 1963, p. 89.

Rodriguez, M. M., Laibson, P., and Kaplan, W.: Exogenous Mycotic Keratitis, Caused by Blastomyces dermititidis. Amer. J. Ophthal. *75*:782–789, 1973.

Ross, H. W., and Laibson, P. R.: Keratomycosis. Amer. J. Ophthal. *74*:438–441, 1972.

Sofot, B. K., et al.: Euphorbia Royleana Latex Keratitis. Amer. J. Ophthal. *74*:634–637, 1972.

Thygeson, P.: Acute Central (Hypopyon) Ulcers of the Cornea. Calif. Med. *69*:18–21, 1948.

Descemet's Membrane Folds (usually follow hypotony, see p. 200)

(usually follow hypotony, see p. 200)

1. Trauma, such as that due to cataract surgery

2. Mechanical cause, such as firm prolonged ocular bandaging or phthisis bulbi with increased corneal curvature

3. Inflammatory condition, such as that following interstitial or herpes simplex keratitis

4. Diabetes (8% to 33%)

5. Ochronosis

6. Toxic
   A. Quinone and hydroquinone—vertical folds
   B. Formaldehyde 26%
   C. Experimental cold injury to cornea
   D. Digitoxin

7. Idiopathic

Henkind, P., and Wise, G. N.: Descemet's Wrinkles in Diabetes. Amer. J. Ophthal. 52:371, 1961.

Rodger, F. C., and Sinclair, H. M.: Metabolic and Nutritional Eye Diseases. Springfield, Ill., Charles C Thomas, 1969, p. 31.

Zagora, E.: Eye Injuries. Springfield, Ill., Charles C Thomas, 1970, pp. 314, 317, 414.

Descemet's Membrane Tears

1. Buphthalmos

2. Conical cornea

3. Myopia with marked anteroposterior diameter

4. Trauma, such as birth injury or contusion

5. Acute hydrops of the cornea, such as that due to kerato-conus

Duke-Elder, S., and Leigh, A. G.: Diseases of the Outer Eye. System of Ophthalmology, Vol. VIII, Part 2. St. Louis, C. V. Mosby Co., 1965, pp. 705–711.

Keratoconus (Conical Cornea) (non-inflammatory ectasia of the cornea in its axial part with considerable visual impairment due to the development of a high degree of irregular myopic astigmatism)

Keratoconus may be associated with:

1. Retinitis pigmentosa

2. Infantile tapetoretinal degeneration of Leber

3. Atopic dermatitis and keratosis plantaris and palmaris

4. Vernal catarrh

5. Mongolism (trisomy 21; Down's syndrome)

6. Blue sclerotics, including van der Hoeve's syndrome of blue sclera (osteogenesis imperfecta) (see blue sclera, p. 211)

7. Aniridia

8. Marfan's syndrome (dystrophia mesodermalis congenita)

9. Apert's syndrome (acrocephalosyndactylism syndrome)

10. Hereditary history

11. Wearing contact lens

12. Ehlers-Danlos syndrome (fibrodysplasia elastica generalisata, cutis hyperelastica)

13. Noonan's syndrome (male Turner's syndrome)—antimongoloid slant, hypertelorism, epicanthal folds, exophthalmos, high myopia, posterior embryotoxon, strabismus

Grayson, M., and Keates, R. H.: Manual of Diseases of the Cornea. Boston, Little, Brown & Co., 1969, p. 293.

Hartstein, J.: Keratoconus That Develops in Patients Wearing Corneal Contact Lenses. Arch. Ophthal. *80*:345, 1968.

Mc Tigue, J. W.: The Human Cornea. Trans. Amer. Ophthal. Soc. *65*:624, 1967.

Schwartz, D. E.: Noonan's Syndrome Associated with Ocular Abnormalities. Amer. J. Ophthal. *73*:955–960, 1972.

Slusher, M. M., Laibson, P. R., and Mulberger, R. D.: Acute Keratoconus in Down's Syndrome. Amer. J. Ophthal. *66*:1137, 1968.

Thomas, C. I.: The Cornea, 2nd ed. Springfield, Ill., Charles C Thomas, 1972.

Staphyloma of Cornea (corneal stretching with incarceration of uveal tissue)

1. Congenital

2. Following corneal ulcer, neuroparalytic keratitis, corneal leprosy, and severe corneal injury

3. Avitaminosis A with keratomalacia

4. Advanced keratoconus (see keratoconus, p. 253)

5. Mucoviscidosis

Grayson, M., and Keates, R. H.: Manual of Diseases of the Cornea. Boston, Little, Brown & Co., 1969.

Thomas, C. I.: The Cornea, 2nd ed. Springfield, Ill., Charles C Thomas, 1972.

Whorl-like Corneal Lesions

1. Vortex dystrophy (cornea verticillata)

2. Chlorpromazine administration

3. Fabry's disease—conjunctival varicosis, swelling of eyelids, angiokeratosis of skin, disturbed sweat sensation

4. Chloroquine toxicity

5. Indomethacin administration

Burns, C. A.: Indomethacin, Reduced Retinal Sensitivity, and Corneal Deposits. Amer. J. Ophthal. 66:825, 1968.
Grayson, M., and Keates, R. H.: Manual of Diseases of the Cornea. Boston, Little, Brown & Co., 1969, p. 296.

Corneal Dermoids (congenital corneal limbal lesions that grow slowly)

The tumors are yellowish, elevated, and variable in size. They consist of fibrofatty tissue covered by epidermal rather than by conjunctival epithelium and may contain ectodermal derivatives such as hair follicles, sebaceous glands, and sweat glands. Trauma, irritation, and puberty hasten their growth.

1. Sporadic

2. Oculoauriculovertebral dysplasia (Goldenhar's syndrome)—epibulbar dermoids, colobomas, abnormally shaped or positioned ears, preauricular fleshy appendages, and unilateral hypoplasia of the mandible

3. Cri du chat syndrome (cry of the cat syndrome)—severe mental/motor retardation, microcephaly, rounded facies, hypertelorism, and a typical cat-like cry

4. Duane's retraction syndrome—enophthalmos and narrowing of palpebral fissure on adduction and widening on abduction

5. Multiple dermoids of the cornea associated with miliary aneurysms of the retina

6. Bloch-Sulzberger syndrome (incontinentia pigmenti)

7. Thalidomide teratogenicities

8. Neurocutaneous syndrome (ectomesodermal dysgenesis)

9. Nevus sebaceous of Jadassohn—antimongoloid lid; coloboma of iris-choroid; nystagmus; esotropia; external oculomotor palsy, unilateral; thickening of bones of orbit; coloboma of lids

Benjamin, S. N., and Allen, H. F.: Classification for Limbal Dermoid Choristomas and Brachial Arch Anomalies. Arch. Ophthal. 87:305–314, 1972.

Gellis, S. S., and Feingold, M.: Atlas of Mental Retardation Syndromes. Washington, D.C., U.S. Government Printing Office, 1968.

Grayson, M., and Keates, R. H.: Manual of Diseases of the Cornea. Boston, Little, Brown & Co., 1969.

Haslam, R. H., and Wirtschafter, J. D.: Unilateral External Oculomotor Palsy and Nevus Sebaceous of Jadassohn. Arch. Ophthal. 87:293–300, 1972.

Marginal Corneal Ulcers

1. Simple marginal ulcers—superficial crescentic gray-colored ulcer
   A. Infection—due to staphylococcus, Koch-Weeks bacillus, diplobacillus of Morax-Axenfeld—usually chronic
   B. Toxic or allergic
   C. Systemic disturbances, such as:
      (1) Influenza
      (2) Brucellosis
      (3) Bacillary dysentery

(4) Acute upper respiratory infection
(5) Lupus erythematosus
(6) Polyarteritis nodosa
(7) Gout
(8) Rheumatoid arthritis—inferior cornea
(9) Periarteritis nodosa

2. Ring ulcers—usually bilateral, circumcorneal injection, and continuous ring or confluent multiple lesions (see ring, corneal, p. 248)
   A. Acute leukemia
   B. Scleroderma
   C. Systemic lupus erythematosus
   D. Influenza
   E. Bacillary dysentery
   F. Polyarteritis nodosa
   G. Wegener's granulomatosis
   H. Rheumatoid arthritis—Sjögren's syndrome
   I. Porphyria
   J. Brucellosis
   K. Gonococcal arthritis
   L. Dengue fever
   M. Tuberculosis
   N. Hookworm infestation
   O. Gold poisoning
   P. Last stages of trachoma, secondary to small circumferential pannus
   Q. Coalescence of several marginal ulcers

Braendstump, P.: Atypical Marginal Ulcers of the Cornea. Acta Ophthal. *19*:163, 1941.
Brown, S. I., and Grayson, M.: Marginal Furrows. Arch. Ophthal. *79*:563–567, 1968.
Ferry, A. P., and Leopold, I. H.: Marginal (Ring) Corneal Ulcer as Presenting Manifestation of Wegener's Granuloma. Trans. Amer. Acad. Ophthal. Otolaryng. *74*:1276–1282, 1970.
Gifford, S. R.: Ring Ulcer of the Cornea. Arch. Ophthal. *27*:231–241, 1942.
Thygeson, P.: Marginal Corneal Infiltrates and Ulcers. Trans. Amer. Acad. Ophthal. Otolaryng. *51*:198–209, 1947.
Wood, W. J., and Nicholson, D. H.: Corneal Ring Ulcer as the Presenting Manifestation of Acute Monocytic Leukemia. Amer. J. Ophthal. *76*:69–72, 1973.

Corneal Problems Associated with Keratotic Skin Lesions

1. Keratosis plantaris and palmaris

2. Keratosis follicularis spinulosa decalvans

3. Ectodermal dysplasia (anhidrotic)

4. Ichthyosis

5. Keratosis follicularis

6. Pityriasis rubra pilaris

Grayson, M., and Keates, R. H.: Manual of Diseases of the Cornea. Boston, Little, Brown & Co., 1969, p. 294.

Corneal Problems Associated with Lid Excrescences

1. Lipid proteinosis

2. Keratosis folliculosis

3. Verruca vulgaris

4. Molluscum contagiosum

Grayson, M., and Keates, R. H.: Manual of Diseases of the Cornea. Boston, Little, Brown & Co., 1969, p. 294.

Corneal Disease Associated with Lenticular Problems

1. Fabry's disease—whorl-like corneal epithelial changes and posterior spoke cataract

2. Mongolism—keratoconus and cataract

3. Myotonic dystrophy—keratoconjunctivitis sicca and cataract

4. Rothmund's syndrome—band keratopathy and posterior spoke cataract

5. Diabetes mellitus—wrinkling of Descemet's membrane and cataract

6. Congenital anomalies

7. Embryopathies—virus (rubella)

8. Steroids—Bowman's membrane haze, ulcers of the cornea, and cataract

9. Wilson's disease—Kayser-Fleischer ring and sunflower cataract

10. Siderosis—pigment in epithelium of lens and endothelium and in front of Descemet's membrane

11. Endothelial dystrophy and anterior polar cataract (Dohlman)

Grayson, M., and Keates, R. H.: Manual of Diseases of the Cornea. Boston, Little, Brown & Co., 1969, p. 295.

Corneal Disease Associated with Retinal Problems

1. Syphilis—interstitial keratitis and chorioretinitis

2. Bietti's marginal crystalline dystrophy with retinitis punctate albescens

3. Leber's infantile tapetoretinal degeneration with keratoconus

4. Atopic keratoconus and retinal detachment

5. Refsum's syndrome—band keratopathy and retinitis pigmentosa

6. Hydrotic ectodermal dysplasia—juvenile macular degeneration

7. Behcet's syndrome—posterior corneal abscess and retinal vascular changes

8. Rubella—microcornea and pigmentary retinal changes

9. Chloroquine—corneal epithelial pigmentation and macular lesions

10. Phenothiazine—epithelial and endothelial pigment and retinal pigmentation

11. Cystinosis—crystals in cornea and pigment in retina

12. Mucopolysaccharidosis—Hurler's (MPS I), Hunter's (MPS II), Sanfilippo's (MPS III), and Scheie's (MPS V)

13. Fabry's disease—whorl-like changes in cornea and vascular changes in retina

14. Cryoglobulinemia—deep corneal opacities and venous stasis

15. Hypercholesterolemia—xanthoma and lipemia retinalis

16. Myotonic dystrophy—keratoconjunctivitis sicca and white streaks on retina

17. Idiopathic hypercalcemia—band keratopathy, optic atrophy, and papilledema

18. Ischemic necrosis—edema of cornea and midperipheral hemorrhages

19. Tuberous sclerosis—corneal deposits and retinal tumors

20. Neurofibromatosis—corneal tumors and retinal tumors

21. Marfan's syndrome—keratoconus and retinitis pigmentosa

22. Ehlers-Danlos—keratoconus and angioid streaks

23. 13-15 Trisomy—malformed cornea and retinal dysplasia

24. Sarcoidosis—corneal opacity and wax-candle lesions

25. Norrie's disease—malformation of sensory cells of retina with deafness, mental retardation, and persistent hyperplastic vitreous associated with corneal nebulae

26. Indomethacin—corneal deposits and reduced retinal sensitivity

Burns, C. A.,: Indomethacin, Reduced Retinal Sensitivity and Corneal Deposits. Amer. J. Ophthal. *66*:825, 1968.
Grayson, M., and Keates, R. H.: Manual of Diseases of the Cornea. Boston, Little, Brown & Co., 1969, p. 297.

Trigger Mechanisms for Recurrent Herpes Simplex Keratitis

1. Fever (most common)

2. Exposure to sunlight (ultraviolet)

3. Menses

4. Gastrointestinal upsets

5. Mechanical trauma

6. Ingestion of food to which patient is allergic

7. Emotional disturbances

8. Corticosteroids (topical)

Kimura, S. J.: Infectious Diseases of the Conjunctiva and Cornea. Symposium of the New Orleans Academy of Ophthalmology. St. Louis, C. V. Mosby Co., 1963, p. 126.

Predisposing Factors in Keratomycosis

1. Trauma

2. Steroids

3. Antibiotics

4. Trauma, steroids, and/or antibiotics

Gingrich, W. D.: Infectious Diseases of the Conjunctiva and Cornea. Symposium of the New Orleans Academy of Ophthalmology. St. Louis, C. V. Mosby Co., 1963, p. 154.

INTRAOCULAR PRESSURE

Contents

Glaucoma Suspect, Infant

1. Epiphora, photophobia, and blepharospasm
2. Corneal edema
3. Corneal enlargement
4. Tears in Descemet's membrane
5. Deep anterior chamber
6. Cupping and atrophy of optic disc
7. Iridodonesis and subluxation of lens
8. Amblyopia ex anopsia

Kolker, A. E., and Hetherington, J.: Becker-Shaffer's Diagnosis and Therapy of Glaucoma, 3rd ed. St. Louis, C. V. Mosby Co., 1970, pp. 259–263.

Conditions Simulating Congenital Glaucoma

1. Inflammation
    A. Syphilitic interstitial keratitis
    B. Intrauterine gonorrhea keratitis
    C. Smallpox and chickenpox viruses—intrauterine
    D. Fetal iritis or uveitis
    E. Blepharitis, keratoconjunctivitis, and keratitis on a chemical, allergic, bacterial, or viral basis

2. Metabolic disorders
    A. Familial lipoidosis
    B. Cystinosis or cystine storage disease

    C. Hurler's disease (MPS I), Morquio-Brailsford disease (MPS IV), Scheie's disease (MPS V), and Maroteaux-Lamy disease (MPS VI)
    D. Porphyria

3. Congenital idiopathic corneal edema

4. Blue sclerotic syndrome (see p. 211)

5. Riley-Day syndrome

6. Megalocornea (see p. 226)

7. Myopia

8. Anterior corneal staphyloma

9. Cornea plana

10. Keratoconus (see p. 253)

11. Keratoectasia

12. Intraocular tumor, such as retinoblastoma or diktyoma

13. Bloch-Sulzberger syndrome (incontinentia pigmenti)

14. Congenital corneal dystrophy

15. Birth injury, such as breaks in Descemet's membrane

16. Trisomy 13-15 syndrome

17. Corneal amyloidosis

18. Corneal xanthomas

19. von Gierke's disease (glycogen disease)

20. Congenital anomalies, such as sclerocornea

Becker, B., and Shaffer, R. N.: Diagnosis and Therapy of Glaucoma, 3rd ed. St. Louis, C. V. Mosby Co., 1970, pp. 263–264.

Geeraets, W. J.: Ocular Syndromes, 2nd ed. Philadelphia, Lea & Febiger, 1969, pp. 221–222.

Howard, R. O., and Abrahams, I. W.: Sclerocornea. Amer. J. Ophthal. 71:1254–1260, 1971.

Kenyon, K. R., et al.: The Systemic Mucopolysaccharidoses. Amer. J. Ophthal. 73:811–833, 1972.

Kwitko, M. L.: Glaucoma in Infants and Children. Mod. Med. Canad. 23:1–8, 1968.

Liebman, S. D., Crocker, A. C., and Geiser, C. F.: Corneal Xanthomas in Childhood. Arch. Ophthal. *76*:220–221, 1966.

McPherson, S. D., Jr., Kiffney, G. T., and Freed, C. C.: Corneal Amyloidosis. Amer. J. Ophthal. *62*:1025, 1966.

Rodger, F. C., and Sinclair, H. M.: Metabolic and Nutritional Eye Diseases. Springfield, Ill., Charles C Thomas, 1969, p. 104.

Ocular and Systemic Anomalies Associated with Congenital Glaucoma

1. Local ocular anomalies
   A. Iridocorneal dysgenesis (anterior chamber cleavage syndrome)
      (1) Posterior embryotoxon of Axenfeld—anterior displacement of Schwalbe's line; iris tissue can be seen crossing the angle, attaching the periphery of the iris to the prominent Schwalbe's line; hypertelorism and skeletal abnormalities
      (2) Rieger's syndrome—hypoplasia of the anterior stromal leaf of the iris, iridotrabecular adhesions, and posterior embryotoxon
      (3) Dense central corneal opacity with iris synechiae
   B. Essential iris atrophy—localized area (or areas) of atrophy begins in the stroma and eventually involves the pigment layers
   C. Aniridia—absence of the iris, never complete; gonioscopy shows a rudimentary iris
   D. Pigmentary glaucoma—idiopathic atrophy of the pigment epithelium of the iris, which is deposited on the lens capsule at the insertion of the zonular fibers, the anterior surface of the iris, the corneal endothelium in the form of Krukenberg's spindle, and in the angle, especially in the trabecular meshwork
   E. Megalocornea (see p. 226)—megalocornea associated with congenital glaucoma is rare

F. Microcornea (see p. 225)—in a hyperopic eye the anterior chamber is often shallow and the angles narrow; an acute attack of glaucoma is possible

G. Microphthalmos (see p. 192)—autosomal dominant and recessive inheritance trait

H. Spherophakia (microphakia) (see p. 348)—lens is small, spherical in shape, and its edges can be identified through the dilated pupil; a high degree of myopia may be present

I. Myopia

J. Retinitis pigmentosa (see p. 421)

K. Coloboma of the iris (see p. 316)

L. Polycoria

M. Sclerocornea

N. Hemangioma of the choroid

O. Glaucoma secondary to local ocular disease
   (1) Retinoblastoma
   (2) Retrolental fibroplasia
   (3) Persistent hyperplastic primary vitreous
   (4) Anterior uveitis (see pp. 329–335)
   (5) Heterochromic iridocyclitis
   (6) Trauma
   (7) Congenital cataract

2. Systemic anomalies
   A. Phakomatoses—disseminated hamartomas that have eye, skin, and brain involvement in common
      (1) Neurofibromatosis (von Recklinghausen's disease)—neurofibromas in various parts of the body, skin pigmentation (café-au-lait spots), and skeletal changes such as pseudoarthrosis. Ocular findings may include ptosis and neurofibroma of the skin of the eyelids and also of the uvea
      (2) Encephalotrigeminal angiomatosis of Sturge-Weber—intracranial angioma associated with facial and choroidal angiomas, which are homolateral and present at birth
      (3) Tuberous sclerosis
      (4) von Hippel-Lindau disease (angiomatosis retinae)

B. Heritable disorders of connective tissue
  (1) Marfan's syndrome—long, thin extremities; diffuse dilatation, and at times dissection of aorta and/or ectopia lentis
  (2) Weil-Marchesani syndrome—brachymorphism and shortness of stature, with round head, pug nose, depressed nasal bridge, and short, pudgy hands and fingers; ectopia lentis
  (3) Homocystinuria—arterial disease, arachnodactylia, ectopia lentis, mental retardation, venous thrombosis, and pulmonary embolism
  (4) Hurler's disease (MPS I)—corneal opacities, true megalocornea, congenital glaucoma, pigmentary retinopathy
C. Lowe's syndrome (oculocerebrorenal syndrome)—systemic acidosis, organic aciduria, decreased ability to produce ammonia in the kidneys, renal rickets, generalized hypotonicity, retardation, glaucoma, and cataracts
D. Pierre Robin syndrome—hypoplasia of the mandible, glossoptosis, cleft palate, high myopia, retinal detachment, glaucoma, cataracts, and microphthalmia
E. Hallerman-Streiff syndrome—dyscephaly, bird-like facies, localized hypotrichosis, localized atrophy of the skin, and bilateral microphthalmos with associated severe congenital glaucoma or cataracts
F. Chromosomal disorders
  (1) Turner's syndrome—infantilism, webbing of the skin of the neck, equinovarus, dwarfism, and amenorrhea
  (2) Trisomy 16-18—failure to thrive, low-set ears, malformed pinnae, mental retardation, hypotonicity, small mouth and mandible, ventricular septal defects, flexion deformities of fingers, partial syndactylia of toes, renal anomalies, congenital glaucoma, optic atrophy, lenticular opacities, corneal opacities, and ptosis
  (3) Trisomy 13-15—malformations of the brain, heart, and viscera; polydactylia, harelip, cleft palate, microphthalmia, retinal dysplasia, iris and

ciliary body colobomas, and persistent hyperplastic primary vitreous

(4) Down's syndrome (mongolism) (trisomy 21)

G. Oculodentodigital syndrome (hereditary oculo-dento-osseous dysplasia)—anomalies of the extremities, mental defects, microphthalmos, coloboma, and glaucoma

H. Dyscraniopygophalangea (Ullrich's syndrome)—cranial deformities, broad nose, small mandible, associated skeletal and visceral abnormalities, bilateral anophthalmos; defects such as microphthalmia, chorioretinal coloboma, complete aniridia, ciliary body hypoplasia, and gross mesodermal abnormalities of the anterior chamber

I. Congenital melanosis oculi—unilateral hyperpigmentation of the uveal tract, sclera, and, occasionally, of the periorbital skin (nevus of Ota)

J. Juvenile xanthogranuloma—widespread yellow- to orange-colored skin nodules that occur shortly after birth; occasionally these lesions occur in the iris and ciliary body and are prone to cause anterior chamber hemorrhage, giving rise to secondary glaucoma

K. Idiopathic infantile hypoglycemia—neonatal hypoglycemia, nasolacrimal duct obstructions, congenital cataracts, squint, cortical blindness, atrophy of the optic disc, congenital glaucoma

L. Congenital rubella syndrome

M. Syphilis

N. Toxoplasmosis

Kwitko, M. L.: Glaucoma in Infants and Children. Mod. Med. Canad. 23:1–8, 1968.

Scheie, H.: Surgical and Medical Management of Congenital Anomalies of the Eye. Transactions of the New Orleans Academy of Ophthalmology. St. Louis, C. V. Mosby Co., 1966, pp. 356–360.

Glaucoma Suspect, Adult

1. Applanation reading 21 mm Hg or higher
2. Schiotz scale reading 4.0/5.5 or 6.25/7.5 or less
3. Visual field changes suggestive of glaucoma
4. Prominent cupping of optic disc
5. Family history of glaucoma
6. Intraocular pressure elevation following use of topical corticosteroids
7. High myopia
8. Thyrotropic exophthalmos
9. Retinal vein occlusion
10. Retinal detachment
11. Krukenberg's spindle and/or dense trabecular pigment band
12. Endothelial dystrophy of cornea
13. Pseudoexfoliation of lens capsule
14. Diabetes mellitus

Kolker, A. E., and Hetherington, J.: Becker-Shaffer's Diagnosis and Therapy of Glaucoma, 3rd ed. St. Louis, C. V. Mosby Co., 1970, pp. 207–210.

Elevated Intraocular Pressure with Normal Optic Disc

1. Hypertension
2. Excessive water intake

3. Hyperthyroid

4. Normal variation

5. Marked emotional stress

6. Mechanical factors in checking intraocular pressure

7. High scleral rigidity (see p. 214)

8. Pre-glaucoma

9. Steroid intake (local, systemic)

Kolker, A. E., and Hetherington, J.: Becker-Shaffer's Diagnosis and Therapy of Glaucoma, 3rd ed. St. Louis, C. V. Mosby Co., 1970, pp. 55–64.

Secondary Open-Angle Glaucoma

1. Due to changes of the lens
   A. Dislocation
   B. Intumescence
   C. Phacolytic or phaco-anaphylactic
   D. Glaucoma capsulare

2. Due to changes in the uveal tract
   A. Iritis and iridocyclitis (see anterior uveitis, pp. 329–335)
   B. Tumor (see pp. 324–328)
   C. Essential iris atrophy
   D. Congenital anomalies, such as posterior embryotoxon or aniridia
   E. Degenerative conditions, such as pigmentary glaucoma
   F. Rubeosis iridis (see rubeosis iridis, p. 318)
   G. Leukemic infiltrates of iris

3. Due to trauma
   A. Massive hemorrhage into the anterior or posterior chamber

    B. Corneal or limbal laceration with iris prolapse into the wound
    C. Iridodialysis or recessed chamber angle
    D. Intraocular foreign body, such as iron, especially in iris
    E. Rupture of lens capsule with lens swelling
    F. Dislocated lens (see p. 349)
    G. Epithelial down-growth

4. Following surgical procedures
    A. Alpha-chymotrypsin induced
    B. Postoperative narrow-angle glaucoma with trabecular damage
    C. Hyphema
    D. Epithelial down-growth
    E. Following retinal detachment surgery

5. Sturge-Weber syndrome

6. Thyrotropic exophthalmos

7. Retrobulbar pressure—infection, tumor, or hemorrhage

8. Steroid-induced glaucoma

9. Elevated episcleral venous pressure—dilated episcleral vessels (see p. 213)

10. Keratitis as metaherpetic

11. Retinitis pigmentosa

12. Epidemic dropsy—consumption of argemone oil

13. Congenital glaucoma

Becker, B., and Shaffer, R. N.: Diagnosis and Therapy of Glaucoma, 3rd ed. St. Louis, C. V. Mosby Co., 1970, pp. 225–249.

Fonken, H. A., and Ellis, P. P.: Leukemic Infiltrates of the Iris. Arch. Ophthal. 76:32, 1966.

Weekers, R., and Delmarcelle, Y.: Pathogenesis of Intraocular Hypertension in Cases of Arteriovenous Aneurysm. Arch. Ophthal. 48:338–343, 1952.

Unilateral Glaucoma

1. Trauma
    A. Contusion
        (1) Angle deformity
        (2) Hyphema
        (3) Scarring and vascularization of the anterior chamber
        (4) Iritis
        (5) Phacolytic glaucoma
        (6) Hemolytic glaucoma
    B. Perforating wound
        (1) Peripheral anterior synechia and scarring of the anterior chamber
        (2) Phacolytic glaucoma
    C. Intraocular foreign body
        (1) Siderosis bulbi
        (2) Chronic inflammation
    D. Chemical burn
        (1) Kerato-iritis
        (2) Phacolytic glaucoma

2. Tumor

3. Neovascularization of iris and chamber angle (see rubeosis iridis, p. 318)

4. Inflammation
    A. Anterior uveitis
        (1) With peripheral anterior synechiae
        (2) With open angle including glaucomatocyclitic crisis
    B. Corneal
        (1) Chronic interstitial keratitis (see p. 244)
        (2) Chemical keratitis
        (3) Chronic keratitis secondary to herpes zoster
        (4) Acute bacterial corneal ulcer

5. Lens changes
    A. Phacolytic reaction

B. Intumescent lens

C. Dislocated lens

6. Uniocular open-angle glaucoma

7. Associated with extradural hemorrhage

8. Carotid-cavernous sinus fistula

9. Many conditions that give bilateral glaucoma with earlier onset in one eye, such as congenital, open-angle, or narrow-angle glaucoma

10. Ophthalmic vein thrombosis

11. Cavernous sinus thrombosis

Boniuk, M.: The Ocular Manifestations of Ophthalmic Vein and Aseptic Cavernous Sinus Thrombosis. Trans. Amer. Acad. Ophthal. Otolaryng. 76:1519–1534, 1972.

de Roetth, A., Jr.: Glaucomatocyclitic Crisis. Amer. J. Ophthal. 69: 370–371, 1970.

Drance, S. M., Wheeley, C., and Pattullo, M.: Uniocular Open-Angle Glaucoma. Amer. J. Ophthal. 65:891, 1968.

Koeppen, A. H., Madonick, M. J., and Barest, M. D.: Acute Unilateral Glaucoma Associated with Extradural Hemorrhage. Amer. J. Ophthal. 63:1696, 1967.

Miles, D. R., and Boniuk, M.: Pathogenesis of Unilateral Glaucoma. Amer. J. Ophthal. 62:493, 1966.

Glaucoma Associated with Displaced Lens

1. Uveitis

2. Pupillary block

3. Peripheral posterior synechiae

4. Anterior chamber angle deformity

5. Phacolytic

6. Anterior chamber recessed angle

Duke-Elder, S.: System of Ophthalmology, Vol. XI. St. Louis, C. V. Mosby Co., 1969, p. 661.

Glaucoma and Elevated Episcleral Venous Pressure

1. Familial glaucoma

2. Obstruction of episcleral veins by caustic agents, radiation, or trachoma

3. Obstruction of vortex veins by inflammation, thrombosis, or mechanical causes

4. Obstruction of orbital veins by phlebitis, pseudotumor, thyroid disease, tumors, or ligation

5. Obstruction of jugular veins by phlebitis

6. Obstruction of superior vena cava by mediastinal tumor or ligation

7. Arteriovenous shunts, including orbital, carotid-cavernous sinus, and internal carotid-jugular vein

Minas, T. F., and Podos, S. M.: Familial Glaucoma Associated with Elevated Episcleral Venous Pressure. Arch. Ophthal. *80*:202–208, 1968.

Podos, S. M., Minas, T. F., and Macri, F. J.: A New Instrument to Measure Episcleral Venous Pressure. Arch. Ophthal. *80*:209–213, 1968.

"Aphakic" Glaucoma (glaucoma in aphakia)

1. Primary open-angle glaucoma

2. Associated with pseudo-exfoliation in aphakia

3. Peripheral anterior synechiae from loss of vitreous, prolapse of iris, incarceration of iris or lens capsule in wound, or absent anterior chamber (see p. 289)

4. Pupillary block

5. Vitreous filling the anterior chamber

6. Immediate postoperative reaction following intracapsular extraction from traumatic iritis or alpha-chymotrypsin use

7. Epithelialization of the anterior chamber

8. Prolonged postoperative inflammation in aphakia in both intracapsular and extracapsular extraction

Chandler, D. A., and Grant, W. M.: Lectures on Glaucoma. Philadelphia, Lea & Febiger, 1965, pp. 234–243.

Kolker, A. E., and Hetherington, J.: Becker-Shaffer's Diagnosis and Therapy of Glaucoma, 3rd ed. St. Louis, C. V. Mosby Co., 1970, pp. 225–243.

Medication That May Cause Glaucoma

1. Aclobrom—propantheline

2. Allegron—nortryptyline hydrochloride

3. Aludrox SA—aluminum hydroxide, magnesium hydroxide, butabarbital, and ambutonium bromide

4. Artane—trihexyphenidyl hydrochloride; benzhexol

5. Ascon—aluminium hydroxide, magnesium trisilicate, and hysocyamine hydrobromide suspension

6. Aventyl—nortryptiline hydrochloride

7. Belladenal—belladonna with phenobarbital

8. Berkomine—imipramine hydrochloride

9. Brontine—dibenzheptropine citrate

10. Butibel—belladonna

11. Cantil—mepenzolate bromide

12. Cogentin—benztropine mesylate

13. Collubarb—aluminium hydroxide, phenobarbital, and atropine sulfate

14. Concordin—protriptyline hydrochloride

15. Dactil—piperidolate hydrochloride

16. Daricon—oxyphencyclimine hydrochloride

17. De-Nol—belladonna leaf with ionized bismuth

18. Deprop—meprobromate with benactyzine hydrochloride

19. Disipal—orphenadrine hydrochloride

20. Donnatal—hyoscyamine sulfate, atropine sulfate, hyoscine hydrobromide, and phenobarbital

21. Donnazyme—pepsin, phenobarbital, hyoscyamine sulfate, atropine sulfate, hyoscine hydrobromide, pancreatin, and bile salts

22. Equanitrate—pentaerythritol tetranitrate with meprobamate

23. Largactil—chlorpromazine hydrochloride

24. Laroxyl—amitriptyline hydrochloride

25. Librax—chlordiazepoxide and clidinium bromide

26. Merbentyl—dicyclomine hydrochloride

27. Monodral—penthienate bromide

28. Neutradonna—aluminium sodium silicate with belladonna equivalent to hyoscyamine

29. Norgesic—orphenadrine citrate with paracetamol

30. Pacatal—mepazine; pecazine

31. Pamine—methscopolamine bromide

32. Pentoxylon—pentaerythritol tetranitrate with alseroxylon

33. Pentrium—chlordiazepoxide with pentaerythritol tetranitrate

10

34. Periactin—cyproheptadine hydrochloride

35. Perideca—cyproheptadine hydrochloride with dexamethasone

36. Perifenil—pentaerythritol tetranitrate with phenelzine sulfate

37. Peritrate—pentaerythritol tetranitrate with phenobarbital

38. Piptal—pipenzolate bromide

39. Placadol—homatropine

40. Portyn—benzilonium bromide

41. Pro-Banthine—propantheline bromide

42. Procol—phenylpropanolamine hydrochloride and diphenylpyraline hydrochloride with isopropamide as the iodide

43. Robinul—glycopyrrolate

44. Saroten—amitriptyline hydrochloride

45. Secergan—phenothiazine methobromide

46. Stelabid—trifluoperazine with isopropamide as the iodide

47. Surmontil—trimipramine

48. Sustac—glyceryl trinitrate

49. Tremonil—methixene hydrochloride

50. Triaminic—phenylpropanolamine hydrochloride, mepyramine maleate, and pheniramine maleate

51. Trinitrin—glyceryl trinitrate of active substance

52. Triogesic—phenylpropanolamine hydrochloride with paracetamol

53. Triotussic—phenylpropanolamine hydrochloride, mepyramine maleate, pheniramine maleate, noscapine, terpin hydrate, and paracetamol

54. Tryptafen—amitriptyline with perphenazine

55. Tryptizol—amitriptyline hydrochloride

56. Tyrimide—isopropamide iodide

57. Vascardin—isosorbide dinitrate
58. Vasomed—aminotrate phosphate
59. Wyovin—dicyclomine hydrochloride

Green, H., and Spencer, J.: Drugs with Possible Ocular Side-Effects. New York, St. Martin's Press, 1969, p. 177.

Hypotony (decreased intraocular pressure)

1. Fistula from intraocular source, including penetrating intraocular trauma or operation and ruptured wall of the globe
2. Phthisis bulbi (see p. 202)
3. Choroidal detachment (see p. 456)
4. Injury to the cervical sympathetic nerve
5. Serous detachment of the retina
6. Myotonic dystrophy
7. Systemic disturbances
    A. Diabetic coma
    B. Uremic coma
    C. Cardiac edema
    D. Extreme or rapid dehydration due to malnutrition, cholera, or diarrhea
    E. Severe abdominal disturbances, such as intestinal perforation or obstruction
    F. Profound anemias
    G. Giant-cell arteritis
    H. Fall in ocular blood pressure due to hypotension, ligation of the carotid artery, carotid occlusion, and pulseless disease (aortic arch syndrome; Takayasu's syndrome)
    I. Postencephalitic syndrome following severe cerebral trauma, barbiturate poisoning, in deep anesthesia, following leukotomy, or on the paralyzed side in cerebral hemiplegia

8. Drugs, such as Eserine, pilocarpine, epinephrine bitartrate, Diamox, and ouabain

9. Detachment of the ciliary body, planned or inadvertent

10. Hyperosmotic agents, such as mannitol or urea

11. Iritis or iridocyclitis

12. Following central retinal vein occlusion

13. Myopia—low scleral rigidity may give false low readings with schiotz but normal readings with applanation

14. Parkinson's disease

15. Herpes zoster

16. Following irradiation with x rays or beta rays

17. Congenital lesions, including microphthalmos, aniridia, and coloboma

18. Concussion trauma

19. Necrosis of anterior segment of the eye

20. Leprosy

21. Idiopathic, including normal variation

Chandler, P. A., and Maumenee, A. E.: A Major Cause of Hypotony. Amer. J. Ophthal. 52:609, 1961.

Cherry, P. M. H.: Rupture of the Globe. Arch. Ophthal. 88:498–507, 1972.

Duke-Elder, S.: System of Ophthalmology, Vol. XI. St. Louis, C. V. Mosby Co., 1969, pp. 726–746.

Lessell, S., Coppeto, J., and Samet, S.: Ophthalmoplegia in Myotonic Dystrophy. Amer. J. Ophthal. 71:1231–1235, 1971.

Pradham, J. S., Shukla, B. R., and Ahuja, O. P.: Shallow Anterior Chamber after Cataract Extraction. Eye Ear Nose Throat Monthly 47:53, 1968.

Slem, G.: Clinical Studies of Ocular Leprosy. Amer. J. Ophthal. 71:431–434, 1971.

Vannas, S., and Raitta, C.: Intraocular Hypotony vs Hypotony after Central Retinal Vein Occlusion. Ann. Ophthal. 2:213–217, 1970.

Walsh, F. B., and Hoyt, W. F.: Clinical Ophthalmology, 3rd ed. Baltimore, Williams & Wilkins Co., 1969, pp. 1850–1853.

ANTERIOR CHAMBER

Contents

Hypopyon (pus in the anterior chamber)

1. Hypopyon ulcer—central corneal ulcer with pus in the anterior chamber (see p. 250)
   A. *Diplococcus pneumoniae*
   B. Streptococcus
   C. *Neisseria gonorrhoeae*
   D. Morax-Axenfeld diplobacillus (*Moraxella lacunata*)
   E. *Proteus vulgaris*
   F. *Pseudomonas aeruginosa*
   G. *Escherichia coli*
   H. Herpes simplex
   I. Herpes zoster
   J. Measles
   K. *Candida albicans*
   L. Chemical, such as latex keratitis

2. Severe acute iridocyclitis

3. Necrosis of intraocular tumors or metastasis

4. Retained intraocular foreign bodies

5. Endophthalmitis—at time of surgical treatment or accidental trauma (see p. 196)
   A. Mucor species
   B. Aspergillosis
   C. Coccidioidomycosis
   D. Bacterial (see 1 above)

6. Accidental intraocular steroid injection (pseudohypopyon)

Fedukowicz, H. B.: External Infections of the Eye. New York, Appleton-Century-Crofts, Inc., 1963.

Newell, F. W.: Ophthalmology, Principles and Concepts. St. Louis, C. V. Mosby Co., 1969.

Schlaegel, T. F., and Wilson, F. M.: Accidental Intraocular Injection of Depot Corticosteroids. Trans. Amer. Acad. Ophthal. Otolaryng. In press.

Sofot, B. K., et al.: Euphorbia Royleana Latex Keratitis. Amer. J. Ophthal. 74:634–637, 1972.

Hyphema (bleeding into the anterior chamber)

1. Trauma
   A. To iris, such as iridodialysis
   B. To ciliary body, such as cyclodialysis
   C. Tear of ciliary body—post-contusion deformity of anterior chamber

2. Overdistention of vessels
   A. Sudden lowering of high intraocular pressure
   B. Obstruction of central retinal vein

3. Fragility of vessel walls
   A. Acute herpes iridocyclitis
   B. Acute gonorrheal iridocyclitis
   C. Acute rheumatoid iridocyclitis

4. Blood derangement
   A. Hemophilia
   B. Anemias
   C. Leukemia
   D. Purpura

5. Metabolic disease
   A. Scurvy
   B. Diabetes

6. Neovascularization of iris (see rubeosis iridis, p. 318)

7. Vascularized tumors of iris (see pigmented and non-pigmented iris lesions, pp. 325 and 326)
   A. Angioma
   B. Lymphosarcoma
   C. Juvenile xanthogranuloma
   D. Retinoblastoma

8. Wound vascularization following cataract extraction

Duke-Elder, S., and Perkins, E. S.: Diseases of the Uveal Tract. System of Ophthalmology, Vol. IX. St. Louis, C. V. Mosby Co., 1966, pp. 19–20.

Hogan, M. J., and Zimmerman, L. E.: Ophthalmic Pathology, 2nd ed. Philadelphia, W. B. Saunders Co., 1962, p. 145.

Swan, K.: Hyphema Due to Wound Vascularization after Cataract Extraction. Arch. Ophthal. *89*:87–90, 1973.

Spontaneous Hyphema

1. Hypertension

2. Intraocular neoplasms

3. Diseases of blood or blood vessels
   A. Leukemia
   B. Hemophilia
   C. Scurvy
   D. Purpura
   E. Malignant lymphoma

4. Severe iritis with or without
   A. Gonococcal infection
   B. Herpes zoster
   C. Diabetes
   D. Behcet's disease

5. Rubeosis iridis (see p. 318)

6. Fibrovascular membranes in retrolental or zonular area
   A. Retrolental fibroplasia
   B. Persistent primary vitreous
   C. Retinoschisis

7. Juvenile xanthogranuloma—yellow nodules of skin

8. Occult trauma or trauma with late effect

9. Hydrophthalmos

10. Vascular anomalies of iris

11. Malignant exophthalmos

12. Delayed following antiglaucomatous operation

13. Iatrogenic

Manor, R. S., and Sachs, W.: Spontaneous Hyphema. Amer. J. Ophthal. *74*:293–296, 1972.

Spontaneous Hyphema in Infants

1. Juvenile xanthogranuloma

2. Retinoblastoma

3. Blood dyscrasias, such as anemia and leukemia

4. Acute rheumatoid iridocyclitis

5. Trauma without history

6. Retrolental fibroplasia

7. Persistent hyperplastic vitreous

8. Retinoschisis

9. Iritis

Duke-Elder, S., and Perkins, E. S.: Diseases of the Uveal Tract. System of Ophthalmology, Vol. IX. St. Louis, C. V. Mosby Co., 1966, pp. 19–20.

Guzak, S. V.: Lymphoma as a Cause of Hyphema. Arch. Ophthal. *84*:229–231, 1970.

Howard, G. M.: Spontaneous Hyphema in Infancy and Childhood. Arch. Ophthal. *68*:615–620, 1962.

Plasmoid Aqueous (aqueous that has a high protein content)

1. Rheumatoid arthritis

2. Serum sickness

3. Infection with gonococcus

4. Following paracentesis or intraocular operation, such as cataract extraction

5. Trauma

Duke-Elder, S., and Perkins, E. S.: Diseases of the Uveal Tract. System of Ophthalmology, Vol. IX. St. Louis, C. V. Mosby Co., 1966.

Newell, F. W.: Ophthalmology, Principles and Concepts. St. Louis, C. V. Mosby Co., 1969, p. 74.

Pigmentation of Trabecular Meshwork

1. In elderly individuals—inferior nasal or faint band circumferential

2. Pseudo-exfoliation of lens with glaucoma—unilateral or bilateral

3. Pigmentary glaucoma

4. Krukenberg's spindle without glaucoma

5. Malignant melanoma—one eye

6. Cyst of pigment layer of iris—unilateral

7. Previous intraocular operation, inflammation, or hyphema—scattered, mostly in lower angle

8. Nevus—dense, isolated patch

9. Open-angle glaucoma—patchy band, whole circumference

10. Following gamma irradiation for malignancy of nasal sinus

Bothman, L.: Glaucoma Following Irradiation. Arch. Ophthal. 23: 1198, 1940.

Chandler, P. A., and Grant, W. M.: Lecture on Glaucoma. Philadelphia, Lea & Febiger, 1965, p. 90.

Pigment Liberation into Anterior Chamber with Dilatation of Pupil

1. Low tension glaucoma

2. Diabetes mellitus

3. Hurler's disease

Kristensen, P.: Pigment Liberation Test in "Low Tension Glaucoma." Acta Ophthal. *45*:594, 1967.

Angle Width of Anterior Chamber (usually determined by gonioscopy)

1. Grade 0—no angle structures visible—narrow angle, complete or partial closure (angle closure)

2. Grade 1—unable to see posterior one half of trabecular meshwork—extremely narrow angle (probably capable of angle closure)

3. Grade 2—part of Schlemm's canal is visible—moderate narrow angle (may be capable of angle closure)

4. Grade 3—posterior portion of Schlemm's canal is visible—moderate open angle (incapable of angle closure)

5. Grade 4—ciliary body is visible—open angle (incapable of angle closure)

Blood in Schlemm's Canal

1. Normal eye

2. Tetralogy of Fallot—increased venous pressure

3. Carotid-cavernous sinus fistula

4. Intraocular inflammation

5. Hypotony (see p. 279)

6. Mediastinal tumors—increased venous pressure

Newell, F. W.: Ophthalmology, Principles and Concepts. St. Louis, C. V. Mosby Co., 1969, p. 34.

Phelps, C. D., et al.: Blood Reflux into Schlemm's Canal. Arch. Ophthal. *88*:625–631, 1972.

Suson, E. B., and Schultz, R. W.: Blood in Schlemm's Canal in Glaucoma Suspects. Arch. Ophthal. *81*:808, 1969.

Deep Anterior Chamber Angle

1. Normal variation

2. Aphakia

3. Myopia

4. Megalocornea or conical cornea including keratoconus (see p. 253)

5. Congenital glaucoma

6. Posterior dislocation of the lens

7. Recession of anterior chamber angle

Newell, F. W.: Ophthalmology, Principles and Concepts. St. Louis, C. V. Mosby Co., 1969.

Narrow Anterior Chamber Angle (may be capable of angle closure glaucoma)

1. Normal variation
2. Predisposition to angle closure
3. Anterior dislocation of the lens
4. Hyperope
5. Spherophakia and microcornea (see p. 348 and p. 225)
6. Postoperative intraocular operation with leaking wound (hypotony p. 279)
7. Choroidal detachment (see p. 456)
8. Pupillary block
9. Loss of aqueous from perforating ulcer, corneal wound, or staphyloma (hypotony, p. 279)
10. Intumescent senile cataract
11. Traumatic cataract that fluffs up
12. Primary hyperplastic primary vitreous
13. Peripheral anterior synechiae (see p. 290)

Newell, F. W.: Ophthalmology, Principles and Concepts. St. Louis, C. V. Mosby Co., 1969.
Scheie, H. G., and Morse, P. H.: Shallow Anterior Chamber as a Sign of Non-surgical Choroidal Detachment. Ann. Ophthal. 6:317–322, 1974.

Irregular Depth of the Anterior Chamber (see narrow anterior chamber, above)

1. Partial dislocation of the lens
2. Tumor of iris or ciliary body

3. Peripheral anterior synechiae on one side of the chamber

4. Iris bombé or pupillary block

5. Ruptured lens capsule with swelling on one side

6. Anatomic narrowing superiorly

7. Subacute angle closure glaucoma

8. Cyclodialysis and traumatic recession of chamber angle

Chandler, P. A., and Grant, W. M.: Lectures on Glaucoma. Philadelphia, Lea & Febiger, 1965, pp. 65–66.

Newell, F. W.: Ophthalmology, Principles and Concepts. St. Louis, C. V. Mosby Co., 1969.

Peripheral Anterior Synechiae (adhesion of iris tissue across the anterior chamber structures in variable amounts noted with gonioscopy)

* = Most important

1. Bridge corneoscleral trabecular meshwork to Schwalbe's line or anterior to Schwalbe's line (uncommon)
    A. Essential atrophy of iris (see p. 322)
    B. Iris bombé from occlusion of pupil
    C. Postoperative flat anterior chamber
    D. Penetrating injury of the cornea
    E. Local adhesion with growth of epithelium into aphakic eye
    F. Anterior chamber cleavage syndrome
        (1) Congenital central anterior synechiae
        (2) Rieger's syndrome—hypoplasia of anterior iris and posterior embryotoxon
        (3) Axenfeld's syndrome—prominent anteriorly displaced Schwalbe's line (posterior embryotoxon) and iridocorneal angle adhesions

*G. Iris or ciliary body tumor pushing iris into contact
　　　　with cornea

　2. Synechiae of iris limited to ciliary band, scleral spur, and
　　　trabecular meshwork (common)
　　　*A. Sequelae to angle closure glaucoma
　　　*B. Intraocular inflammation
　　　*C. Neovascular glaucoma—rubeosis iridis with shrinkage
　　　　　of fibrovascular membrane (see p. 318)

Chandler, P. A., and Grant, W. M.: Lectures on Glaucoma. Phila-
　　delphia, Lea & Febiger, 1965, pp. 276–279.
Kolker, A. E., and Hetherington, J.: Becker-Shaffer's Diagnosis and
　　Therapy of the Glaucomas, 3rd ed. St. Louis, C. V. Mosby Co.,
　　1970, pp. 197–206.
Newell, F. W.: Ophthalmology, Principles and Concepts. St. Louis,
　　C. V. Mosby Co., 1969.
Reese, A. B., and Ellsworth, R.: The Anterior Chamber Cleavage
　　Syndrome. Arch. Ophthal. 75:307, 1966.

Neovascularization of Anterior Chamber Angle (newly formed vessels extend into the trabecular meshwork)

* = Most important

　1. Proximal vascular disease
　　　A. Aortic arch syndrome
　　　B. Carotid occlusive disease
　　　C. Carotid ligation
　　　D. Carotid cavernous fistula
　　　E. Cranial arteritis

　2. Ocular vascular disease
　　　*A. Central retinal vein thrombosis
　　　*B. Central retinal artery thrombosis

　3. Retinal diseases
　　　*A. Diabetes mellitus

B. Leber's miliary aneurysms
C. Coats' disease
D. Eales' disease
E. Sickle cell retinopathy
F. Retinal hemangioma
G. Persistent hyperplastic primary vitreous
H. Retrolental fibroplasia
I. Retinoblastoma
J. Norrie's disease
K. Retinal detachment
L. Melanoma of choroid
M. Glaucoma, chronic

4. Iris tumors
   A. Melanoma
   B. Metastatic carcinoma
   C. Hemangioma

5. Postinflammatory
   A. Uveitis, chronic
   B. Retinal detachment operation
   C. Fungal endophthalmitis
   D. Radiation

Schulze, R. R.: Rubeosis Iridis. Amer. J. Ophthal. 63:487, 1967.

Iris Processes (pectinate ligaments in the anterior chamber angle)

* = Most frequent

1. Achondroplasia, diastrophic dwarfism, cartilage-hair hypoplasia, and spondyloepiphyseal dysplasia

2. Marfan's syndrome

3. Legg-Perthes disease

4. Mucopolysaccharides

5. Congenital scoliosis

6. Myopic patients

*7. Normal, especially brown-eyed persons

Burian, H. M., von Noorden, G. K., and Ponseti, I. V.: Chamber Angle Anomalies in Systemic Connective Tissue Disorders. Arch. Ophthal. *64*:671–680, 1960.

Lichter, P. R.: Iris Processes in 340 Eyes. Amer. J. Ophthal. *68*: 872–878, 1969.

Rosenthal, A. R., Ryan, S. J., and Horowitz, P.: Ocular Manifestations of Dwarfism. Trans. Amer. Acad. Ophth. Otolaryng. *76*: 1500–1518, 1972.

von Noorden, G. K., and Schultz, R. O.: A Gonioscopic Study of the Chamber Angle in Marfan's Syndrome. Arch. Ophthal. *64*: 929–934, 1960.

Cholesterolosis of the Anterior Chamber (cholesterol crystals in the anterior chamber; usually in a blind eye following trauma, but may be associated with hyphema or secondary glaucoma)

Associated with
1. Congenital microphthalmic eye
2. Traumatic cataract
3. Lens subluxation
4. Retinal detachment
5. Vitreous hemorrhage
6. Mature or hypermature cataract
7. Chronic uveitis
8. Vascular disorders

Wand, M., and Garn, R. A.: Cholesterolosis of the Anterior Chamber. Amer. J. Ophthal. *78*:143–144, 1974.

PUPIL

Contents

Mydriasis (dilated pupil) (usually greater than 5 mm)

1. Physiologic
   A. Larger pupils in women than in men
   B. Larger pupils in myopes than in hypermetropes
   C. Larger pupils in blue irides than in brown irides
   D. Larger pupils in adolescents and middle-aged than in very young or old
   E. Voluntary dilatation (rare) by respiratory suspension and acceleration of heart beat
   F. Surprise, fear, pain, strong emotion, or vestibular stimulation
   G. General anesthesia of stages I, II, and IV
   H. Autosensory pupillary reflex—stimulation of middle ear
   I. Auditory pupillary reflex—tuning fork adjacent to ear
   J. Vestibular pupillary reflex—stimulation of labyrinth by heat, cold, or rotation
   K. Vagotonic pupillary reflex—stimulation on deep inspiration

2. Drugs and toxins
   A. Sympathomimetic drugs, such as phenylephrine
   B. Parasympatholytic drugs, such as atropine sulfate, cyclopentolate (Cyclogyl), tropicamide (Mydriacyl), aftershave lotion
   C. Toxins of *Clostridium botulinum* and tetanus
   D. Bromides (usually potassium or sodium)
   E. Cannabis (marihuana)
   F. Paraldehyde overdose
   G. Adrenergic agents, such as nasal sprays, or asthma therapy in newborns
   H. Para-aminosalicylic acid
   I. Antimalarials, including quinine and quinacrine (Atabrine)
   J. Chlorpromazine (Compazine)
   K. Salicylates (alkalosis)
   L. Antihistaminics
   M. Topical anesthetics
   N. Lead

O. Carbon monoxide
P. Organic phosphorus
Q. Chloral hydrate and barbiturate overdose
R. Bovine milk protein in infants with allergic malabsorption
S. Topical steroids

3. Ocular causes
   A. Iris atrophy
   B. Glaucoma, usually acute
   C. Glaucocyclytic crisis
   D. Paralytic mydriasis, following trauma
   E. Iris sphincter rupture
   F. Intraocular foreign body
   G. Complications of photocoagulation
   H. Amaurotic mydriasis—blind eye has larger pupil than the seeing eye
   I. Larger pupil in amblyopic eye
   J. Congenital mydriasis (rare) with absence of sphincter muscle
   K. Aniridia (pseudomydriasis)

4. Lesions of ciliary ganglion causing internal ophthalmoplegia, e.g., dilated pupil and absent accommodation (see p. 337)
   A. Varicella
   B. Congenital lesion
   C. Herpes zoster
   D. Early lesion of acute or chronic ophthalmoplegia

5. Acute or chronic ophthalmoplegias (see p. 142 or 144)

6. Third nerve lesion—also ptosis and ophthalmoplegia on affected side (see third nerve palsy, p. 134)

7. Lesions anterior to lateral geniculate body

8. Coma due to alcohol ingestion, eclampsia, diabetes, uremia, epilepsy, apoplexy, or meningitis—the pupils are equally dilated and do not constrict with light stimulation

9. Midbrain tumors, such as pinealoma, in which dilated pupils, paralysis of vertical gaze (especially upward gaze), and retraction nystagmus are manifest

10. Epidural or subdural hematoma

11. Paralytic parasympathetic lesions

12. Irritative sympathetic lesion—pupillary dilatation, widening of palpebral aperture, and slight exophthalmos
    A. Idiopathic
    B. Irritative lesion, such as tumor, encephalitis, or syringomyelia of the hypothalamus, midbrain, medulla, or cervical cord
    C. Thoracic lesions, such as cervical rib, aneurysms of the thoracic vessels, mediastinal tumors, or tubercular pleurisy
    D. Cervical lesions, including nasopharyngeal tumors, thyroid swelling, or cervical nodes
    E. Rabies
    F. Trauma
    G. Visceral disease
    H. Aortic dilatation or exudative endocarditis (Roque's sign)
    I. Acute abdominal conditions, such as appendicitis, cholecystitis, or colitis (Moskowskij's sign)
    J. Psychiatric patients with pressure over McBurney's point (Meyer's phenomenon)
    K. Buried wisdom tooth

13. Tumors, injury, or hemorrhage of frontoparietal, parietal, temporal, or temporo-occipital area—contralateral mydriasis and ipsilateral defect in the visual field

14. Fractured skull

15. Adie's syndrome—unilateral, usually female in third decade, decreased tendon reflexes, slow reaction to light, 2.5% methacholine chloride (Mecholyl Chloride) causes miosis

16. "Springing pupil" (seesaw anisocoria)—one pupil temporarily becomes larger than the other
    A. Horner's syndrome
    B. Psychic stimuli
    C. Progressive, generalized degeneration of the cervical spinal cord (syringomyelia)

D. Congenital vascular malformation of the cervicodorsal spinal cord
E. Neurosyphilis
F. Veronal poisoning
G. Normal

17. Pupillary escape (Marcus Gunn sign)—direct and consensual light reactions are present, but the contraction is not maintained under bright illumination so that the pupil dilates slowly; swinging flashlight test demonstrates pupillary escape
   A. Optic neuritis, intraocular or retrobulbar
   B. Retinal detachment
   C. Optic atrophy
   D. Direct pressure on the intraorbital or intracranial part of the optic nerve due to a mass lesion
   E. Occlusion of central retinal artery or vein or of the branches of either
   F. Incipient prechiasmal optic nerve compression
   G. Other widespread organic disease of the retina

18. Idiopathic

19. Ross' syndrome—tonic pupil, progressive segmental hypohidrosis, hyporeflexia

20. Acute autonomic neuropathy

21. Acute pandysautonomia

Duke-Elder, S., and Scott, G. I.: System of Ophthalmology, Vol. XII. St. Louis, C. V. Mosby Co., 1971, pp. 616–630.
Grant, W. M.: Toxicology of the Eye, 2nd ed. Springfield, Ill., Charles C Thomas, 1973.
Haddad, H. M.: Adverse Effects of Ophthalmic Agents in Pediatrics. In Leopold, I. H. (Ed.): Ocular Therapy: Complications and Management. St. Louis, C. V. Mosby Co., 1967, pp. 46–62.
Hallet, M., and Cogan, D. G.: Episodic Unilateral Mydriasis in Otherwise Normal Patients. Arch. Ophthal. 84:130–136, 1970.
Huber, A.: Eye Symptoms in Brain Tumors, 2nd ed. St. Louis, C. V. Mosby Co., 1971, p. 13.
Kearns, T. P.: The Neuro-ophthalmologic Examination. The University of Miami Neuro-ophthalmology Symposium. Springfield, Ill., Charles C Thomas, 1964, pp. 8–14.

Knight, C. L., Hoyt, W. F., and Wilson, C. B.: Syndrome of Incipient Prechiasmal Optic Nerve Compression. Arch. Ophthal. *87*: 1–11, 1972.

Levatin, P.: Pupillary Escape in Disease of the Retina or Optic Nerve. Arch. Ophthal. *62*:768, 1959.

Liu, H. Y., Giday, Z., and Moore, B. F.: Certain Bovine Milk Protein Inducible Eye Signs in Patients with Allergic Malabsorption. J. Pediat. Ophthal. *10*:7–11, 1973.

Massey, J. Y., Roy, F. H., and Bornhofen, J. H.: Ocular Manifestations of Reye Syndrome. Arch. Ophthal. *91*:441–444, 1974.

Newell, F. W.: Ophthalmology, Principles and Concepts. St. Louis, C. V. Mosby Co., 1969, p. 220.

Newsome, D. A., et al.: "Steroid-induced" Mydriasis and Ptosis. Invest. Ophthal. *10*:424–429, 1971.

Smolin, G.: Unilateral Intermittent Pupillary Dilation. Arch. Ophthal. *81*:705, 1969.

Wolter, J. R.: Mydriasis Due to Parasympathetic Denervation as a Result of After-shave Lotion in the Eye. J. Pediat. Ophthal. *9*: 179–182, 1972.

Zinn, K. M.: The Pupil. Springfield, Ill., Charles C Thomas, 1972.

Fixed, Dilated Pupil

1. Midbrain damage—vascular accidents, tumors, degenerative and infectious diseases
   A. Dorsal (Edinger-Westphal nucleus and its connections)—rare, involves both pupils, pupillary near vision reaction often retained, and often associated with supranuclear vertical gaze palsy
   B. Ventral (fascicular part of third nerve)—associated with other neurologic deficits, such as Nothnagel's syndrome, Benedikt's syndrome, Weber's syndrome—unlikely to spare the extraocular components of the third nerve

2. Damage to the third nerve (from interpeduncular fossa to ciliary ganglion)
   A. Basal aneurysms
   B. Supratentorial space-occupying masses, causing displacement of the brain stem or transtentorial herniation of the uncus—stuporous or comatose

C. Basal meningitis—often bilateral internal ophthalmoplegia
D. Ischemic oculomotor palsy ("diabetic ophthalmoplegia")—usually spares the pupillary fibers
E. Parasellar tumor (e.g., pituitary adenoma, meningioma, craniopharyngioma, nasopharyngeal carcinoma, or distant metastases)
F. Parasellar inflammation (e.g., "Tolosa-Hunt," temporal arteritis, herpes zoster)

3. Damage to the ciliary ganglion or short ciliary nerves—results in Adie's tonic pupil
    A. Viral ciliary ganglionitis or involvement of the ciliary nerves, such as from herpes zoster
    B. Orbital trauma or tumor
    C. Choroidal trauma or tumor
    D. Blunt trauma to the globe may injure the ciliary plexus at the iris root (traumatic iridoplegia)

4. Damage to the iris
    A. Degenerative or inflammatory diseases of the iris
    B. Posterior synechiae
    C. Acute rise of intraocular pressure (hypoxia of sphincter)
    D. Blunt injury to the globe with sphincter damage (traumatic iridoplegia)
    E. Pharmacologic blockade by atropinic substances

5. Total blindness, including cortical blindness (p. 531)

Newell, F. W.: Ophthalmology, Principles and Concepts. St. Louis, C. V. Mosby Co., 1969.
Thompson, H. S., Newsome, D. A., and Loewenfeld, I. E.: The Fixed Dilated Pupil. Arch. Ophthal. 86:21–27, 1971.
Zinn, K. M.: The Pupil. Springfield, Ill., Charles C Thomas, 1972.

Miosis (small pupil) (usually less than 2 mm)

1. Physiologic
    A. Smaller pupil in men than in women
    B. Smaller pupil in hypermetropes than in myopes

C. Smaller pupil in brown irides than in blue irides
D. Smaller pupil in very young or old than in adolescents and middle-aged
E. Sleep, fatigue, coma
F. Stage III anesthesia
G. Orbicularis reflex

2. Drugs, including
   A. Topical parasympathomimetic (cholinergic) drugs, such as pilocarpine, methacholine (Mecholyl), carbachol (Doryl), acetylcholine, nicotine (small concentration), physostigmine (Eserine), neostigmine (Prostigmin), edrophonium (Tensilon), echothiophate (Phospholine), demecarium (Humorsol), and isoflurophate (DFP), and insecticides including TEPP, HETP, and OMPA
   B. Sympatholytic drugs, such as hexamethonium, nicotine (large concentration), pentolinium, guanethidine (Ismelin), Bretylium Tosylate (Darenthin), reserpine, alpha methyldopa (Aldomet), MAO inhibitors, Dibenzyline, phentolamine (Regitine), tolazoline (Priscoline)
   C. Histamine
   D. Morphine—opiates given to mother produce transient newborn miosis
   E. Acute alcoholism

3. Ocular Causes
   A. Corneal irritation, such as keratitis or corneal injury
   B. Iris irritation, such as iritis
   C. Conjunctival irritation
   D. Rapid hypotony with intraocular injury or intraocular operation
   E. Retinitis pigmentosa
   F. Dislocated lenses
   G. Long-term use of miotics
   H. Congenital miosis due to absent dilator muscle
   I. Posterior iris synechiae, usually irregular

4. Spastic miosis—bilateral miosis with total or partial loss of the light reaction but intact near reaction

A. Acute pontine angle lesion, such as hemorrhage or tumor associated with disturbed conjugate gaze
B. Epidemic encephalitis
C. Purulent meningitis
D. Infections of the cavernous sinus or superior orbital fissure (see p. 135)
E. Lesions of the orbit
F. Facial tetanus
G. Severe hypoxia
H. Arteriosclerotic and degenerative diseases of the cerebrum
I. Alcoholism
J. Myotonic dystrophy
K. Diabetes mellitus

5. "Cluster headache" or histamine cephalgia—ptosis; miosis; red, watering eye on side of headache

6. Raeder's paratrigeminal syndrome—ipsilateral miosis and pain—may be associated with third nerve paralysis or corneal anesthesia
   A. Idiopathic
   B. Migraine
   C. Meningioma
   D. Post-trauma
   E. Extracranial aneurysm of internal carotid

7. Horner's syndrome—relative miosis, slight ptosis with narrowing of palpebral fissure and slight enophthalmos (see p. 55)

8. Parkinsonism

9. First tonic stage of epileptic fit

10. Psychogenic diseases, such as schizophrenia, dementia precox, or hysteria

11. Argyll Robertson pupil—small, irregular, reacts better to accommodation than to light
    A. Syphilis
    B. Diabetes mellitus
    C. Chronic alcoholism

D. Different kinds of encephalitis

E. Multiple sclerosis

F. Senile and degenerative diseases of the central nervous system

G. Midbrain tumors, such as pinealomas and craniopharyngioma

H. Friedreich's ataxia

I. Malaria

J. Syringomyelia

K. Carbon disulfide poisoning

L. Herpes zoster, usually mydriasis

M. Pressure on third cranial nerve trunk by cerebral aneurysm

N. Trauma to skull or orbit

O. Aberrant regeneration of the third nerve

12. Refsum's syndrome—ophthalmoplegia, ataxia, deafness, and polyneuritis

Duke-Elder, S., and Scott, G. I.: System of Ophthalmology, Vol. XII. St. Louis, C. V. Mosby Co., 1971, pp. 630–635, 657–666.

Haddad, H. M.: Adverse Effects of Ophthalmic Agents in Pediatrics. *In* Leopold, I. H. (Ed.): Ocular Therapy: Complications and Management. St. Louis, C. V. Mosby Co., 1967, pp. 46–62.

Kearns, T. P.: The Neuro-Ophthalmologic Examination. The University of Miami Neuro-Ophthalmology Symposium. Springfield, Ill., Charles C Thomas, 1964, pp. 8–14.

Newell, F. W.: Ophthalmology, Principles and Concepts. St. Louis, C. V. Mosby Co., 1969, pp. 219–220.

Roy, F. H., Hanna, C., Brown, L. E., and Clifton, E. C.: Irreversible Miosis Following Long-Term Echothiophate (Phospholine) Iodide Use. J. Pediat. Ophthal. 7:20–23, 1970.

Spaeth, G. L.: Ocular Manifestations of the Lipidoses. *In* Tasman, W. (Ed.): Retinal Diseases in Children. New York, Harper & Row, 1971, pp. 181–187.

Walsh, F. B., and Hoyt, W. F.: Clinical Neuro-ophthalmology, Vol. I, 3rd ed. Baltimore, Williams & Wilkins Co., 1969, pp. 505, 510.

Zinn, K. M.: The Pupil. Springfield, Ill., Charles C Thomas, 1972.

Mecholyl Test (miosis following topical ocular instillation of 2.5% methacholine chloride [Mecholyl] due to denervation hypersensitivity)

1. Small proportion of normal population, both adults and newborns

2. Tonic pupil (Adie's syndrome)

3. Familial dysautonomia (Riley-Day syndrome)

4. Hereditary amyloidosis

5. Generalized paresis with fixed, dilated pupils

6. Tabes dorsalis patients with Argyll Robertson-like pupils

7. Cri du chat syndrome (crying cat syndrome)

de Haas, E. B. H.: Adie's Syndrome. Arch. Ophthal. *61*:866–884, 1959.

Goldberg, M. F., Payne, J. W., and Brunt, P. W.: Ophthalmologic Studies of Familial Dysautonomia. Arch. Ophthal. *80*:732, 1968.

Hedges, T. R.: The Tonic Pupil, Familial Incidence, Recognition, and Progression. Arch. Ophthal. *80*:21, 1968.

Howard, R. O.: Ocular Abnormalities in the Cri du Chat Syndrome. Amer. J. Ophthal. *73*:949–954, 1972.

Zinn, K. M.: The Pupil. Springfield, Ill., Charles C Thomas, 1972.

Paradoxical Pupillary Reaction (either [1] the pupil dilates with near vision or constricts in distant vision or [2] the pupil dilates on exposure to light or constricts when the light is withdrawn)

1. Syphilis

2. General paralysis

3. Tumors of quadrigeminal region

4. Sleeping individuals, some of whom had been taking barbiturates

5. Trauma

6. Lesion distal to the ciliary ganglion

7. Sensitization of iris muscles to circulating autonomic drugs

Freeman, M. I., Burde, R. M., and Gay, A. J.: A Case of True Paradoxical Pupillary Reaction. Arch. Ophthal. 75:740, 1966.

Walsh, F. B., and Hoyt, W. F.: Clinical Neuro-ophthalmology, 3rd ed. Baltimore, Williams & Wilkins Co., 1969, p. 524.

Anisocoria (an inequality of the pupils of 1 mm or greater)

1. Physiologic
   A. Familial
   B. Non-familial—normal variation (small percentage of the population)
   C. Anisometropia—larger pupil with the more myopic eye
   D. Tournay's reaction—with the eyes turned sharply to the side, dilatation of the pupil of the abducting eye and miosis of pupil of the adducting eye
   E. Lateral illumination of one eye gives more miosis in that eye than in the other

2. Ocular conditions
   A. Cornea, such as keratitis or abrasion
   B. Iris, such as iritis, synechiae, iris atrophy, or iris sphincter rupture
   C. Opacities of the cornea, lens, or vitreous
   D. Amblyopia

E. Glaucoma
F. Retina or optic nerve disease
G. Amaurotic eye (blind)
H. Ocular trauma
I. Artificial eye
J. Spastic miosis

3. Central nervous system
   A. Horner's syndrome (see p. 55)
   B. Pontine lesions
   C. Aberrant third nerve regeneration
   D. Third nerve lesions
   E. Cervical rib (ipsilateral constricted pupil)
   F. Tabes dorsalis
   G. Aneurysm of the aorta or carotid artery
   H. Cerebrovascular accidents
   I. Wernicke's hemianopic pupil
   J. Adie's (tonic) pupil
   K. Encephalitis (mild cases)
   L. Trigeminal neuralgia

4. Unilateral mydriasis (see p. 296)

5. Unilateral miosis (see p. 301)

Duke-Elder, S., and Scott, G. I.: System of Ophthalmology, Vol. XII. St. Louis, C. V. Mosby Co., 1971, pp. 613–636.
Paton, D., and Goldberg, M. F.: Injuries of the Eye, the Lids, and the Orbit. Philadelphia, W. B. Saunders Co., 1968, p. 4.
Sharpe, J. A., and Glaser, J. S.: Tournay's Phenomenon. Amer. J. Ophthal. 77:250–255, 1974.
Zinn, K. M.: The Pupil. Springfield, Ill., Charles C Thomas, 1972.

Irregularity of the Pupil

1. Congenital coloboma of the iris, usually below

2. Adherent leukoma as one part of iris is pulled up to corneal scar, peripheral anterior synechiae (see p. 290), or corneal laceration with prolapse of iris

3. Glaucoma—oval, dilated pupil

4. Operation—as sector iridectomy or peripheral iridectomy

5. Iritis—usually small but pupil may be any shape with anterior or posterior synechiae

6. Tumors of iris or ciliary body

7. Injury of the iris

8. Argyll Robertson pupil—small, irregular, reacts better to accommodation than to light—same type as seen in diabetics (pseudotabetic pupil)

9. Segmental iris atrophy (see p. 322)

10. Vitreous or zonule into corneal laceration

11. Optic atrophy due to causes such as syphilis, quinine poisoning, and internal ophthalmoplegia of vascular or traumatic origin

12. Medication, with faster reaction of one sector of iris than of another—miosis or mydriasis

Duke-Elder, S.: System of Ophthalmology, Vol. IX. St. Louis, C. V. Mosby Co., 1966, pp. 650, 665–694.

Duke-Elder, S., and Scott, G. I.: System of Ophthalmology, Vol. XII. St. Louis, C. V. Mosby Co., 1971, pp. 689–690.

Newell, F. W.: Ophthalmology, Principles and Concepts. St. Louis, C. W. Mosby Co., 1969, pp. 219–220.

Hippus (visible, rhythmic but irregular pupillary oscillations, deliberate in time, and 2 mm or more excursion. It has no localizing significance.)

1. Normal

2. Presence of total third cranial nerve palsy

3. Hemiplegia

4. Multiple sclerosis

5. Meningitis (acute)

6. Cerebral syphilis, tabes and general paralysis

7. Myasthenia gravis

8. Tumors of corpora quadrigemina

9. Epileptics

10. Cheyne-Stokes breathing

11. Disseminated sclerosis

12. Cerebral tumors

13. Incipient cataracts

14. Neurasthenia (nervous exhaustion, Beard's disease)

15. Barbiturate poisoning

16. Paraldehyde poisoning

Duke-Elder, S., and Scott, G. I.: System of Ophthalmology, Vol. XII. St. Louis, C. V. Mosby Co., 1971, pp. 637–638.
Zinn, K. M.: The Pupil. Springfield, Ill., Charles C Thomas, 1972.

11

Tonohaptic Pupil (long latent period preceding both contraction to light and re-dilatation followed in each instance by a short but prompt movement)

1. Catatonic state
2. Schizoid state
3. Introverted persons of the schizophrenic group
4. Post-encephalitic condition
5. Parkinsonism
6. Diabetes insipidus
7. Diabetes mellitus
8. Dystrophia adiposogenitalis (Frohlich's syndrome) or pituitary cachexia (Simmond's disease)
9. Pigmentary retinal dystrophy

Duke-Elder, S., and Scott, G. I.: System of Ophthalmology, Vol. XII. St. Louis, C. V. Mosby Co., 1971, pp. 688–689.

Leukokoria (white pupil—see lesions confused with retinoblastoma, p. 424)

1. Retinoblastoma
2. Cataract (congenital)
3. Nematode endophthalmitis (*T. canis*)
4. Coats' disease
5. Persistent hyperplastic primary vitreous
6. Retrolental fibroplasia
7. Retinal dysplasia (massive retinal fibrosis)

8. Vitreous organization following unsuspected penetrating wounds

9. Organized vitreous hemorrhage

10. Falciform fold of retina

11. Angiomatosis of retina

12. Retrolental membrane associated with Bloch-Sulzberger syndrome (incontinentia pigmenti)

13. Exudative retinitis or chorioretinitis or both

14. Diktyoma

15. Congenital retinal detachment

16. Norrie's disease

17. Juvenile retinoschisis

18. Metastatic endophthalmitis

19. Tumors other than retinoblastoma

20. Coloboma of choroid and optic disc

21. Medullation of nerve fiber layer

22. Traumatic chorioretinitis

23. High myopia with advanced chorioretinal degeneration

Barishak, Y. R., and Stein, R.: The Differential Diagnosis in Leucocoria. J. Pediat. Ophthal. 9:95–97, 1972.

Gitter, K. A., Meyer, D., White, R. H., Ortolon, G., and Sarin, L. K.: Ultrasonic Aid in the Evaluation of Leukocoria. Amer. J. Ophthal. 65:190, 1968.

Hansen, A. C.: Norrie's Disease. Amer. J. Ophthal. 66:328–332, 1968.

Hogan, M. F., and Zimmerman, L. E.: Ophthalmic Pathology, 2nd ed. Philadelphia, W. B. Saunders Co., 1962, p. 523.

Howard, G. M., and Ellsworth, R. M.: Differential Diagnosis of Retinoblastoma: A Statistical Survey of 500 Children. Amer. J. Ophthal. 60:610, 1965.

Jones, S. T.: Retrolental Membrane Associated with Bloch-Sulzberger Syndrome (Incontinentia Pigmenti). Amer. J. Ophthal. 62: 330, 1966.

Manschot, W. A.: Pathology of Hereditary Juvenile Retinoschisis. Arch. Ophthal. 88:131–138, 1972.

Long Ciliary Processes Extending into the Dilated Pupillary Space

1. Retrolental fibroplasia (RLF)
2. Persistent hyperplastic primary vitreous (PHPV)
3. Norrie's disease
4. Falciform detachment of the retina
5. Incontinentia pigmenti (Bloch-Sulzberger syndrome)
6. Retinal dysplasia of Reese
7. 13-15 Trisomy (trisomy D)
8. Extreme mydriasis
9. Surgical coloboma
10. Aniridia
11. Anterior rotation of ciliary processes
    A. Plateau iris
    B. Angle closure
    C. Anterior choroidal separation
    D. After scleral buckling operation
    E. From adherence to limbal scar
    F. Cyst or tumor behind iris
    G. Dislocated lens

Chandler, P. A., and Grant, W. M.: Lectures on Glaucoma. Philadelphia, Lea & Febiger, 1965, pp. 78–81.

Hansen, A. C.: Norrie's Disease. Amer. J. Ophthal. 66:320–332, 1968.

Howard, G. M., and Ellsworth, R. M.: Differential Diagnosis of Retinoblastoma: A Statistical Survey of 500 Children. Amer. J. Ophthal. 60:610, 1965.

Persistent Pupillary Membrane

* = Most important
1. Physiologic
2. Hereditary
3. Fetal iritis
*4. Use of oxygen therapy in premature nursery

Hornblass, A.: Persistent Pupillary Membrane and Oxygen Therapy in Premature Infants. Ann. Ophthal. 3:95–99, 1971.

Decentered Pupillary Light Reflex

1. Positive angle kappa—pseudo-exotropia
2. Negative angle kappa—pseudo-esotropia
3. Eccentric fixation—deep unilateral amblyopia
4. Ectopic macula—macular displacement by retinal scarring or strands, such as retrolental fibroplasia
5. Ectopic pupil

Von Noorden, G. K., and Maumenee, A. E.: Atlas of Strabismus, 2nd ed. St. Louis, C. V. Mosby Co., 1973, pp. 36–39.

Pupillary Block Following Cataract Extraction

1. Leaky wound

2. Postoperative iridocyclitis

3. Posterior vitreous detachment associated with pooling or retrovitreal aqueous

4. Dense, impermeable anterior hyaloid membrane

5. Air pupillary block

6. Non-perforating iridectomy

7. Swollen lens material behind the iris

8. Subchoroidal hemorrhage

9. Free vitreous block

Jaffe, N. S.: The Vitreous in Clinical Ophthalmology. St. Louis, C. V. Mosby Co., 1969, p. 169.

IRIS

Contents

Aniridia (absence of iris, partial or complete)

1. Rieger's syndrome (hypodontia and iris dysgenesis)

2. Associated with autosomal dominant inheritance with 85% penetrance and aplasia of the macula

3. Associated with autosomal recessive inheritance with fully developed macula

4. Sporadic occurrence with nephroblastoma (Wilms' tumor)

5. Homocystinuria

6. Traumatic

Gellis, S. S., and Feingold, M.: Atlas of Mental Retardation. Washington, D.C., U.S. Government Printing Office, 1968.

Presley, G. D., Stinson, I. N., and Sidbury, J. B.: Homocystinuria. Amer. J. Ophthal. *66*:884, 1968.

Sorsby, A.: Ophthalmic Genetics, 2nd ed. New York, Appleton-Century-Crofts Inc., 1970.

Coloboma of Iris (failure of fusion of fetal fissure in optic vesicle, usually inferior or inferonasal)

1. Hurler's syndrome (MPS I)

2. Nevoid basal cell carcinoma syndrome

3. Oculoauriculovertebral dysplasia syndrome (Goldenhar)

4. Rieger's syndrome

5. Rubinstein-Taybi syndrome

6. Linear sebaceous nevi syndrome

7. Treacher Collins syndrome

8. Trisomy 13-15 (D trisomy) syndrome

9. Trisomy 17-18 syndrome

10. Ellis-van Creveld (chondroectodermal dysplasia) syndrome

11. Hemifacial microsomia (otomandibular dysostosis) syndrome

12. Associated with microphthalmos—autosomal dominant inheritance

13. Sporadic

14. Maternal vitamin A deficiency

15. Associated with persistence of primary vitreous and retinal dysplasia

16. Partial deletion of chromosome of group D

17. Maternal use of thalidomide

18. Cat eye syndrome—imperforate anus, preauricular fistula, hypertelorism, antimongoloid lid slant, small acrocentric (G group) extra chromosome

19. Chromosome and partial short arm deletion syndrome (Wolf's syndrome)—iris and/or retinal coloboma, hypertelorism, epicanthus, strabismus, microcephaly, hydrocephalus, seizures

20. Associated with hyperchromic heterochromia (see p. 320)

21. Nevus sebaceous of Jadassohn—antimongoloid lid; dermoid limbus; nystagmus; esotropia; external oculomotor palsy, unilateral; thickening of bones of the orbit; coloboma of lids

22. Focal dermal hypoplasia syndrome (Goltz's syndrome)— papillomas of the lids, strabismus, uveal colobomas, microphthalmia, and usually female

23. Idiopathic

Drews, R. C., and Pico, G.: Heterochromia Associated with Coloboma of the Iris. Amer. J. Ophthal. 72:827, 1971.

Francois, J.: Diagnosis of Blindness in the Infant. Ann. Ophthal. 2:533–554, 1970.

Geeraets, W. J.: Ocular Syndromes, 2nd ed. Philadelphia, Lea & Febiger, 1969.

Gellis, S. S., and Feingold, M.: Atlas of Mental Retardation. Washington, D.C., U.S. Government Printing Office, 1968.

Goodman, R. M., and Gorlin, R. J.: The Face in Genetic Disorders. St. Louis, C. V. Mosby Co., 1970, pp. 38, 70.

Haslam, R. H., and Wirtschafter, J. D.: Unilateral External Oculomotor Nerve Palsy and Nevus Sebaceous of Jadassohn. Arch. Ophthal. 87:293–300, 1972.

Peterson, R. A.: Schmid-Fraccaro Syndrome ("Cat's Eye" Syndrome) Partial Trisomy of G Chromosome. Arch. Ophthal. 90:287–291, 1973.

Sorsby, A.: Ophthalmic Genetics, 2nd ed. New York, Appleton-Century-Crofts, Inc., 1970, pp. 22, 112.

Rubeosis Iridis (neovascularization [new-formed blood vessels] on the iris)

* = Most important

1. Proximal vascular disease
   A. Aortic arch syndrome (pulseless disease; Takayasu's syndrome)
   B. Carotid occlusive disease
   C. Carotid ligation
   D. Carotid-cavernous fistula
   E. Cranial arteritis

2. Ocular vascular disease
   *A. Central retinal vein thrombosis
   *B. Central retinal artery thrombosis
   C. Long posterior ciliary artery occlusion
   D. Reversed flow through the ophthalmic artery

3. Retinal diseases
   *A. Diabetes mellitus
   B. Leber's miliary aneurysms
   C. Coats' disease
   D. Eales' disease
   E. Sickle cell retinopathy
   F. Retinal hemangioma
   G. Persistent hyperplastic primary vitreous
   H. Retrolental fibroplasia
   I. Retinoblastoma
   J. Norrie's disease
   K. Retinal detachment
   L. Melanoma of choroid
   M. Glaucoma, chronic

4. Iris tumors
   A. Melanoma
   B. Metastatic carcincma
   C. Hemangioma

5. Postinflammatory
   A. Uveitis, chronic
   B. Retinal detachment operation
   C. Fungal endophthalmitis (see p. 196)
   D. Radiation

6. Vascular tufts at the pupillary margin
   A. Myotonic dystrophy
   B. Cataract
   C. Diabetes mellitus
   D. Respiratory failure
   E. Ocular hypotony

Cobb, B., Shilling, J. S., and Chisholm, I. H.: Vascular Tufts at the Pupillary Margin in Myotonic Dystrophy. Amer. J. Ophthal. 69: 573–582, 1970.

Huckman, M. S., and Haas, J.: Reversal Flow through the Ophthalmic Artery as a Cause of Rubeosis Iridis. Amer. J. Ophthal. 74: 1094–1099, 1972.

Schulze, R. R.: Rubeosis Iridis. Amer. J. Ophthal. 63:487, 1967.

Wolter, J. R.: Double Embolism of the Central Retinal Artery and One Long Posterior Ciliary Artery Followed by Secondary Hemorrhagic Glaucoma. Amer. J. Ophthal. 73:651–657, 1972.

Hyperemia of the Iris (dilatation of pre-existing vessels of the iris)

1. Corneal ulcer
2. Foreign body on the cornea
3. Iritis
4. Iridocyclitis
5. Uveitis
6. Injury, intraocular
7. Scleritis

O'Brien, C. S.: Ophthalmology, Notes for Students. Iowa City, Athens Press, 1930, p. 312.

Heterochromia (difference of color in the two irides)

1. Hypochromic heterochromia—abnormal eye with iris of lighter color than that of the fellow eye
   A. Horner's syndrome—paralysis of sympathetic nerves to dilator pupillae (congenital or early in life)
   B. Fuch's heterochromia—mild iridocyclitis, with ciliary injection, often with cataract and sometimes glaucoma
   C. Glaucomacyclitic crisis (Posner-Schlossman syndrome)
   D. Diffuse iris atrophy (unilateral), including that due to trauma, inflammation, or senility (see iris atrophy, p. 322)
   E. Infiltration of non-pigmented tumor into iris (see non-pigmented iris tumors, p. 326)
   F. Hypopigmentation carried as dominant trait

G. Parry-Romberg syndrome (progressive hemifacial atrophy)
H. Chediak-Higashi syndrome
I. Klein-Waardenburg syndrome
J. Congenital, sporadic, and/or familial
K. Status dysraphicus (Bremer's syndrome)

2. Hyperchromic heterochromia—abnormal eye with iris of darker color than that of the fellow eye
   A. Retention of intraocular iron foreign body—siderosis
   B. Malignant melanoma of the iris or other pigmented tumors of the iris, page 325
   C. Monocular melanosis in which there are excess chromatophores in the stroma of the iris (melanosis bulbi)
   D. Anterior chamber hemorrhage, prolonged (see p. 283)
   E. Perforating injuries or contusion of the globe occurring before the subject is ten years of age
   F. Associated with microcornea (see p. 225)
   G. Ectropion uvea
   H. Severe contusion with hypertrophy of the superficial layers of the stroma of the iris
   I. Neurofibromatosis
   J. Nevi of iris
   K. Klein-Waardenburg syndrome
   L. Congenital, sporadic, and/or familial
   M. Status dysraphicus (Bremer's syndrome)
   N. Neovascular, such as rubeosis iridis or hyperemia of iris, unilateral (see p. 318)
   O. Associated with coloboma
   P. Iris abscess
3. Dark central pupillary margin, pale pigment around its circumference
   A. Hereditary osteo-onychodysplasia (HOOD)
   B. Normal iris

Drews, R. C., and Pico, G.: Heterochromia Associated with Coloboma of the Iris. Amer. J. Ophthal. 72:827, 1971.
Flickinger, R. R., and Spivey, B. E.: Lester's Line in Hereditary Osteo-onychodysplasia. Arch. Ophthal. 82:700–703, 1969.
Gass, J. D. M.: Iris Abscess Simulating Malignant Melanoma. Arch. Ophthal. 90:300–302, 1973.

Geeraets, W. J.: Ocular Syndromes, 2nd ed. Philadelphia, Lea & Febiger, 1969.

Gladstone, R. M.: Development and Significance of Heterochromia of the Iris. Arch. Neurol. *21*:184–192, 1969.

Goldberg, M. F.: Waardenburg's Syndrome with Fundus and other Anomalies. Arch. Ophthal. *76*:797, 1966.

Newell, F. W.: Ophthalmology, Principles and Concepts. St. Louis, C. V. Mosby Co., 1969.

Schlaegel, T. F.: Essentials of Uveitis. Boston, Little, Brown & Co., 1969, pp. 273–274.

Iris Atrophy

1. Posterior pigment layer is swollen and degenerated
   A. Diabetes mellitus
   B. Hurler's disease

2. Due to old age

3. Postinflammatory—iritis due to such diseases as tuberculosis, syphilis, herpes zoster, and smallpox

4. Ischemia
   A. Trauma
   B. Hemoglobin SC disease

5. Glaucomatous atrophy
   A. Acute—atrophy and/or iridoschisis
   B. Chronic—stromal and epithelial

6. Neurogenic—tabes with stromal atrophy

7. Xeroderma pigmentosa, including skin lesions

8. Essential (progressive) atrophy

9. Due to quinine use

10. Takayasu 's syndrome (aortic arch syndrome; pulseless disease)

11. Complication of retinal detachment operation

12. Complication of light coagulation and beta radiation

13. Norrie's disease

Duke-Elder, S., and Perkins, E. S.: Diseases of the Uveal Tract. System of Ophthalmology, Vol. IX. St. Louis, C. V. Mosby Co., 1966, p. 686.

Galinos, S., et al.: Hemoglobin SC Disease Associated with Iris Atrophy. Invest. Ophthal. *11*:627, 1972.

Geeraets, W. J.: Ocular Syndromes, 2nd ed. Philadelphia, Lea & Febiger, 1969.

Knox, D. L., Palmer, C. A. L., and English, F.: Iris Atrophy after Quinine Amblyopia. Arch. Ophthal. *76*:359, 1966.

Norton, E. W. D.: Complications of Retinal Detachment Surgery. Symposium on Retina and Retinal Surgery. Transactions of New Orleans Academy of Ophthalmology. St. Louis, C. V. Mosby Co., 1969, p. 230.

Schwartz, L. W., et al.: Iris Atrophy in Sickle Cell Disease. Amer. J. Ophthal. *77*:247–249, 1974.

Iridodonesis (tremulous iris)

1. Dislocation of the lens

2. Aphakia following cataract extraction

3. Hypermature senile cataract

4. Hydrophthalmos or buphthalmos

O'Brien, C. S.: Ophthalmology, Notes for Students. Iowa City, Athens Press, 1930, p. 312.

Tumors Arising from the Pigment Epithelium of the Iris

1. Hyperplasia
   A. Primary (congenital)
      (1) At pupillary margin
      (2) At margins of colobomas
   B. Acquired
      (1) Region of sphincter—migrating epithelial cells appear in stroma as clump cells (equivocal origin)
      (2) Cells can reach anterior surface of iris and proliferate (velvety black in appearance)
   C. Secondary
      (1) Intraocular inflammation—pigmented cells proliferate around the pupillary margin onto anterior iris surface
      (2) Long-standing glaucoma
         a. Proliferation around the pupillary margin onto anterior iris surface
         b. Migration through stroma to anterior surface at collarette
      (3) Trauma (including operation)—proliferation of pigment epithelium on anterior surface of iris, across pupil, or on posterior surface of cornea
      (4) Strong cholinesterases—hyperplasia often associated with cystic formation

2. Neoplasia
   A. Benign—well-differentiated epithelial cells, usually pigmented, often with pseudoacinar arrangement and cysts. May have limited locally invasive properties
   B. Malignant
      (1) Carcinoma
      (2) Papillary cystadenoma
      (3) Local invasion, cellular atypia, intraocular metastases
      (4) Medulloepithelioma, embryonal type (diktyoma)

Morris, D. A., and Henkind, P.: Neoplasms of the Iris Pigment Epithelium. Amer. J. Ophthal. 66:31, 1968.

Pigmented Lesions of the Iris

1. Malignant melanoma of the iris

2. Anterior staphyloma

3. Exudative mass in the anterior chamber

4. Stromal mass in the anterior chamber

5. Corneal or scleral perforation

6. Cyst—congenital, spontaneous, or traumatic, including post-operative

7. Nodular thickening and scarring of the iris

8. Foreign body of iris, including iron with siderosis

9. Ectropion uvea

10. Segmental melanosis oculi, including congenital melanosis and oculodermal melanocytosis (nevus of Ota)

11. Fuch's syndrome of heterochromic cyclitis with the darker normal iris considered to contain a diffuse melanoma

12. Neurofibromatosis with increased pigmentation of the iris

13. Hemosiderosis due to contusions with hyphema or injuries and disease in the posterior portion of the eye with recurrent bleeding

14. Nevi of the iris

15. Leiomyoma or leiomyosarcoma of the iris

16. Pigment epithelial tumors of the iris

17. Uveitis, such as that due to conglomerate tuberculous lesions of the stroma or sarcoid involvement of the iris

18. Metastatic carcinomas arising in the lung, breast, gastro-intestinal tract, thyroid gland, prostate gland, kidney, or testicle

19. Leukemic infiltrates and malignant lymphomas

20. Hemangioma of the iris with pigmentation due to hemorrhage

21. Pigmentary glaucoma

22. Juvenile xanthogranuloma

23. Epithelioma of the ciliary body

24. Ectopic lacrimal gland tissue

Ferry, A. P.: Lesions Mistaken for Malignant Melanoma of the Iris. Arch. Ophthal. *74*:9, 1965.

Gass, J. D. M.: Iris Abscess Simulating Malignant Melanoma. Arch. Ophthal. *90*:300–302, 1973.

Hogan, M. J.: Clinical Aspects, Management, and Prognosis of Melanomas of the Uvea and Optic Nerve. Ocular and Adnexal Tumors, New and Controversial Aspects. St. Louis, C. V. Mosby Co., 1964, pp. 203–302.

Naumann, G., and Green, W. R.: Spontaneous Non-pigmented Iris Cysts. Arch. Ophthal. *78*:496, 1967.

Zimmerman, L. E.: Pathologic Considerations in Iris Tumors. *In:* Turtz, A. I. (Ed.): Proceedings of the Centennial Symposium Manhattan Eye, Ear and Throat Hospital, Vol. I. St. Louis, C. V. Mosby Co., 1969, pp. 18–27.

Non-pigmented Lesions of the Iris

1. Metastatic carcinoma of the iris arising from the lungs, breast, gastrointestinal tract, thyroid gland, prostate gland, kidney, or testicle

2. Amelanotic melanoma

3. Hemangioma of the iris

4. Seeding of tumor, such as retinoblastoma, from the posterior segment

5. Juvenile xanthogranuloma—may be associated with cutaneous xanthomatous lesions, recurrent hyphema, and diffuse infiltration of the iris

6. Iris cyst

7. Tuberculosis
   A. Acute miliary—small grayish-yellow or reddish nodules
   B. Tuberculoma—white-gray lesion
   C. Hyalinized or fibrotic scar (Michel's flecks)

8. Leprosy
   A. Leprotic pearls—minute white spots on surface of iris
   B. Lepromas of the iris

9. Syphilis
   A. Papules (condylomas)—multiple, small, vascular, yellowish lesions
   B. Gummas—solitary, large, avascular, white lesion

10. Sarcoid nodules—multiple, discrete, irregularly distributed over the iris

11. Iris nodules
    A. Ectodermal (Koeppe nodules)—pupillary margin and gray with ocular inflammation
    B. Mesodermal (Busacca nodules)—anterior surface of iris in collarette region

12. Exudative mass in the anterior chamber

13. Foreign body

14. Leiomyoma or leiomyosarcoma of the iris

15. Forward extension of diktyoma

16. Neurofibroma and neuroglioma

17. Fibrosarcoma

18. Teratoma

19. Endothelioma

Bennett, T., and D'Amico, R. A.: Epithelial Inclusion Cyst of Iris after Keratoplasty. Amer. J. Ophthal. 77:87–89, 1974.
Duke-Elder, S.: System of Ophthalmology, Vol. IX. St. Louis, C. V. Mosby Co., 1966.
Ferry, A. P.: Lesions Mistaken for Malignant Melanoma of the Iris. Arch. Ophthal. 74:9, 1965.
Heath, P.: Tumors of the Iris; Classification and Clinical Follow-up. Trans. Amer. Ophthal. Soc. 62:51–85, 1964.

Hogan, M. J.: Clinical Aspects, Management, and Prognosis of Melanomas of the Uvea and Optic Nerve. Ocular and Adnexal Tumors, New and Controversial Aspects. St. Louis, C. V. Mosby Co., 1964, pp. 203–302.

Manz, H. J., et al.: Neuroectodermal Tumor of Anterior Lip of the Optic Cup. Arch. Ophthal. *89*:382–386, 1973.

Roy, F. H., and Hanna, C.: Spontaneous Congenital Iris Cyst. Amer. J. Ophthal. *72*:97–108, 1971.

Schwartz, L. W., Rodrigues, M. M., and Hallett, J. W.: Juvenile Xanthogranuloma Diagnosed by Paracentesis. Amer. J. Ophthal. 77:243–246, 1974.

Spencer, W. H., and Jesberg, D. O.: Glioneuroma (Choristomatous Malfunction of the Optic Cup Margin). Arch. Ophthal. *89*:387–391, 1973.

Conditions Simulating Anterior Uveitis or Iritis

1. Hereditary deep dystrophy of cornea

2. Hyalinized keratitic precipitate

3. Pigment floaters in the anterior chamber, especially after mydriasis

4. Scleroderma of the scalp

5. Fuch's syndrome, probably degenerative rather than inflammatory

6. Iridoschisis—splitting of iris

7. Brushfield's spots

8. Neurofibromas of the iris

9. Malignant lymphomas or leukemia

10. Reticulum cell sarcoma

11. Juvenile xanthogranuloma of the iris (nevoxanthoendothelioma)

12. Malignant melanoma

13. Retinoblastoma

14. Siderosis bulbi

15. Pseudoexfoliation of the lens capsule (glaucoma capsulare)

16. Metastatic tumor, such as bronchogenic carcinoma

Schlaegel, T. F.: Essentiails of Uveitis. Boston, Little, Brown & Co., 1969, pp. 267–276.
Talegaonkar, S.: Anterior Uveal Tract Metastasis. Brit. J. Ophthal. 53:123–126, 1969.

Iritis (Anterior Uveitis)*—Major Types (listed in order of frequency)

1. Peripheral uveitis (cyclitis)

2. Ankylosing spondylitis

3. Herpes simplex

4. Herpes zoster

5. Sarcoid

6. Tuberculosis

7. Endophthalmitis phacoanophylactica

8. Syphilis

9. Unknown

10. Anterior and posterior uveitis
    A. Toxoplasmosis
    B. Peripheral uveitis (cyclitis)
    C. Unknown

    D. Syphilis
    E. Tuberculosis
    F. Sarcoidosis
    G. Vogt-Koyanagi-Harada syndrome

*From Schlaegel, T. F.: Essentials of Uveitis. Boston, Little, Brown & Co., 1969, Columns 1 and 2 of Table 1–1, p. 2.

Iritis (Anterior Uveitis) in Children

1. Iridocyclitis
    A. Still's syndrome
    B. Ankylosing spondylitis
    C. Behçet's syndrome
    D. Trauma
    E. Sarcoidosis
    F. Unknown

2. Chronic cyclitis (peripheral uveitis)

3. Fuch's heterochromic cyclitis

4. Keratouveitis
    A. Herpes simplex
    B. Herpes zoster

5. Anterior and posterior uveitis
    A. Vogt-Koyanagi-Harada syndrome
    B. Sarcoidosis
    C. Sympathetic ophthalmia

Kimura, S. J., and Hogan, M. J.: Uveitis in Children: Analysis of 274 Cases. Trans. Amer. Ophthal. Soc. 62:173, 1964.

Non-granulomatous Uveitis

1. Physical insult
   A. Exogenous
   B. Endogenous
2. Toxic insults
   A. Autointoxication—ptomaines, protein split products, etc., from food poisoning
   B. Bacterial endotoxins
   C. Viral toxins
   D. Toxins from disintegrating helminths
   E. Reticulum cell sarcoma of brain
3. Immediate hypersensitive reaction
   A. Airborne allergens
   B. Foods
   C. Drugs
   D. Protein antigens (anaphylaxia)
4. Delayed hypersensitive reaction
   A. Bacterial antigens
   B. Viral antigens
5. Doubtful entities, non-granulomatous uveitis
   A. Uveitis associated with collagen diseases
   B. Heterochromic iridocyclitis
   C. Gouty iritis
   D. Amebiasis
   E. Diabetic iritis
   F. Secondary to metabolic disease, such as biliary cirrhosis and systemic xanthomatosis
   G. Sarcoid
6. Mixed granulomatous and non-granulomatous
   A. Lens-induced uveitis
   B. Peripheral uveitis

Duke-Elder, S.: System of Ophthalmology Vol. IX. St. Louis, C. V. Mosby Co., 1966, p. 524.
Gamel, J. W., and Allansmith, M. R.: Metastatic Staphylococcal Endophthalmitis Presenting as Chronic Iridocyclitis. Amer. J. Ophthal. 77:454–458, 1974.

Martins, J. C.: Corticosteroid-induced Uveitis. Amer. J. Ophthal. 77:433–437, 1974.

Neault, R. W., et al.: Uveitis Associated with Isolated Reticulum Cell Sarcoma of the Brain. Amer. J. Ophthal. 73:431–436, 1972.

Schlaegel, T. F.: Essentials of Uveitis. Boston, Little, Brown & Co., 1969.

Woods, A. C.: Endogenous Inflammations of the Uveal Tract. Baltimore, Williams & Wilkins Co., 1961, p. 138.

Granulomatous Uveitis

1. Proven or probable etiology
   A. Associated with non-pyogenic systemic infections
      (1) Syphilis (*Treponema pallidum*)
      (2) Tuberculosis (*Mycobacterium tuberculosis*)
      (3) Leprosy (*Mycobacterium leprae*)
      (4) Leptospirosis (*Leptospira canicola, L. icterohaemorrhagiae, L. pomona*)
      (5) Brucellosis (*Brucella melitensis, B. abortus, B. suis*)
   B. Protozoan infections
      (1) Trypanosomiasis (*Trypanosoma cruzi, T. gambiense*)
      (2) Toxoplasmosis (*Toxoplasma gondii*)
      (3) Amebiasis (*Entamoeba coli, E. histolytica, Endolimax nana, Acanthamoeba hartomonella*)
   C. Fungal infections
      (1) Actinomycosis
      (2) Blastomycosis
      (3) Coccidioidomycosis
      (4) Aspergillosis
      (5) Mucormycosis (phycomycosis)
      (6) Histoplasmosis (*Histoplasma capsulatum*)
      (7) Candidiasis (moniliasis)
      (8) Cryptococcosis (*Cryptococcus neoformans* or *Torula histolytica*)
      (9) Sporotrichosis (*Sporotrichum schenckii*)
      (10) Nocardiosis

D. Helminth infestations
  (1) Nematodes
    a. Onchocerciasis (*Onchocerca volvulus*)
    b. Ancylostomiasis (*Toxocara canis, Ancylostoma duodenale, Ancylostoma caninum, Necator americanus*)
  (2) Cestodes
    a. Cysticercosis (*Cysticercus cellulosae*)
    b. Teniasis (*Taenia echinococcus*)
  (3) Diptera larvae (exogenous)
  (4) Ascaridiosis (*Ascaris lumbricoides*)

2. Recognized clinical and histopathologic entity, of unknown cause
  A. Sympathetic ophthalmia
  B. Sarcoidosis

3. Nonspecific granulomatous uveitis, of unknown cause including granulomatous ileocolitis

4. Mixed granulomatous and non-granulomatous
  A. Lens-induced uveitis
  B. Peripheral uveitis

5. Viral uveitis
  A. Proven or probable
    (1) Herpes simplex
    (2) Herpes zoster
    (3) Vaccinia
    (4) Cytomegalic inclusion disease
  B. Suspected
    (1) Behçet's syndrome
    (2) Vogt-Koyanagi-Harada syndrome

Bell, R., and Font, R. L.: Granulomatous Anterior Uveitis Caused by Coccidioides immitis. Amer. J. Ophthal. *74*:93–98, 1972.
Schlaegel, T. F.: Essentials of Uveitis. Boston, Little, Brown & Co., 1969.
Woods, A. C.: Endogenous Inflammations of the Uveal Tract. Baltimore, Williams & Wilkins Co., 1961, pp. 22–23.

Characteristics of Granulomatous and Non-granulomatous Inflammation in Anterior Uvea

Sympto-matology	Granulomatous Uveitis	Non-granulomatous Uveitis	
		Due to Acute, Self-limited Insult	Due to Chronic or Oft-repeated Insult
Clinical onset	Slow and insidious, chronic and protracted; often remissions and exacerbations	Acute, usually self-limited (1–6 weeks)	Acute or insidious, usually protracted or chronic over months
Inflammation	Low-grade ciliary inflammation; acute only when there is a secondary allergic reaction	Acute, intense ciliary inflammation	Usually low-grade or intermittent inflammation
Keratitic deposits	Heavy, often "mutton-fat" epithelioid cell deposits	Pinpoint lymphoid cell deposits	Pinpoint lymphocytic cell deposits
Aqueous	Few cells; fibrin only if there is a superimposed allergic reaction; usually weak aqueous flare	Many cells; often fibrin; intense flare in active stages	Moderate number of cells; rarely fibrin; low-grade or absent flare
Nodules	Frequent—Koeppe, Busacca, stromal	None	None

Characteristics of Granulomatous and Non-granulomatous Inflammation in Anterior Uvea (Continued)

Sympto-matology	Granulomatous Uveitis	Non-granulomatous Uveitis	
		Due to Acute Self-limited Insult	*Due to Chronic or Oft-repeated Insult*
Iris changes	Slight edema; organic thickening from cellular infiltration	Edema; blurring of iris pattern; acute capillary dilatation frequent	Slight blurring of iris pattern; slight capillary dilatation; pigmentary degeneration
Posterior synechiae	Heavy, organized adhesions form slowly, usually difficult or impossible to break	None, or easily broken fibrinous adhesions in early attacks; become organized only after repeated attacks	Slowly forming but may become organized
Organic damage	If disease is unchecked usually progressive damage from onset of first attack, fibrosis, posterior synechiae, occlusio pupillae, secondary glaucoma, capsular clouding and phthisis bulbi	Usually none in early attacks; band keratitis, posterior synechiae, secondary glaucoma, cataracts, and phthisis bulbi may occur after repeated attacks	Gradually increasing irreversible changes, such as in recurrent acute attacks

Woods, A. C.: Endogenous Inflammations of the Uveal Tract. Baltimore, Williams & Wilkins Co., 1961, p. 317.

Pigmented Ciliary Body Lesions

1. Post-traumatic pigmentary migration

2. Ciliary body cyst

3. Peripheral uveal detachment

4. Malignant melanoma

5. Melanocytoma of ciliary body

Shields, J. A., Green, W. R., and McDonald, P. R.: Uveal Pseudo-melanoma Due to Post-Traumatic Pigmentary Migration. **Arch. Ophthal.** *89*:519–522, 1973.

Neuroepithelial Tumors of the Ciliary Body

1. Congenital
   A. Glioneuroma
   B. Medulloepithelioma
      (1) Benign
      (2) Malignant
   C. Teratoid medulloepithelioma
      (1) Benign
      (2) Malignant

2. Acquired
   A. Pseudoadenomatous hyperplasia
   B. Adenoma
      (1) Solid
      (2) Papillary
      (3) Pleomorphic

C. Adenocarcinoma
   (1) Solid
   (2) Papillary
   (3) Pleomorphic

Spencer, W. H., and Jesberg, D. O.: Glioneuroma (Choristomatous Malfunction of the Optic Cup Margin). Arch. Ophthal. *89*:387–391, 1973.
Zimmerman, L. E.: Verhoeff's Teratoneuroma. A Critical Reappraisal in Light of New Observations and Current Concepts of Embryonic Tumors. Amer. J. Ophthal. *72*:1039–1057, 1971.

Internal Ophthalmoplegia (paresis of ciliary body with loss of power of accommodation and pupil dilatation due to lesion of ciliary ganglion [see paresis of accommodation, p. 354, and mydriasis, p. 296])

* = Most important

*1. Cycloplegic ocular medication—most common

2. Infections, including chickenpox, measles, diphtheria, syphilis, scarlet fever, pertussis, smallpox, influenza, herpes zoster, botulism, sinusitis, and viral hepatitis

3. Congenital—rare

4. Increased intracranial pressure

5. Trauma to eye or orbit

6. May be early lesion of acute or chronic ophthalmoplegia

7. Acute porphyria—frequently bilateral

8. Aneurysm of the posterior communicating artery at its junction with the internal carotid—unilateral

9. Vogt-Koyanagi-Harada syndrome

10. During acute illness—transient

11. Retrobulbar injections of alcohol

12. Metastatic tumors of choroid

13. Transcleral diathermy

14. Adie's syndrome

15. Nasopharyngeal carcinoma—early

Duke-Elder, S., and Scott, G. I.: System of Ophthalmology, Vol. XII. St. Louis, C. V. Mosby Co., 1971, pp. 698–706.

Levy, N. S., Kramer, S. G., and de Borros, T.: Pupillary and Accommodative Abnormalities in the Vogt-Koyanagi-Harada Syndrome. Amer. J. Ophthal. 69:582–588, 1970.

Payne, J. W., and Adamkiewicz, J.: Unilateral Internal Ophthalmoplegia with Intracranial Aneurysm. Amer. J. Ophthal. 68:349, 1969.

Walsh, F. B., and Hoyt, W. F.: Clinical Neuro-ophthalmology, 3rd ed. Baltimore, Williams & Wilkins Co., 1969, p. 497.

LENS

Contents

Anterior Subcapsular Cataract

1. Atopic—eczema cataract

2. Electric cataract

3. Advanced diabetic cataract with other changes

4. Hypermature cataract with other changes

5. Pemphigus foliaceous cataract

6. Endocrine cataract
   A. Werner's syndrome—dwarfism, premature balding and graying, and skin atrophy
   B. Rothmund's syndrome—cutaneous lesions, dwarfism, exophthalmic eyes, beaked nose, and large head

7. Congenital anterior polar lens changes
   A. Anterior polar (pyramidal) cataract
   B. Capsular flakes
   C. Circular capsular or subcapsular cataracts

8. Due to treatment with echothiophate iodine (Phospholine Iodide)

9. Due to myotonic dystrophy

10. Due to intraocular copper and iron

11. Due to chronic head-banging

12. Due to coughing

13. Due to trauma, such as contusion

14. Due to Thorazine ingestion

15. Due to naphthalene ingestion

16. Due to concentrated zinc chloride

Axelsson, U., and Holmberg, A.: The Frequency of Cataract after Miotic Therapy. Acta Ophthal. *44*:421, 1966.

Bemporad, J. R., Sours, J. A., and Spatter, J. R.: Cataracts Following Chronic Headbanging A Report of Two Cases. Amer. J. Psychiat. *125*:245–249, 1968.

Fraunfelder, F. T., and Hanna, C.: Electric Cataracts. Arch. Ophthal. 87:179–183, 1972.

Haik, G. M.: Symposium on Diseases and Surgery of the Lens. St. Louis, C. V. Mosby Co., 1957, pp. 43–84.

Hanna, C., and Potts, J. L.: Anterior Sub-Capsular Cataract Resulting from a Blow to the Eye. J. Arkansas Med. Soc. 66:284–286, 1970.

Houle, R. E., and Grant, W. M.: Zinc Chloride Keratopathy and Cataracts. Amer. J. Ophthal. 75:992–996, 1973.

Jampol, L. M., et al.: Anterior Polar Cataracts. Amer. J. Ophthal. 78:95–97, 1974.

Rosen, E.: Atopic Cataract. Springfield, Ill., Charles C Thomas, 1959, pp. 33–43.

Simon, K. A.: Diabetes and Lens Changes in Myotonic Dystrophy. Arch. Ophthal. 67:312, 1962.

Sugar, H. S., Kobernick, S. D., and Weingarten, J. E.: Hematogenous Ocular Siderosis of Local Cause. Amer. J. Ophthal. 64:749, 1967.

Central Lens Opacity—Nucleus and Cortex

1. Nuclear sclerosis

2. Galactosemia

3. Congenital rubella syndrome

4. Congenital zonular (lamellar) cataract
   A. Tetany cataract (hypoparathyroidism)
   B. Trauma
   C. Iritis
   D. Perforating injuries
   E. Idiopathic

5. Embryonal nuclear cataract

6. Paradichlorobenzene (mothballs)

Haik, G. M.: Symposium on Diseases and Surgery of the Lens. St. Louis, C. V. Mosby Co., 1957, pp. 43–84.

Havener, W. H.: Drugs Used in the Management of Cataracts. In Symposium on Ocular Pharmacology and Therapeutics. Transactions of New Orleans Academy of Ophthalmology. St. Louis, C. V. Mosby Co., 1970, p. 206.

12

Posterior Subcapsular Cataract

1. Complicated cataract
   A. Anterior segment involvement, such as that due to:
      (1) Acute and chronic corneal ulcer
      (2) Iridocyclitis
      (3) Chronic anterior uveitis
      (4) Acute or chronic glaucoma
   B. Posterior segment involvement such as that due to:
      (1) Chronic posterior uveal inflammation
      (2) Long-standing retinal detachment
      (3) High myopia
      (4) Hereditary retinal lesions
      (5) Persistent hyperplastic primary vitreous

2. Senile posterior cortical cataract

3. Cataract resulting from ionizing radiation, such as that encountered in x-ray, radium, or neutron therapy

4. Cataract due to diabetes mellitus

5. Cataract resulting from blunt ocular trauma

6. Dinitrophenol cataract, busulfan (Myleran), triparanol (MER-29)

7. Cataracts due to treatment with steroids (topical or systemic)

8. Congenital posterior polar lens changes
   A. Spurious posterior capsular cataract (Mittendorf's dot)
   B. Posterior polar cataract—persistent fibrovascular sheath of lens with or without secondary cataract
   C. Posterior lenticonus

9. Glassblowers' (heat) cataract

10. Congenital amaurosis of Leber

11. Cataract due to Fabry's disease

12. Cataract resulting from high-energy microwave radiation—questionable

13. Associated with neurofibromatosis
14. Kyrle's disease—hyperkeratosis follicularis et parafollicularis in cutem penetrans
15. Werner's syndrome—dwarfism, premature balding and graying, skin atrophy, beaked nose
16. Myotonic dystrophy

Bullock, J. D., and Howard, R. O.: Werner's Syndrome. Arch. Ophthal. *90*:53–56, 1973.

Grace, E.: Diffuse Angiokeratosis (Fabry's Disease). Amer. J. Ophthal. *62*:139–145, 1966.

Grant, W. M.: Toxicology of the Eye. Springfield, Ill., Charles C Thomas, 1966, p. 87.

Haik, G. M.: Symposium on Diseases and Surgery of the Lens. St. Louis, C. V. Mosby Co., 1957, pp. 43–94.

Lee, D. K., and Abbott, M. L.: Familial Central Nervous System Neoplasia. Arch. Neurol. *20*:154–160, 1969.

Oglesby, R. B., et al.: Cataracts in Rheumatoid Arthritis Patients Treated with Corticosteroids. Arch. Ophthal. *66*:519–523, 1961.

Schoppert-Kimmijser, J., Henkes, H. E., and Von den Bosch, J.: Amaurosis Congenita (Leber). Arch. Ophthal. *61*:211, 1959.

Telles, N. C., Carpenter, R. L., and Toker, D. L.: Microwave Injury. Arch. Ophthal. *84*:127–128, 1970.

Tessler, H., Apple, D. J., and Goldberg, M. F.: Ophthalmologic Findings in a Kindred with Kyrle's Disease (Hyperkeratosis Follicularis et Parafollicularis in Cutem Penetrans). Invest. Ophthal. *11*:626, 1972.

Wilson, F. M., Grayson, M., and Pieroni, D.: Corneal Changes in Ectodermal Dysplasia: Case Report, Histopathology, and Differential Diagnosis. Amer. J. Ophthal. *75*:17–27, 1973.

Syndromes Associated with Congenital Cataracts*

1. Lowe's syndrome (oculocerebrorenal syndrome)—systemic acidosis, organic aciduria, decreased ability to produce ammonia in the kidneys, renal rickets, generalized hypotonicity, mental retardation, and congenital glaucoma

*This section from Scheie, H. G., and Schaffer, D. B.: Congenital Cataracts. In New Orleans Academy of Ophthalmology: Symposium on Surgical and Medical Management of Congenital Anomalies of the Eye. St. Louis, The C. V. Mosby Co, 1968, pp. 325–327, with modifications.

2. Alport's syndrome—chronic nephritis, deafness, and anterior lenticonus

3. Congenital cataract with oxycephaly (tower skull)—optic atrophy, exophthalmos, proptosis, strabismus, and nystagmus

4. Craniofacial dysostosis (Crouzon's disease)—acrocephaly, beak-shaped nose, hypoplastic maxilla, short upper lip, and protruding lower lip

5. Apical malformations associated with cataracts—abnormalities of the hands and feet such as polydactylia, syndactylia, comptodactylia and arachnodactylia

6. Congenital stippled epiphysis (Conradi's syndrome)—small calcified areas of the tarsal and carpal bones, and epiphysis of the long bones; craniofacial maldevelopment, congenital heart defects, and cutaneous anomalies may be present

7. Bonnevie-Ullrich syndrome—pterygium coli (webbed neck), laxity and hyperelasticity of the skin, muscular hypertonia, facial and ocular paralysis, lymphangiectatic edema, and multiple developmental skeletal anomalies

8. Hallerman-Streiff syndrome—dyscephaly, bird-like facies, proportionately short stature, localized hypotrichosis, localized atrophy of skin, lateral microphthalmos and congenital glaucoma

9. Congenital hemolytic icterus

10. Oligophrenia—mental debility, imbecility, and idiocy
    A. Sjögren's syndrome—mental retardation with imbecility and idiocy and bilateral congenital cataract
    B. Marinesco-Sjögren syndrome—this syndrome is similar to Sjögren's syndrome except that the patients also have cerebellar heredoataxia

11. Trisomy syndrome
    A. Trisomy 13-15—malformation of brain, heart, viscera, polydactylia, harelip, cleft palate, microphthalmia, retinal dysplasia, and iris and ciliary body colobomas
    B. Trisomy 16-18—failure to thrive, low-set ears, mal-

formed pinnae, mental retardation, hypertonicity, small mouth and mandible, ventricular septal defects, optic atrophy, and congenital glaucoma

    C. Mongolism (trisomy 21)—mongoloid facies, Brushfield spots, and snowflake cataract

12. Myotonic dystrophy—atrophy of the muscles of the face, upper extremities, and thighs; frontal baldness, endocrinopathies, and cardiac abnormalities

13. Dermatologic disorders
    A. Acquired conditions
        (1) Atopic dermatitis
        (2) Werner's syndrome (scleropoikiloderma)—dwarfism, premature balding and graying, skin atrophy
    B. Congenital conditions
        (1) Rothmund's syndrome (infantile poikiloderma)—this syndrome occurs in the first year of life and consists of infantile poikiloderma, cataracts, and hypogenitalism
        (2) Schaefer's syndrome (congenital dyskeratosis)—congenital dyskeratosis, alopecia, thick nails, microcephaly, oligophrenia, and congenital cataracts
        (3) Congenital ichthyosiform erythroderma—thickened, red, scaly skin that usually undergoes lichenification
        (4) Siemens' syndrome (congenital atrophy of the skin)—atrophy or hypoplasia of the skin and congenital cataracts
        (5) Bloch-Sulzberger syndrome (incontinentia pigmenti)—patchy, slate-gray discoloration of the skin, pseudoglioma, optic atrophy, strabismus, congenital cataracts, alopecia, and dental abnormalities
        (6) Ectodermal dysplasia—anhidrosis, hypotrichosis, absence or underdevelopment of the teeth, and microphthalmos
        (7) Jadassohn-Lewandowski syndrome (pachyonychia congenita)—thick, up-curved overgrown

nails; keratosis and hyperhidrosis of palms and soles; autosomal dominant inheritance

(8) Monilethrix—rare autosomal dominant, lanugo brain, follicular hyperkeratosis, dental anomalies

14. Nieden's syndrome—generalized telangiectases, aortic stenosis and organic disease of the heart

15. Albright's hereditary osteodystrophy (pseudohypoparathyroidism)

16. Cerebrohepatorenal syndrome

17. Hypercalcemia (infantile) with mental retardation (supravalvular aortic stenosis syndrome)

18. Laurence-Moon-Biedl syndrome—dwarfism, hypogonadism, retinitis pigmentosa, and polydactylia

19. Osteopetrosis (Albers-Schönberg disease; marble bone disease)

20. Pierre Robin syndrome

21. Congenital rubella syndrome—deafness, retinopathy, thrombocytopenia, cardiac defects

22. Treacher Collins syndrome (mandibulofacial dysostosis)

23. Gorlin-Goltz syndrome (multiple basal cell nevi syndrome)—glaucoma, strabismus, hypertelorism

24. Cockayne's syndrome (dwarfism with retinal atrophy and deafness)—mental retardation, optic atrophy

25. Turner's syndrome (only one X chromosome instead of two, thus a total of 45 chromosomes instead of 46)—ptosis, cataract, strabismus, epicanthus, blue sclera, color blindness, and corneal nebulae

26. Male Turner's syndrome—myopia, retinal detachment, and glaucoma

27. Homocystinuria—discoloration of lens, optic atrophy, spherophakia, aniridia, retinal detachment

28. Herpes simplex virus

29. Galactosemia-transferase deficiency, "oil droplet" cataract

30. Galactokinase deficiency, nuclear or "oil droplet"

31. Infantile hypoglycemia (male)—complicated pregnancy, mental retardation, small for gestational age, bilateral lamellar cataracts

32. Hutchinson-Gilford syndrome (progeria of children)

33. Varicella infection

34. Smith-Lemli-Opitz syndrome—microcephaly, micrognathia, polydactyly and syndactyly, hypospadius and cryptorchidism, mental retardation, congenital pyloric stenosis

35. Francois' dyscephalic syndrome—dyscephaly, bird-like head, dental anomalies, proportional dwarfism, hypotrichosis, skin atrophy, microphthalmos, nystagmus, strabismus

36. Meckel's syndrome—autosomal recessive with developmental abnormalities incompatible with life, and anophthalmos or microphthalmia

37. Ring chromosome in the D group (13-15)—microphthalmos, epicanthus, blepharophimosis, cataracts

38. Chromosome 18 short arm deletion—webbed neck, ptosis, cataracts, hypertelorism, strabismus

39. Morquio-Brailsford syndrome (MPS IV)

40. Conradi's syndrome

Beutler, E., et al.: Galactokinase Deficiency as Cause of Cataracts. New Eng. J. Med. *288*:1203–1206, 1973.

Bilchik, R. C., et al.: Anomalies with Ring D Chromosome. Amer. J. Ophthal. *73*:83–89, 1972.

Cibis, A., and Burde, R. M.: Herpes Simplex Virus-Induced Congenital Cataracts. Arch. Ophthal. *85*:220–223, 1971.

Cotlier, E., and Rice, P.: Cataracts in the Smith-Lemli-Opitz Syndrome. Amer. J. Ophthal. *72*:955–959, 1971.

Duke-Elder, S., and Scott, G. I.: System of Ophthalmology, Vol. XII. St. Louis, C. V. Mosby Co., 1971, pp. 340–341.

Francois, J., and Pierard, J.: The Francois Dyscephalic Syndrome and Skin Manifestations. Amer. J. Ophthal. *71*:1241–1250, 1971.

Geeraets, W. J.: Ocular Syndromes, 2nd ed. Philadelphia, Lea & Febiger, 1969.

Gellis, S. S., and Feingold, M.: Atlas of Mental Retardation. Washington, D.C., U.S. Government Printing Office, 1968.

Khodadoust, A., and Paton, D.: Turner's Syndrome in a Male. Arch. Ophthal. 77:630, 1967.

Lessell, S., and Forbes, A. P.: Eye Signs in Turner's Syndrome. Arch. Ophthal. 76:211, 1966.

Levenson, J. E., Crandall, B. F., and Sparkes, R. S.: Partial Deletion Syndromes of Chromosome 18. Ann. Ophthal. 3:756–760, 1971.

MacRae, D. W., et al.: Ocular Manifestations of the Meckel Syndrome. Arch. Ophthal. 88:106–113, 1972.

Merin, S., and Crawford, J. S.: Hypoglycemia and Infantile Cataract. Arch. Ophthal. 86:495–498, 1971.

Oberman, A. E., et al.: Galactokinase Deficiency Cataracts in Identical Twins. Amer. J. Ophthal. 74:887–892, 1972.

Prestley, G. D., Stinson, I. W., and Sidbury, J. B.: Homocystinuria. Amer. J. Ophthal. 66:884, 1968.

Robb, R. M.: Cataracts Acquired Following Varicella Infection. Arch. Ophthal. 87:352–354, 1972.

Roy, F. H., Dungan, T., and Inlow, C.: Infantile Hypercalcemia and Supravalvular Aortic Stenosis. J. Pediat. Ophthal. 8:188–194, 1971.

Scheie, H.: Surgical and Medical Management of Congenital Anomalies of the Eye. Transactions of New Orleans Academy of Ophthalmology. St. Louis, C. V. Mosby Co., 1966, pp. 325–327.

Wilson, F. M., Grayson, M., and Pieroni, D.: Corneal Changes in Ectodermal Dysplasia: Case Report, Histopathology, and Differential Diagnosis. Amer. J. Ophthal. 75:17–27, 1973.

Microphakia or Spherophakia (small lens or highly spherical lens)

1. Associated with lenticular myopia as recessive inheritance trait

2. Rubella syndrome

3. Marfan's syndrome

4. Reticular dystrophy of the retinal pigment epithelium

5. Homocystinuria

348

6. Lowe's syndrome (renal rickets)

7. Hyperlysinemia

8. Alport's syndrome—hereditary renal disease, cataracts, arcus juvenilus

Chavis, R. M., and Groshong, T.: Corneal Arcus in Alport's Syndrome. Amer. J. Ophthal. *75*:793–794, 1973.

Deutman, A. F., and Rumke, A. M. L.: Reticular Dystrophy of Retinal Pigment Epithelium. Arch. Ophthal. *82*:4–9, 1969.

Smith, T. H., Holland, M. G., and Woody, N. C.: Ocular Abnormalities in Association with Hyperlysinemia. Trans. Amer. Acad. Ophthal. Otolaryng. *75*:355–360, 1971.

Sorsby, A.: Ophthalmic Genetics, 2nd ed. New York, Appleton-Century-Crofts, Inc., 1970.

Zimmerman, L. E., and Font, R. L.: Congenital Malformations of the Eye; Some Recent Advances in Knowledge of the Pathogenesis and Histopathological Characteristics. J.A.M.A. *196*:684–692, 1966.

Dislocated Lens

1. Marfan's syndrome—usually superior displacement of lens

2. Marchesani's syndrome—usually superior displacement of lens

3. Dwarfism, genetic type

4. Scleroderma

5. Trauma as in Frenkel's syndrome (ocular contusion syndrome)

6. Homocystinuria—usually downward displacement of lens

7. Syphilis

8. Recession of anterior chamber angle

9. Spontaneous (degenerative)

10. Surgical accidents (iatrogenic)

11. Spherophakia (see p. 348)

12. Autosomal recessive abnormality without other defects—usually ectopic pupils

13. Associated ocular findings
    A. High myopia
    B. Congenital glaucoma
    C. Aniridia
    D. Megalocornea
    E. Coloboma of iris and choroid

14. Ehlers-Danlos syndrome

15. Rieger's syndrome

16. Mandibulofacial dysostosis

17. Hyperlysinemia

18. Sulfite oxidase deficiency

Cross, H. E., and Jensen, A. D.: Ocular Manifestations in the Marfan Syndrome and Homocystinuria. Amer. J. Ophthal. 75:405–420, 1973.

Geeraets, W. J.: Ocular Syndromes, 2nd ed. Philadelphia, Lea & Febiger, 1969, p. 224.

Jarrett, W. H.: Dislocation of the Lens. Arch. Ophthal. 78:289, 1967.

Kirkham, T.: Mandibulofacial Dysostosis with Ectopic Lentis. Amer. J. Ophthal. 70:947–949, 1970.

Laster, L., et al.: A Previously Unrecognized Disorder of Metabolism of Sulfur-Containing Compounds: Abnormal Urinary Excretion of S-Sulfo-L-Cysteine, Sulfite and Thiosulfate in a Severely Retarded Child with Ectopic Lentis. J. Clin. Invest. 46:1082, 1967.

Rizzuti, A. B.: Complications in the Surgical Management of the Displaced Lens. Int. Ophthal. Clin. 5:3–54, 1965.

Smith, T. H., Holland, M. G., and Woody, N. C.: Ocular Abnormalities in Association with Hyperlysinemia. Trans. Amer. Acad. Ophthal. Otolaryng. 75:355–360, 1971.

Spaeth, G. D., and Barber, G. W.: Homocystinuria—Its Ocular Manifestations. J. Pediat. Ophthal. 3:42–48, 1966.

Exfoliation of the Lens Capsule (superficial layers of the lens capsule split off and float in the aqueous as a fine membrane)

1. Senile exfoliation

2. Toxic exfoliation
   A. Atrophic eyes
   B. Prolonged iridocyclitis
   C. Lodgement of metallic foreign body, such as iron or copper

3. Traumatic
   A. Perforating injury
   B. Contusions with suspensory ligament separated from a dislocated lens

4. Heat exposure, such as that experienced by glass-blowers

Duke-Elder, S.: System of Ophthalmology, Vol. XI. St. Louis, C. V. Mosby Co., 1969, pp. 42–45.

Iridescent Crystalline Deposits in Lens

1. Idiopathic

2. Hypothyroid (cretinism)

3. Hypocalcemia
   A. Postoperative—removal of thyroid and accidental parathyroid removal
   B. Idiopathic hypoparathyroidism
   C. Pseudohypoparathyroidism (hypoparathyroid cretinism) or with hyperphosphatemia (Albright's disease)

D. Pseudopseudohypoparathyroidism   (brachymetacarpal dwarfism)

4. Myotonic dystrophy

Duke-Elder, S.: System of Ophthalmology, Vol. XI. St. Louis, C. V. Mosby Co., 1969, pp. 175–176, 182, 186.

Lenticular Disease Associated with Corneal Problems

1. Fabry's disease—whorl-like corneal epithelial changes and posterior spoke cataract

2. Mongolism—keratoconus and cataract

3. Myotonic dystrophy—keratoconjunctivitis sicca and cataract

4. Rothmund's syndrome—band keratopathy and posterior spoke cataract

5. Diabetes mellitus—wrinkling of Descemet's membrane and cataract

6. Congenital anomalies

7. Embryopathies—virus (rubella)

8. Steroids—Bowman's membrane haze and ulcers of the cornea and cataract

9. Wilson's disease—Kayser-Fleischer ring and sunflower cataract

10. Siderosis—pigment in epithelium of lens and endothelium and in front of Descemet's membrane

11. Endothelial dystrophy and anterior polar cataract (Dohlman)

Grayson, M., and Keates, R. H.: Manual of Diseases of the Cornea. Boston, Little, Brown & Co., 1969, p. 295.

Aphakia (absence of the lens in usual position behind iris)

1. Congenital absence of lens—rare
2. Injury to lens capsule with gradual absorption of the lens material
3. Following cataract extraction
4. Dislocation of the lens into vitreous cavity, anterior chamber, or subconjunctival area

Hanna, C., Fraunfelder, F. F., and King, Y. Y.: Extraocular Traumatic Luxation of the Lens. J. Arkansas Med. Soc. *66*:210, 1969.
O'Brien, C. S.: Ophthalmology, Notes for Students. Iowa City, Athens Press, 1930, p. 319.

Spasm of Accommodation (increased tone of ciliary body with increased convexity of crystalline lens) (see acquired myopia, p. 516)

1. Fatigue cramp of overworked ciliary muscle; most frequent with compound hyperopia and mixed astigmatism associated with anisometropia
2. Reflex irritation, such as in trigeminal neurologia
3. Cholinergic drugs, such as pilocarpine or Phospholine Iodide
4. Ocular inflammation, such as ciliary muscle irritant
5. Drugs
   A. Morphine

B. Hydrastin
C. Alcohol
D. Digitalis group
E. Sulfonamides and carbonic anhydrase inhibitors
F. After large doses of vitamin B_1
G. Organic arsenicals, such as arsphenamine

6. Irritative lesions of brain stem and oculomotor trunk, such as epidemic encephalitis, tabes, meningitis, influenza, scleritis, or orbital inflammation

7. Contusion injury to the globe or head

8. Sympathetic paralysis

9. Infectious, such as diphtheria, helminthic infestations, or sinus disease

10. Cyclic oculomotor palsy or spasm (see p. 110)

11. Pineal tumor

Duke-Elder, S., and Scott, G. I.: System of Ophthalmology, Vol. XII. St. Louis, C. V. Mosby Co., 1971, pp. 706–709.
Walsh, F. B., and Hoyt, W. F.: Clinical Neuro-ophthalmology, 3rd ed. Baltimore, Williams & Wilkins Co., 1969, pp. 549–551.

Paresis of Accommodation (partial or total loss of the physiologic ability to change shape of the lens and thus the focus of the eye [see mydriasis, p. 296]; this ability is related to age [see acquired hyperopia, p. 518])

1. Presbyopia—gradual decrease in amplitude of accommodation related to age

2. Accommodative insufficiency
   A. Asthenic individuals

B. Illness or debilitation including intestinal toxemia, tuberculosis, influenza, whooping cough, measles, and tonsillar and dental infections
   C. Anemia
   D. Overwork
   E. Whiplash injury

3. Ciliary body aplasia—with or without pupillary and iris abnormalities

4. Iridocyclitis—acute and chronic

5. Glaucoma with atrophy of ciliary body

6. Choroidal metastasis with suprachoroidal extension

7. Trauma, such as tears in iris sphincter, tears at root of iris, or recession of the anterior chamber angle with posterior displacement of the ciliary attachment and ocular hypotension

8. Rupture of zonular fibers and partial subluxation of lens

9. Myotonic dystrophy

10. Drugs
   A. Cycloplegics, such as atropine, scopolamine, and homatropine
   B. Parkinsonism drugs, such as Artane, or lystrone
   C. Antihistamines—slight
   D. Ganglionic blocking agents action on ciliary ganglion
   E. Central nervous system stimulants
   F. Massive doses of tranquilizing drugs, such as phenothiazine derivatives

11. Neurogenic causes
   A. Infectious conditions
      (1) Epidemic encephalitis
      (2) Anterior poliomyelitis
      (3) Exanthemas and acute infections, such as scarlet fever, mumps, measles, influenza, typhoid fever, dengue fever, viral hepatitis, amebic dysentery, and malaria
      (4) Herpes zoster

(5) Syphilis
(6) Tuberculosis
(7) Leprosy
(8) Focal infections, such as from teeth or nasal sinuses
B. Toxic conditions
  (1) Alcohol
  (2) Lead
  (3) Arsenic
  (4) Carbon monoxide
  (5) Diphtheritic paralysis
  (6) Botulism
  (7) Extensive burn
  (8) Snake venom
C. Degenerative conditions
  (1) Congenital hereditary ophthalmoplegia
  (2) Progressive congenital ophthalmoplegia
  (3) Hereditary ataxia
  (4) Myotonic dystrophy
  (5) Myasthenia gravis
D. Metabolic conditions
  (1) Acute hemorrhagic anterior polioencephalitis of Wernicke
  (2) Diabetes mellitus
  (3) Lactation
  (4) Following pregnancy
E. Isolated internal ophthalmoplegia (see p. 337 or Adie's syndrome, p. 338)
F. Isolated failure of near reflex, such as with inverse Argyll Robertson pupil
G. Lesions of parasympathetic nuclei in midbrain
  (1) Encephalitis
  (2) Pineal tumor
  (3) Other signs of mesencephalic disease, including multiple sclerosis, infectious polyneuropathy, and vascular lesions
  (4) Syphilis—bilateral
H. Trauma to head or neck
  (1) Cerebral concussion
  (2) Craniocervical extension injuries

Duke-Elder, S., and Scott, G. I.: System of Ophthalmology, Vol. XII. St. Louis, C. V. Mosby Co., 1971, pp. 698–706.

Marmor, M. F.: Transient Accommodative Paralysis and Hyperopia in Diabetes. Arch. Ophthal. 89:419–421, 1973.

Roca, P. D.: Ocular Manifestations of Whiplash Injuries. Ann. Ophthal. 4:63–73, 1972.

Romano, P. E., and Stark, W. J.: Pseudomyopia as a Presenting Sign in Ocular Myasthenia Gravis. Amer. J. Ophthal. 75:872–875, 1973.

Walsh, F. B., and Hoyt, W. F: Clinical Neuro-ophthalmology, 3rd ed. Baltimore, Williams & Wilkins Co., 1969, pp. 544–550.

Weintraub, M. O., Ribner, J. A., and Gallagher, B. B.: Transient Internal Ophthalmoplegia. Arch. Ophthal. 86:595–598, 1971.

VITREOUS

Contents

Pseudodetachment of the Vitreous (conditions simulating detachment of the vitreous)

1. Membranous formations within the vitreous associated with uveitis and hemorrhage
2. The outline of the ascending portion of Cloquet's canal just anterior to the disc
3. An enormous cavity in the vitreous body with a relatively thin posterior wall

Jaffe, N. S.: The Vitreous in Clinical Ophthalmology. St. Louis, C. V. Mosby Co., 1969, pp. 83–98.

Anterior Vitreous Detachment (the anterior vitreous may be separated from the posterior lens or posterior zonular fibers)

1. Retrolenticular—usually caused by vitreous shrinkage
    A. Trauma
    B. Hemorrhage
    C. Senescence
    D. Inflammation
    E. Retinal detachment

2. Retrozonular
    A. Vitreous shrinkage
    B. Ciliary body tumor
    C. Blood
    D. Exudate

3. Retrolenticular and retrozonular combined occurs with rupture of the hyaloideocapsular ligament

Jaffe, N. S.: The Vitreous in Clinical Ophthalmology. St. Louis, C. V. Mosby Co., 1969, pp. 83–98.

Posterior Vitreous Detachment (vitreous separated from the retina)

1. Complete posterior detachment
    A. Simple detachment—occurs in young persons
        (1) Exudate from chorioretinitic focus
        (2) Hemorrhage between the vitreous and the retina
        (3) Retraction of the cortical vitreous caused by exudate within the vitreous
        (4) Vitreous hemorrhage in a young individual with vitreous shrinkage due to thrombosis of central retinal vein, retinitis proliferans, central serous retinopathy, and trauma
    B. Complete posterior detachment with collapse
        (1) Senescent changes are primary cause
        (2) Uveitis
        (3) Trauma
        (4) Hemorrhage
    C. Funnel-shaped posterior detachment
        (1) Perforating injuries of globe
        (2) Retinitis proliferans
        (3) Massive vitreous detachment
    D. Atypical complete posterior detachment—residual adherence of vitreous to a peripheral retinal area
        (1) Focus of chorioretinitis
        (2) Following cataract extraction with loss of vitreous
        (3) Following perforating wounds
2. Partial posterior detachment (unusual)
    A. Superior detachment—primarily a senescent change; generally forerunner of posterior vitreous detachment with collapse
    B. Partial posterior detachment (not infrequent)
        (1) Preretinal hemorrhage
        (2) Retinitis proliferans
    C. Partial lateral or partial inferior detachment
        (1) Focus of choroiditis
        (2) Circumscribed retinal periphlebitis
        (3) Intraocular foreign body

Boniuk, M., and Burton, G. L.: Unilateral Glaucoma Associated with Sickle-Cell Retinopathy. Trans. Amer. Acad. Ophthal. Otolaryng. *68*:316–328, 1964.

Jaffe, N. S.: The Vitreous in Clinical Ophthalmology. St. Louis, C. V. Mosby Co., 1969, pp. 83–98.

	Complete, Simple Posterior Vitreous Detachment	*Complete Posterior Vitreous Detachment with Collapse*
Age	Young	Old or myopes of any age
Etiology	Inflammation, hemorrhage, trauma	Senescence
Refractive error	Unimportant	Myopia in younger patients
Prior vitreous degeneration	None	Fibrillary degeneration and cavities
Vitreous cells	Cells and vitreous precipitates (VP)	None
Rocking movements of vitreous	Rare	Frequent
Retinal breaks	None	10 to 15%
Hemorrhages	Rare	10 to 15%
Vitreoretinal traction	Rare	10 to 15%
Prepapillary opacity	Yes	Yes
Onset	Slowly progressive	Rapid
Shape of posterior vitreous border	Spherical	Collapsed

Jaffe, N. S.: The Vitreous in Clinical Ophthalmology. St. Louis, C. V. Mosby Co., 1969, p. 96.

Vitreous Hemorrhage

1. Associated with retinal break or tear with or without retinal detachment and avulsed retinal vessels

2. Sickle cell disease—SA, SS, or SC

3. Thalassemia

4. Eales' disease

5. Blood disease—retinal hemorrhage breaking into vitreous
   A. Anemias
      (1) Pernicious anemia
      (2) Hypochromic anemias
      (3) Aplastic anemias
      (4) Hemolytic anemias
   B. Polycythemia vera
   C. Thrombocytopenic purpura
   D. Hemophilia associated with trauma
   E. Leukemias
   F. Dysproteinemias—macroglobulins and cryoglobulins
   G. Multiple myeloma

6. Collagen disease
   A. Disseminated lupus erythematosus
   B. Polyarteritis nodosa
   C. Dermatomyositis
   D. Scleroderma

7. Thromboangiitis obliterans

8. Coats' disease

9. Angiomatosis retinae (von Hippel-Lindau disease)

10. Terson's syndrome of associated vitreous and subarachnoid hemorrhage

11. Malignant melanoma

12. Arsenic toxicity

13. Purtscher's disease (traumatic retinal angiopathy)

14. Diabetes mellitus

15. Hemorrhages in the newborn
    A. Persistent vessels of the hyaloid system
    B. Hemorrhagic disease of the newborn—factor VII and prothrombin deficiency
    C. Retinal hemorrhage of newborn breaking through to vitreous cavity

16. Trauma

17. Associated with uveitis

18. Intraocular foreign body

19. Complete posterior vitreous detachment with collapse (see p. 361)

20. Hypertension

21. Cicatricial stage of retrolental fibroplasia

22. Juvenile retinoschisis

23. Hemorrhagic disciform degeneration

24. Intraocular tumor

25. Neovascularization following vascular occlusion

26. Persistent hyaloid artery

27. From retinal hemorrhage (see p. 408)

28. Iatrogenic—globe perforation associated with strabismus operation

29. Drusen of optic disc

30. Indomethacin reaction

Chopman, R. A.: Suspected Adverse Reaction to Indomethacin. Canad. Med. Assoc. J. 95:1156, 1966.

Ellsworth, R.: Tumors of the Retina. In Tasman, W. (Ed.): Retinal Diseases in Children. New York, Harper & Row, 1971, pp. 50–51.

Faris, B. M., and Brockhurst, R. J.: Retrolental Fibroplasia in the Cicatricial Stage. Arch. Ophthal. 82:60–65, 1969.

Gottlieb, F., and Castro, J. L.: Perforation of the Globe during Strabismus Surgery. Arch. Ophthal. 84:151–157, 1970.

Jaffe, N. S.: The Vitreous in Clinical Ophthalmology. St. Louis, C. V. Mosby Co., 1969, pp. 251–276.

Robertson, D. M., Curtin, V. T., and Norton, E. W. D.: Avulsed Retinal Vessels with Retinal Breaks. Arch. Ophthal. *85*:669–672, 1971.

Ruiz, R. S.: Diagnosis and Management of Vitreous Hemorrhage. Southern Med. J. *63*:9–11, 1970.

Sanders, T. E., Gay, A. J., and Newman, M.: Hemorrhagic Complications of Drusen of the Optic Disc. Amer. J. Ophthal. *71*:204–217, 1971.

Vitreous Opacities

1. Single opacities
    A. Anterior hyaloid remnant (Mittendorf's dot)—25% normal eyes, dot on posterior lens surface
    B. Hyaloid remnants, uncommon
    C. Foreign body—history of trauma or operation
    D. Dislocated lens (see p. 349)
    E. Parasitic cysts
        (1) Hydatid disease (echinococcosis)—rare, children and young adults, tropical
        (2) Cysticercosis—rare
    F. Vitreous detachment—common in older or myopic persons

2. Scattered opacities
    A. Vitreous degeneration—older and myopic persons
    B. Heterochromic uveitis—20 to 50 years old; 3% of all uveitis, iris atrophy, lens changes
    C. Snowball opacities—rare, associated with pars planitis or sarcoidosis
    D. Amyloid disease—rare, older persons
    E. Myelomatosis—rare, 50 to 70 years old, bone pain, anemia
    F. Red blood cells—see vitreous hemorrhage (p. 363)
    G. White blood cells—inflammatory disease

H. Pigment cells—post-traumatic (hematogenous), senile, or melanotic
I. Tumor cells—retinoblastoma in older child
J. Tissue cells—epithelial, histiocytic, glial
K. Protein coagula—plasmoid vitreous
    (1) Cyclitis
    (2) Chorioretinitis
    (3) Choroidal tumors
    (4) Contusions
L. Crystalline deposits
    (1) Asteroid bodies
    (2) Synchysis scintillans
M. Coagula of the colloid basis of the gel

3. Opaque sheets in the vitreous
    A. Normal posterior capsule—often following extracapsular cataract extraction or needling
    B. Soemmerring's ring following extracapsular cataract extraction or needling
    C. Elschnig's pearls after extracapsular cataract extraction or needling
    D. Vitreous adhesion to cataract section after cataract extraction with vitreous loss

4. Pseudoglioma (see p. 310)—leukokoria

Byers, B., and Kimura, S. J.: Uveitis after Death of a Larva in the Vitreous Cavity. Amer. J. Ophthal. 77:63–66, 1974.
Duke-Elder, S.: System of Ophthalmology, Vol. III, Part 2. St. Louis, C. V. Mosby Co., 1963, pp. 764–765.
Duke-Elder, S.: System of Ophthalmology, Vol. XI. St. Louis, C. V. Mosby Co., 1969, pp. 322–323.
Perkins, E. S., and Dobree, J. H.: The Differential Diagnosis of Fundus Conditions. St. Louis, C. V. Mosby Co., 1972, pp. 10–23.

Beads in Vitreous (snowballs in vitreous)

1. Severe uveitis

2. Retinoblastoma

3. Sarcoid

4. Pars planitis

5. Behçet's syndrome

Schlaegel, T. F.: The Uvea. Arch. Ophthal. *85*:624–635, 1971.

Asteroid Hyalosis vs Synchysis Scintillans

	Asteroid Hyalosis	*Synchysis Scintillans*
Age of patient	Elderly	Usually young
Bilaterality	Usually unilateral	May be bilateral more often
Incidence	Rare	Extremely rare
Appearance	Spherical white bodies	Flat, angular crystals
Motility	Moves with vitreous structure and returns to original position	Moves freely and falls to floor of vitreous cavity
Chemistry	Calcium soaps	Cholesterol crystals
Associated ocular disease	None; diabetes mellitus?	Secondary to other ocular disease or trauma

Jaffe, N. S.: The Vitreous in Clinical Ophthalmology. St. Louis, C. V. Mosby Co., 1969, p. 226.

Complications Following Operative Vitreous Loss

1. Inflammatory complications
   A. Irritable eye
   B. Recurrent or persistent uveitis
   C. Vitreitis with vitreous opacities

2. Wound complications
   A. Epithelial invasion or downgrowth
   B. Fibrous downgrowth
   C. Fistula or gaping of wound
   D. Infection and endophthalmitis
   E. Excessive astigmatism

3. Corneal complications
   A. Corneal edema
   B. Bullous keratopathy
   C. Corneal opacification

4. Secondary glaucoma
   A. Vitreous obstruction of anterior chamber angle
   B. Pupillary block (iridohyaloid adhesions, anterior hyaloid displacement, uveitis)
   C. Iris and vitreous adherence to wound (peripheral anterior synechiae)

5. Fibroblastic and traction phenomena
   A. Pupillary membrane
   B. Pupillary distortion—"peaked" or updrawn
   C. Macular edema
   D. Retinal detachment
   E. Optic neuritis or papilledema
   F. Vitreous hemorrhage
   G. Posterior vitreous detachment

Jaffe, N. S.: The Vitreous in Clinical Ophthalmology. St. Louis, C. V. Mosby Co., 1969, p. 121.
Turtz, A. I.: Vitrectomy. Ann. Ophthal. 4:929–959, 1972.

Postoperative Vitreous Retraction (usually manifested by circular equatorial retinal fold or star-shaped retinal fold)

1. Perforating diathermy and excessively strong or repeated applications of superficial diathermy, which may cause vitreous hemorrhage or thermal injury to the vitreous. Impairment of chorioretinal blood circulation may result in exudation and hemorrhage into the vitreous

2. Giant breaks allowing a large area of direct contact between the choroid and the vitreous

3. Venous stasis caused by the compression of vortex veins by the indentation resulting from a buckling procedure

4. Accidental perforation of the sclera at operation which may be associated with hemorrhage and loss of vitreous resulting in a pathologic formation of new membrane

Jaffe, N. S.: The Vitreous in Clinical Ophthalmology. St. Louis, C. V. Mosby Co., 1969, pp. 190–191.

Vitreous Cyst (cystic structure in the vitreous body)

1. Congenital (developmental)—may be associated with hyaloid remnants
2. Acquired
   A. Infectious cyst, such as with toxoplasmosis
   B. Parasitic cysts
      (1) Hydatid disease (echinococcosis)—rare, children and young adults, tropical
      (2) Cysticercosis—rare
   C. Nematode cyst

Bullock, J. D.: Developmental Vitreous Cysts. Arch. Ophthal. *91*: 83–84, 1974.

RETINA

Contents

13

Anatomic Classification of Macular Diseases

1. Vitreoretinal surface
   A. Preretinal hemorrhage and sub-internal limiting membrane hemorrhage
   B. Vitreous traction on the macula
   C. Contraction of the inner surface of the retina

2. Nerve fiber-ganglion cell layers
   A. Hereditary cerebromacular degenerations
      (1) Sphingolipidoses
         a. Tay-Sachs disease (GM_2-gangliosidosis type I)
         b. Sandhoff's disease (GM_2-gangliosidosis type II)
         c. Niemann-Pick disease
         d. Lactosyl ceramidosis
         e. Metachromatic leukodystrophy
         f. Gaucher's disease
      (2) Mucolipidoses
         a. Farber's lipogranulomatosis
         b. Sea-blue histiocyte syndrome (chronic Niemann-Pick disease)
         c. Generalized gangliosidosis (GM_1-ganglosidosis type I)
         d. Mucolipidosis I (lipomucopolysaccharidosis)
      (3) Goldberg's disease (unclassified syndrome with features of mucopolysaccharidoses, sphingolipidoses; and mucolipidoses)
      (4) Other
         a. Jansky-Bielschowsky disease (late infantile)
         b. Batten-Mayou, Vogt-Spielmeyer disease (juvenile)
   B. Vitreoretinal dystrophies
      (1) Macular degeneration in juvenile sex-linked retinoschisis
      (2) Goldmann-Fayre recessive vitreoretinal dystrophy

3. Nerve fiber-ganglion cell-inner plexiform-inner nuclear-outer plexiform layers
   A. Ischemia secondary to inadequate perfusion of retinal vessels (branch occlusion of artery or vein)
   B. Senile macular degeneration (inner type?)

4. Outer plexiform layer
   A. Cystoid macular degeneration
      (1) With retinal vascular leakage
         a. Postoperative (Irvine-Gass)
         b. Acute non-granulomatous iridocyclitis
         c. Acute cyclitis
         d. Peripheral posterior segment inflammation (pars planitis)
         e. Vascular anomalies
         f. Hypertension
         g. Diabetes
         h. Low-grade venous obstruction
         i. Radiation retinopathy
      (2) Without obvious retinal vascular leakage
         a. Vitreous traction on the macula
         b. Serous detachment of sensory epithelium
         c. Serous detachment of pigment epithelium
         d. Hemorrhagic detachment of macula
         e. Choroidal tumors
         f. Senile?
   B. Lipid deposits in macula secondary to vascular disease in retina
      (1) Stellate retinopathy (see p. 382)
         a. Hypertensive retinopathy
         b. Diabetic retinopathy
         c. Coats' disease
         d. Trauma—ocular or cerebral
         e. Retinal artery or vein occlusion
         f. Retinal periphlebitis
         g. Juxtapapillary choroiditis
         h. Papilledema
         i. Angiomatosis retinae
         j. Papillitis

         k. Acute febrile illness, such as measles, influenza, meningitis, erysipelas, psittacosis, Behçet's disease

         l. Chronic infections, such as tuberculosis or syphilis

         m. Coccidioidomycosis

         n. Parasitic infection, such as that due to teniae, Giardia, Ancylostoma

         o. Idiopathic

      (2) Circinate retinopathy

         a. Senile vascular disease

         b. Venous obstruction

         c. Diabetic retinopathy

         d. Coats' disease

         e. Retinal detachment

         f. Anemia

         g. Leukemia

         h. Idiopathic (primary)

      (3) Diabetic retinopathy

5. Outer nuclear or rod and cone layers (neuroepithelium, sensory epithelium)

    A. Congenital hereditary vision defects (see p. 549)

      (1) Trichromatism (anomalous)

      (2) Dichromatism

      (3) Monochromatism

    B. Hereditary macular dystrophies

      (1) Stargardt's disease (atrophic macular dystrophy with fundus flavimaculatus)

      (2) Dominant progressive foveal dystrophy (dominant Stargardt's disease)

      (3) Progressive cone dystrophy

      (4) Central retinopathia pigmentosa (inverse pigmentary dystrophy)

    C. Olivopontocerebellar degeneration

    D. Solar burn (idiopathic foveomaculopathy)

6. Pigment epithelium

    A. Hereditary macular dystrophies

      (1) Vitelliform dystrophy (Best's)

      (2) Fundus flavimaculatus

  (3) Dominant drusen (Doyne's honeycomb degeneration, Hutchinson-Tay, Malattia leventinese)
  (4) Reticular dystrophy (Sjögren)
  (5) Butterfly-shaped pigment dystrophy (Deutman)
  (6) Albipunctate dystrophy
  (7) Sjögren-Larsson syndrome
 B. Inflammatory lesions
  (1) Rubella
  (2) Acute posterior multifocal placoid pigment epitheliopathy
 C. Toxic lesions
  (1) Chloroquine
  (2) Phenothiazine
  (3) Sparsomycin
  (4) Ethambutol
  (5) Indomethacin
  (6) Griseofulvin?
 D. Drusen (senile, degenerative)
 E. Refsum's syndrome—ophthalmoplegia, ataxia, deafness, polyneuritis
 F. Myotonic dystrophy

7. Bruch's membrane
 A. Angioid streaks associated with (see p. 452):
  (1) Pseudoxanthoma elasticum (Groenblad-Strandberg)
  (2) Senile elastosis of skin
  (3) Osteitis deformans (Paget's disease)
  (4) Fibrodysplasia hyperelastica (Ehlers-Danlos)
  (5) Sickle cell disease
  (6) Acromegaly
 B. Senile fracture of Bruch's membrane (a type of angioid streaks?)
 C. Traumatic fracture of Bruch's membrane

8. Pigment epithelium-Bruch's membrane choriocapillaris
 A. Degenerative lesions
  (1) Disciform macular degeneration (senile, juvenile)
  (2) Pseudo-inflammatory macular dystrophy of Sorsby
  (3) Senile macular degeneration (outer type)

      (4) Adult hereditary cerebromacular degeneration (Kufs?)

      (5) Congenital cystic macular degeneration?

B. Serous detachment of neuroepithelium or pigment epithelium associated with:

      (1) Idiopathic leak from choriocapillaris

      (2) Hemangioma of choroid

      (3) Malignant melanoma

      (4) Pit of optic disk

      (5) Hypotony

      (6) Leukemic infiltrates of choroid

      (7) Terminal illness

      (8) Trauma

      (9) Uveitis

      (10) Optic neuritis

      (11) Papilledema

      (12) Acute hypertension

      (13) Vitreous traction

      (14) Angioid streaks

      (15) Harada's disease

      (16) *Toxocara canis*

      (17) Myopic choroidal degeneration

      (18) Metastatic carcinoma

      (19) Choroidal nevus

      (20) Collagen vascular disease

      (21) Hemorrhagic or organized disciform detachment

C. Lipoid proteinosis (Urbach-Wiethe)

9. Choroid

A. Degenerative lesions

      (1) Central areolar choroidal atrophy

      (2) Myopic choroidal atrophy

      (3) Helicoid peripapillary chorioretinal atrophy?

B. Inflammatory lesions

      (1) Histoplasmosis

C. Vascular occlusive lesions

10. Miscellaneous

A. Retinal inflammations (multilayer alterations that may involve the macula)

      (1) *Toxoplasma gondii*

        (2) *Toxocara canis*
        (3) Septic emboli
            a. Candida
            b. Bacteria
    B. Congenital anomalies of the macula
        (1) Aplasia
        (2) Hypoplasia
        (3) Heterotopia
        (4) Colobomas
        (5) Aberrant macular vessels

Betten, M. G., Bilchik, R. C., and Smith, M. E.: Pigmentary Retinopathy of Myotonic Dystrophy. Amer. J. Ophthal. *72*:7203, 1971.
Duke-Elder, S.: Diseases of the Retina. System of Ophthalmology. Vol. X. St. Louis, C. V. Mosby Co., 1967, pp. 125–127.
Maumenee, A. E., and Emery, J. M.: An Anatomic Classification of Diseases of the Macula. Amer. J. Ophthal. *74*:594–599, 1972.

Pseudomacular Edema

1. Exudative senile maculopathy—serous and/or hemorrhagic detachment of the macular retina in individuals 50 years of age or older, including "giant cyst of macula"

2. Serous detachment of retinal pigment epithelium

3. Central serous retinopathy

Gass, J. D. M.: Pathogenesis of Disciform Detachment of Neuroepithelium. Amer. J. Ophthal. *63*:573–711, 1967.
Zweng, H. C., Little, H. L., and Peabody, R. R.: Laser Photocoagulation of Macular Lesions. Trans. Amer. Acad. Ophthal. Otolaryng. *72*:377–388, 1968.

Macular Edema (loss of foveal depression with ophthalmoscope and outline of multiple cystoid spaces retroilluminated with slit lamp. Often a yellow exudate lies deep within or beneath the retina in the foveal area)

1. Following trauma to globe (commotio retinae)

2. Associated with pit of optic nerve

3. Associated with uveitis, either anterior or posterior

4. Hypotony following intraocular operation (see p. 379), including cataract operation, vitreous operation, and aphakic keratoplasty

5. Drugs, such as hydrochlorothiazide (Hydro-Diuril, Esidrix)

6. Electrical injuries to the retina

7. Central angiospastic retinopathy

8. Topical epinephrine

9. Hemangioma of choroid

10. von Hippel's angiomatosis of retina

11. Telangiectasis of retina

12. Vein occlusion (see p. 406), including branch vein occlusion

13. Diabetic exudative retinopathy

14. Pars planitis (peripheral uveitis)

15. Hunter's syndrome (MPS II)

16. Sun eclipse injury, photocoagular or laser (early)

17. Intraretinal nematode

18. Oral contraceptives

19. Vitreous operation or vitreous loss

20. Retinitis pigmentosa

21. Fabry's disease (ceramide trihexoside lipidosis)

22. Subacute sclerosing panencephalitis (Dawson's disease)

23. Radiation retinopathy

Ballantyne, A. J., and Michaelson, I. C.: The Fundus of the Eye, 2nd ed. Baltimore, Williams & Wilkins Co., 1972.

Blankenship, G. W., and Okun, E.: Retinal Tributary Vein Occlusion. Arch. Ophthal. 89:363–368, 1973.

Gass, J. D. M.: Pathogenesis of Disciform Detachment of Neuroepithelium. Amer. J. Ophthal. 63:573–711, 1967.

Gass, J. D. M.: A Fluorescein Angiographic Study of Macular Dysfunction Secondary to Retinal Vascular Disease. Arch. Ophthal. 80:535–617, 1968.

Gass, J. D. M.: Stereoscopic Atlas of Macular Diseases. St. Louis, C. V. Mosby Co., 1970, pp. 148–172.

Goren, S. B.: Retinal Edema Secondary to Oral Contraceptives. Amer. J. Ophthal. 64:447–449, 1967.

Grant, W. M.: Toxicology of the Eye, 2nd ed. Springfield, Ill., Charles C Thomas, 1974.

Landers, M. B., III, and Klintworth, G. K.: Subacute Sclerosing Panencephalitis. Arch. Ophthal. 86:156–163, 1971.

Newell, F. W.: Ophthalmology, Principles and Concepts. St. Louis, C. V. Mosby Co., 1969, p. 240.

Patz, A., et al.: Macular Edema—an Overlooked Complication of Diabetic Retinopathy. Trans. Amer. Acad. Ophthal. Otolaryng. 77:OP34–42, 1973.

Rubin, M. L., et al.: Intraretinal Nematode: Case Report. Trans. Amer. Acad. Ophthal. Otolaryng. 72:855–866, 1968.

Spaeth, G. L.: Ocular Manifestations of the Lipidoses. In Tasman, W. C. (Ed.): Retinal Diseases in Children. New York, Harper & Row, 1971, pp. 149–153.

West, C. E., Fitzgerald, C. R., and Servell, J. H.: Cystoid Macular Edema Following Aphakic Keratoplasty. Amer. J. Ophthal. 75:77–81, 1973.

Macular Pucker (tiny folds often arranged in a stellate manner around the macula and usually associated with a pre-retinal membrane)

1. Vitreous blood

2. Total retinal detachment

3. Detachment of the macula

4. Multiple retinal operations

5. Multiple perforations

6. Loss of formed vitreous at operation

7. Following posterior vitreous separation, such as trauma to the eye and whiplash injury

Daily, L.: Macular and Vitreal Disturbances Produced by Traumatic Vitreous Rebound. Southern Med. J. 63:1197–1198, 1970.

Jaffee, N. S.: Macular Retinopathy After Separation of Vitro-retinal Adherence. Arch. Ophthal. 78:585–591, 1967.

Tanenbaum, H. L., et al.: Macular Pucker Following Retinal Detachment Surgery. Arch. Ophthal. 83:286–293, 1970.

Macular Star or Stellate Retinopathy (exudates in a star-formation radiating around the macula in the nerve-fiber layer)

1. Hypertension

2. Ocular or cerebral trauma

3. Obstruction of the artery or vein supplying the macular area

4. Retinal periphlebitis

5. Juxtapapillary choroiditis

6. Papillitis (see p. 477)

7. Papilledema (see p. 482)

8. Acute febrile illness, such as measles, influenza, meningitis, erysipelas, psittacosis, Behçet's disease

9. Chronic infections, such as tuberculosis or syphilis

10. Coccidioidomycosis

11. Parasitic infection, such as that due to teniae, Giardia, Ancylostoma

12. Idiopathic

Duke-Elder, S.: Diseases of the Retina. System of Ophthalmology, Vol. X. St. Louis, C. V. Mosby Co., 1967, pp. 125–127.

Cherry-Red Spot in Macula (rule out macular hemorrhage)

1. Sphingolipidoses
   A. Tay-Sachs disease (GM_2-gangliosidosis I)
   B. Niemann-Pick disease
   C. Gaucher's disease
   D. Infantile metachromatic leukodystrophy

2. Mucolipidoses
   A. Generalized gangliosidosis (GM_1-gangliosidoses I and II)
   B. MLS I (lipomucopolysaccharidosis)
   C. Farber's disease

3. Vogt-Spielmeyer cerebral degeneration

4. Occlusion of central retinal artery (see p. 395)

5. Temporal arteritis

6. Cryoglobulinemia

7. Hurler's syndrome

8. Myoclonic syndrome

9. Severe hypertension

10. Quinine toxicity

11. Traumatic retinal edema (commotio retinae; Berlin's edema)

12. Macular retinal hole with surrounding detachment

13. β-Galactosidase deficiency (MPS VII)

Emery, J. M., et al.: GMI-Gangliosidosis: Ocular and Pathological Manifestations. Arch. Ophthal. *85*:177–187, 1971.

Goldberg, M. F., et al.: Macular Cherry Red Spot, Corneal Clouding and β-Galactosidase Deficiency: Clinical, Biochemical, and Electron Microscopic Study of New Autosomal Recessive Storage Disease. Arch. Intern. Med. *128*:387–398, 1971.

Haessler, F. H.: Eye Signs in General Disease. Springfield, Ill., Charles C Thomas, 1960, pp. 90–91.

Kenyon, K. R., and Sensenbrenner, J. A.: Mucolipidosis II (I-cell Disease): Ultrastructure Observations of Conjunctiva and Skin. Invest. Ophthal. *10*:555–567, 1971.

Quigley, H. A., and Goldberg, M. F.: Conjunctival Ultrastructure in Mucolipidosis III (Pseudo-Hurler Polydystrophy). Invest. Ophthal. *10*:568–580, 1971.

Spaeth, G. L.: Ocular Manifestations of the Lipidoses. *In* Tasman, W. (Ed.): Retinal Diseases in Children. New York, Harper & Row, 1971, p. 171.

Walsh, F. B., and Hoyt, W. F.: Clinical Neuro-ophthalmology, 3rd ed. Baltimore, Williams & Wilkins Co., 1969,

Macular Hemorrhage (see retinal hemorrhage, pp. 408 and 409)

1. High myopia (Fuch's spot)
2. Disciform degeneration of the macula—may be surrounded by hemorrhage
3. Inflammation, such as that due to histoplasmosis
4. Angioid streaks
5. Familial

Ballantyne, A. J., and Michaelson, I. C.: Textbook of the Fundus of the Eye, 2nd ed. Baltimore, Williams & Wilkins Co., 1972.
Kalina, R. E., and Kaiser, M.: Familial Retinal Hemorrhages. Amer. J. Ophthal. 74:252–255, 1972.

Macular Cyst (must be differentiated from macular hole with Hruby lens or contact lens and slit lamp)

1. Cystic degeneration—common following trauma, uveitis, and vascular disease
2. Parasitic and mycotic cysts
3. Histoplasmosis
4. Amebiasis
5. Hydatid disease (echinococcosis)—rare, tropical areas, contact with dogs; subretinal or vitreal cyst, movement if in vitreous, unilateral
6. Cysticercosis—subretinal cyst; head with hooklets may be seen

Perkins, E. S., and Dobree, J. H.: The Differential Diagnosis of Fundus Conditions. St. Louis, C. V. Mosby Co., 1972, pp. 100–101, 116–117.

Macular Holes (must be differentiated from macular cyst with Hruby lens or contact lens and slit lamp)

1. Trauma

2. From:
   A. Edema (see macular edema, p. 380)
      (1) Inflammatory
      (2) Toxic
      (3) Vascular
      (4) Following papilledema
   B. High myopia
   C. Senility
   D. Ischemic, such as with retinal detachment or choroidal tumor—the macula is separated from choriocapillaris
   E. Degenerative conditions of the retina and retinal dystrophy
   F. Trauma
   G. Radiation injury
   H. Glaucoma
   I. Posterior senile retinoschisis
   J. High tension electric shock
   K. Central serous retinopathy
   L. Posterior retinal detachment associated with optic pits

3. Detachment of posterior vitreous from macula with focal traction

4. Dawson's disease—subacute sclerosing panencephalitis

5. Foveomacular retinitis—usually young males

Aaberg, T. M., Blair, C. J., and Gass, J. D. M.: Macular Holes. Amer. J. Ophthal. 69:555–562, 1970.
Ballantyne, A. J., and Michaelson, I. C.: Textbook of the Fundus of the Eye, 2nd ed. Baltimore, Williams & Wilkins Co., 1972.
Feman, S. S., Hepler, R. S., and Straatsma, B. R.: Rhegmatogenous Retinal Detachment Due to Macular Hole. Arch. Ophthal. 91:371–372, 1974.
Gass, J. D. M.: Stereoscopic Atlas of Macular Disease. St. Louis, C. V. Mosby Co., 1970, pp. 195–199.

Howard, G. M., and Campbell, C. J.: Surgical Repair of Retinal Detachments Caused by Macular Holes. Arch. Ophthal. *81*:317–321, 1969.

Kerr, L. M., and Little, H. L.: Foveomacular Retinitis. Arch. Ophthal. *76*:498–504, 1966.

Margheris, R. R., and Schepens, C. L.: Macular Breaks. Amer. J. Ophthal. *74*:219–240, 1972.

Nelson, D. A., et al.: Retinal Lesions in Subacute Sclerosing Panencephalitis. Arch. Ophthal. *84*:613–621, 1970.

Siam, A. L.: Macular Hole with Central Retinal Detachment in High Myopia with Posterior Staphylomata. Brit. J. Ophthal. *53*:62–63, 1969.

Elevated Macular Lesion

1. Malignant melanoma

2. Central serous detachment of retina

3. Angiospastic retinopathy

4. Chorioretinitis especially histoplasmosis and toxoplasmosis

5. Dawson's disease (subacute sclerosing panencephalitis)

Nelson, D. A., et al.: Retinal Lesions in Subacute Sclerosing Panencephalitis. Arch. Ophthal. *84*:613–621, 1970.

Newell, F. W.: Ophthalmology, Principles and Concepts. St. Louis, C. V. Mosby Co., 1969, p. 236.

Heterotopia of the Macula (abnormal location of the macula in relation to the optic disc. The eye with the ectopic macula tends to deviate in the same direction as the macular displacement. Visual fields show displacement of blind spot and cover-uncover test shows no shift of fixation)

1. Congenital

2. Inflammatory

3. Chorioretinitis

4. Incomplete or abortive form of retrolental fibroplasia

Stern, S. D., and Arenberg, I. K.: Heterotopia of the Macula with Associated Retinal Detachment. J. Pediat. Ophthal. 6:198–202, 1969.

White or Yellow Flat Macular Lesion and Pigmentary Change

1. Post-traumatic—pigmentary disturbance; cysts or hole at macula

2. Postinflammatory—chorioretinal atrophy with pigment clumping at center and periphery of lesion

3. Coloboma of macula—atrophic area at macula often associated with coloboma of disc; sclera may be ectatic

4. Radiation injuries—common after solar eclipse; punched-out appearance

5. Fuchs' dark spot—pigmented spot associated with other signs of degenerative myopia

6. Toxic retinopathies—patients treated with chloroquine and phenothiazine derivatives; bull's-eye pigmentation at macula

7. Stellate retinopathy (see p. 382)—star-shaped exudates

8. Hard exudates and circinate retinopathy (see p. 420)

9. Colloid bodies—common, discrete yellow spots beneath retina

10. Doyne's honeycomb choroiditis—rare; honeycomb pattern of yellow patches at posterior pole; degenerative changes at macula

11. Fundus flavimaculatus—yellow patches at posterior pole; degenerative changes at macula

12. Heredomacular dystrophies
    A. Best's disease—up to 7 years of age; egg-yolk lesion at macula, later absorbed to leave atrophic scar
    B. Stargardt's disease—8 to 14 years of age; variable appearance in different families; bilateral lesions showing some degree of symmetry
    C. Behr's disease—adults, similar to Stargardt type
    D. Presenile and senile—pigmentary changes followed by atrophy, bilateral and symmetrical

13. Central choroidal sclerosis—rare, atrophic retina with sclerosed choroidal vessels showing clearly

14. Central areolar choroidal atrophy—rare, exudate and edema followed by sharply defined atrophic area with white strands of choroidal vessels

15. Pseudoinflammatory macular dystrophy—rare, initially edema and exudates followed by scarring with pigmentary disturbance and atrophic patches

16. Gaucher's disease—rare, ring-shaped macular lesions, lipid deposits in cornea and conjunctiva

17. Diffuse leukoencephalopathy—rare, white deposits in periphery and macular area

18. Sjögren-Larsson syndrome—rare, infants, bilateral macular degeneration, mental deficiency

19. Angioid streaks (see p. 452)

20. Geographic choroiditis (acute multifocal placoid pigment epitheliopathy)—rare, map-like pigmentary disturbance at posterior pole or more widespread over posterior fundus

Perkins, E. S., and Dobree, J. H.: The Differential Diagnosis of Fundus Conditions. St. Louis, C. V. Mosby Co., 1972, pp. 95–115.

Pigmentary Changes in the Macula

1. Hereditary macular degeneration without cerebral or other disease
   A. Best
   B. Stargardt
   C. Behr
   D. Senile

2. Primary pigmentary retinopathy (retinitis pigmentosa)

3. Secondary pigmentary retinopathy following trauma or inflammation (see p. 421)

4. Batten's cerebral degeneration with macular changes (juvenile amaurotic familial idiocy)

5. Metabolic disease associated with pigmentary retinopathy
   A. A-beta-lipoproteinemia
   B. A-lipoproteinemia deficiency
   C. Refsum's disease
   D. Vitamin A
   E. Hepatic disease
   F. Hurler's, Hunter's, Sanfilippo's, and Scheie's mucopolysaccharidoses

6. Intoxications
   A. Chloroquine
   B. Chloropromazine

7. Inflammation
   A. Toxoplasmosis
   B. Trauma

Spaeth, G. L.: Ocular Manifestations of the Lipidoses. *In* Tasman, W. (Ed.): Retinal Diseases in Children. New York, Harper & Row, 1971, pp. 127–206.

Macular Wisps and Foveolar Splinter (noted in focal illumination with Goldmann contact lens, invisible ophthalmoscopically)

1. Spontaneous senile posterior vitreous detachment

2. Old, healed chorioretinitis

3. Direct and indirect ocular concussion

4. Whiplash injury

5. Retinitis pigmentosa

6. Juvenile macular degeneration

7. Foveomacular retinitis

8. Following absorption of small prefoveal hemorrhage

Daily, L.: Foveolar Splinter and Macular Wisps. Arch. Ophthal. *83*:406–411, 1970.
Daily, L.: Further Observations on Foveolar Splinter and Macular Wisps. Arch. Ophthal. *90*:102–103, 1973.

Retinal Vascular Tortuosity

1. Normal variation with fullness

2. Congenital

3. Hereditary hemorrhagic telangiectasis (Osler's disease)—tortuosity and varicosity

4. Hypertension

5. Racemose hemangioma of retina, angiomatosis retinae without obvious tumor formation, or von Hippel-Lindau syndrome

6. Sickle cell disease

7. Chronic respiratory insufficiency, such as in cystic fibrosis and familial dysautonomia (Riley-Day syndrome)

8. Polycythemia with vessel fullness

9. Eales' disease

10. Macroglobulinemia

11. Cryoglobulinemia

12. Visceral larva migrans

13. Premature birth

14. Maroteaux-Lamy syndrome (mucopolysaccharidosis type VI)

15. Fabry's disease

16. Coats' disease

17. Cri du chat (crying cat) syndrome—epicanthus, hypertelorism, antimongoloid lid, optic atrophy

18. Leukemia

19. Aortic coarctation

20. Chronic simple glaucoma

21. Myopic patients

22. Choked disc

Ballantyne, A. J., and Michaelson, I. C.: Textbook of the Fundus of the Eye, 2nd ed. Baltimore, Williams & Wilkins Co., 1972.

Goldberg, M. G., Payne, J. W., and Brunt, P. W.: Ophthalmologic Studies of Familial Dysautonomia, the Riley-Day Syndrome. Arch. Ophthal. *80*:732–743, 1968.

Goldberg, M. F., Pollack, I. P., and Green, W. R.: Familial Retinal Arteriolar Tortuosity with Retinal Hemorrhage. Amer. J. Ophthal. *73*:183–191, 1972.

Howard, R. O.: Ocular Abnormalities in the Cri du Chat Syndrome. Amer. J. Ophthal. *73*:949–954, 1972.

O'Connor, P. R.: Visceral Larva Migrans of the Eye. Arch. Ophthal. *88*:526–529, 1972.

Aneurysmal Dilatation of Retinal Vessels (string of beads)

1. Loaiasis (*Loa loa*)

2. Diabetes mellitus

3. Macroglobulinemia

Schlaegel, T. F.: Essentials of Uveitis. Boston, Little, Brown & Co., 1969, p. 299.

Ophthalmodynamometry (blood pressure of retinal artery. A difference between eyes of about 15% of the diastolic readings is significant)

1. High ophthalmodynamometry values
   A. Progressive intracranial arterial occlusion syndrome
   B. Basilar-vertebral occlusion
   C. Bilateral distal internal carotid occlusion—unusual

2. Low ophthalmodynamometry values
   A. Reduced on side of an occluded internal carotid artery
   B. Both sides reduced with orthostatic hypotension

3. False positive or variable readings
   A. Cardiac abnormalities, such as atrial fibrillation, heart block, or extrasystoles
   B. Measurements of ophthalmic artery pressure of less than 20 g on the instrument
   C. Abnormally high or low intraocular pressure or asymmetry between the two eyes
   D. Variation in systemic blood pressure between readings
   E. Marked asymmetry of retinal vessels in the two eyes
   F. Poor patient cooperation

Goldstein, J. E., Peczon, J. D., and Cogan, D. G.: Intraocular Pressure and Ophthalmodynamometry. Arch. Ophthal. 74:175–176, 1965.

Hollenhorst, R. W.: Carotid and Vertebral-Basilar Arterial Stenosis and Occlusion: Neuroophthalmologic Considerations. Trans. Amer. Acad. Ophthal. Otolaryng. 66:166–180, 1962.

Smith, J. L., Zieper, I. H., and Cogan, D. G.: Observations on Ophthalmodynamometry. J.A.M.A. 170:1403–1407, 1959.

Swietliczko, I., Szapiro, J., and Polis, Z.: Value of Retinal Artery Pressure Determination in the Diagnosis of Internal Carotid Artery Thrombosis: the Role of the Carotid Compression Test. Amer. J. Ophthal. 52:862–866, 1961.

Walsh, F. B., and Hoyt, W. F.: Clinical Neuro-ophthalmology, 3rd ed. Baltimore, Williams & Wilkins Co., 1969, pp. 1817–1819, 1877.

Zappia, R. J., et al.: Progressive Intracranial Arterial Occlusion Syndrome. Arch. Ophthal. 86:455–458, 1971.

Pulsation of Retinal Arteriole (high pulse pressure)

1. Aortic regurgitation

2. Hyperthyroidism

3. Intraocular blood pressure higher than diastolic blood pressure

Haessler, F. H.: Eye Signs in General Disease. Springfield, Ill., Charles C Thomas, 1960, pp. 79–82.
Newell, F. W.: Ophthalmology, Principles and Concepts. St. Louis, C. V. Mosby Co., 1969, p. 251.

Retinal Artery Occlusion (sudden blindness; on ophthalmoscopic examination, a diffuse retinal pallor and a cherry-red spot in the macula are noted)

1. Embolism—cardiac or pulmonary sources
    A. In young persons—due to postrheumatic vegetations, cardiac catheterization, or valvotomy
    B. In the elderly—due to atheroma of carotid artery
    C. Cardiac myxoma
    D. Iatrogenic trauma induced by angiography
    E. Amniotic fluid embolization

2. Atherosclerosis of common carotid artery (ophthalmodynamometry employed for diagnosis)

3. Ischemia
    A. Massive hemorrhage, such as that occurring in hematemesis, gastrointestinal bleeding, or surgical procedures
    B. Generalized shock
    C. Heart failure (rare)
    D. Too rapid lowering of blood pressure in hypertensive subjects

E. Carotid occlusion

F. Pulseless disease (aortic arch syndrome)—widespread vascular occlusion, including bilateral carotid occlusion

G. Occlusion of carotid artery by ligation in treatment for intracranial aneurysm or fistula

H. Essential hypotension

I. Following retinal detachment operation

J. Following orbital floor fractures or repair

K. Orbital hemorrhage following retrobulbar injection

4. Inflammation

A. Temporal arteritis

B. Takayasu's disease (pulseless disease)

C. Arteriole vasculitis, such as periarteritis nodosa

D. Rocky Mountain spotted fever

5. Following ocular trauma with secondary glaucoma in youths with sickle-trait hemoglobinopathy

6. Sickle cell disease

7. Syphilis

Acacio, I., and Goldberg, M. F.: Peripapillary and Macular Vessel Occlusions in Sickle Cell Anemia. Amer. J. Ophthal. 75:861–866, 1973.

Cogan, D. G.: Neurology of the Visual System, 3rd ed. Springfield, Ill., Charles C Thomas, 1968, pp. 31–46.

Fischbein, F. I.: Ischemic Retinopathy Following Amniotic Fluid Embolization. Amer. J. Ophthal. 67:351–357, 1969.

Krausher, M. F., Seelenfreund, M. H., and Freilich, D. B.: Closure of the Central Retinal Artery During Orbital Hemorrhage Following Retrobulbar Injection. Trans. Amer. Acad. Ophthal. Otolaryng. 78:OP65–70, 1974.

Michaelson, P. E., and Pfaffenbach, D.: Retinal Arterial Occlusion in Youths with Sickle-Trait Hemoglobinopathy. Amer. J. Ophthal. 74:494–497, 1972.

Nickolson, D. H., and Guyzk, S. V.: Visual Loss Complicating Repair of Orbital Floor Fractures. Arch. Ophthal. 86:369–375, 1971.

Presley, G. D.: Fundus Changes in Rocky Mountain Spotted Fever. Amer. J. Ophthal. 67:263–267, 1969.

Sarin, L. K., and McDonald, P. R.: Changes in the Posterior Pole Following Successful Re-attachment of the Retina. Trans. Amer. Acad. Ophthal. Otolaryng. 74:75–80, 1970.

Smith, J. L.: Acute Blindness in Early Syphilis. Arch. Ophthal. 90:256–258, 1973.

Localized Arterial Narrowing

1. Retinal atrophy following:
    A. Trauma
    B. Inflammation
    C. Degeneration
    D. Treatment with diathermy, light or cryopexy

2. Any vascular retinopathy

Perkins, E. S., and Dobree, J. H.: The Differential Diagnosis of Fundus Conditions. St. Louis, C. V. Mosby Co., 1972, pp. 80–81.

Generalized Arterial Narrowing

1. Local causes
    A. Apparent narrowing
        (1) High hypermetropia—common, small disc, narrow vessels, sometimes pseudopapilledema
        (2) Congenital microphthalmos—rare, hypermetropia, often cataract
        (3) Aphakia—cataract operation, dislocated lens, etc.
    B. Trauma
        (1) Avulsion of optic nerve—rare, secondary optic atrophy
        (2) Fracture involving bony optic canal—rare, secondary optic atrophy
        (3) Following retro-ocular injection—rare, secondary optic atrophy
        (4) Orbital hemorrhage following retro-ocular injection or orbital operation—rare, secondary optic atrophy

        (5) Carotid ligation for carotid-cavernous fistula, etc.—rare, secondary optic atrophy

        (6) Following angiography—rare, secondary optic atrophy

        (7) Siderosis bulbi—metallic intraocular foreign body

  C. Infection and edema

        (1) Orbital cellulitis—exophthalmos, restricted ocular movements

        (2) Following thyrotropic exophthalmos—ocular muscle paresis, lid retraction

  D. Degenerations, such as progressive cone-rod degeneration

  E. Primary tapetoretinal degenerations, such as retinitis pigmentosa

2. Systemic disease

  A. Arteriosclerosis

        (1) In involutionary sclerosis—50% of population older than 70 years of age, generalized arteriolar narrowing, diminished light reflexes

        (2) In arteriosclerotic disease

            a. Arteriosclerotic central artery occlusion—common, arteriovenous crossing signs, focal arteriolar constriction

            b. Embolus from atheromatous plaque, etc.—common, sudden onset, visible white embolus

  B. Hypertensive conditions

        (1) Essential hypertension—retinal hemorrhages, cotton-wool spots, arteriovenous crossing signs, etc.

        (2) Malignant hypertension—retinal hemorrhages, cotton-wool spots, edema of disc

        (3) Toxemia of pregnancy—rare, sometimes hemorrhages, cotton-wool spots, edema of disc, serous detachment

        (4) Coarctation of aorta—rare, hypertensive changes vary greatly in degree

        (5) Pheochromocytoma—rare, hypertensive changes vary greatly in degree

(6) Adrenal tumor, hyperaldosteronism—rare, hypertensive changes vary greatly in degree

(7) Cushing's tumor (adrenocortical hyperfunction)—rare, hypertensive changes vary greatly in degree

(8) Motor neuron disease of cervicothoracic cord—hypertension may occur after prolonged artificial pulmonary ventilation

C. Other forms of vascular disease

    (1) Retinal ischemia—hypotension following severe or recurrent bleeding, unilateral blindness in 15% of patients

    (2) Temporal arteritis (cranial arteritis, giant-cell arteritis)—common, 55 years or older, mean age at onset 70 years, sudden blindness at onset

    (3) Polyarteritis nodosa—multiple signs involving choroid, retina, cornea, episclera, and ocular muscles

    (4) Proliferative diabetic retinopathy—arterial narrowing occurs in 17% of patients with proliferative diabetic retinopathy, mainly in cicatricial stage

    (5) Cardiac arrest—thread-like arterioles, segmentation of blood column, generalized retinal pallor, pallor of disc, sometimes cherry-red spot on macula

    (6) Raynaud's disease—young adults, more common in women

D. Renal disease

    (1) Acute glomerulonephritis—preceding illnesses, including scarlet fever, streptococcal tonsillitis, otitis media, erysipelas, subacute bacterial endocarditis, polyarteritis nodosa, and many others

    (2) Chronic glomerulonephritis—often symptomless and found on routine examination

    (3) Pyelonephritis and pyelitis—commonest causes of renal failure

E. Diseases of the central nervous system

    (1) Migraine—arterial spasm, rare complication of common disease, vasomotor instability

           (2) Syphilitic neuroretinitis—rare, manifestation of secondary syphilis

           (3) Viral neuroretinitis (rare complication)

           (4) Tay-Sachs disease (amaurotic familial idiocy)—relatively common, opaque white area surrounds cherry-red spot at macula, vessels gradually become attenuated with progressive optic atrophy

           (5) Jansky-Bielschowsky disease (amaurotic familial idiocy, late form)—rare; pallor of posterior pole and cherry-red spot, not as clearly differentiated as in infantile form

           (6) Myotonic dystrophy

    F. Toxic causes

           (1) Chloroquine, hydroxychloroquine, quinacrine, amodiaquine

           (2) Lead—rare, in adults, such as industrial disease, in children from lead toys

           (3) Quinine—rare—may follow large doses (abortifacient) or normal dose in sensitive subjects

Berson, E. L., Gouras, P., and Gunkel, R. D.: Progressive Cone-Rod Degeneration. Arch. Ophthal. *80*:68, 1968.

Godtfredsen, E., and Jensen, S. F.: Dystrophic Myotonica and Retinal Dystrophy. Acta Ophthal. *47*:565–569, 1969.

Haessler, F. H.: Eye Signs in General Disease. Springfield, Ill., Charles C Thomas, 1960, pp. 72–82.

Perkins, E. S., and Dobree, J. H.: The Differential Diagnosis of Fundus Conditions. St. Louis, C. V. Mosby Co., 1972, pp. 72–80.

Periarteritis Retinalis Segmentalis (white plaques arranged in segments encircling the arteries like a cuff, and localized to one or more arterial branches)

1. Periarteritis nodosa

2. Temporal arteritis

3. Lupus erythematosus

Rask, A. J.: Peri-arteritis Retinalis Segmentalis. Acta Ophthal. *47*: 234–237, 1969.

Sheathing of Retinal Veins (white or gray envelopes around veins. Retinal and/or vitreous hemorrhage and exudates may be present.)

1. Disc only—developmental

2. Disc and retina—papillitis or papilledema

3. Peripheral sheathing
   A. Diabetes mellitus
   B. Hypertension
   C. Eales' disease—common in young males; exudates around veins and sheathing; retinal hemorrhages, venous engorgement and tortuosity, and distortion; new vessels in affected areas leading to recurrent sub-hyaloid and vitreous hemorrhages
   D. Tuberculin or BCG vaccination—rare, sectorial or generalized changes, such as in Eales' disease
   E. Septicemia and bacteremia—rare, venous engorgement, usually with multiple hemorrhages and focal sheathing
   F. Syphilis (secondary)—bilateral generalized venous engorgement with sheathing and hemorrhages
   G. Brucellosis—rare, tortuosity and sheathing of veins, vitreous haze, retinal hemorrhages
   H. Rickettsial infections—peripheral or central perivascular involvement, venous engorgement and sheathing associated with retinal hemorrhages
   I. Infectious mononucleosis—peripheral or central perivascular involvement, venous engorgement and sheathing associated with retinal hemorrhages
   J. Viral infections, including
      (1) Herpes zoster ophthalmicus
      (2) Herpes simplex
      (3) Cytomegalic inclusion disease
      (4) Influenza
      (5) Rift Valley fever
   K. Filariasis—hemorrhages and exudates
   L. Behçet's disease
   M. Sarcoidosis

N. Candidiasis
O. Coccidioidomycosis
P. Amebiasis

4. Peripheral sheathing without secondary retinopathy—multiple sclerosis

5. Wide and usually dense sheathing of dilated and tortuous veins, suggestive of myelogenous leukemia

Duke-Elder, S., and Dobree, J. H.: System of Ophthalmology, Vol. X. St. Louis, C. V. Mosby Co., 1967, pp. 218–236, 248, 256.
Haessler, F. H.: Eye Signs in General Disease. Springfield, Ill., Charles C Thomas, 1960, pp. 85–86.
Perkins, E. S., and Dobree, J. H.: The Differential Diagnosis of Fundus Conditions. St. Louis, C. V. Mosby Co., 1972, pp. 63–65, 90–93.
Schaegel, T. F.: Essentials of Uveitis. Boston, Little, Brown & Co., 1969, p. 29.

Absent Venous Pulsations (spontaneous venous pulsations absent at venules on the disc)

1. Normal individuals

2. Impending central vein occlusion (see p. 406)

3. Papilledema (see p. 482)

Newell, F. W.: Ophthalmology, Principles and Practice. St. Louis, C. V. Mosby Co., 1969, p. 251.

Dilated Retinal Veins (normally arteriole-venule ratio is 2:3, with increase in this ratio the retinal veins may be dilated)

1. Congenital
   A. Congenital tortuosity of retinal vessels—rare, sometimes associated with coarctation of aorta
   B. Fabry's disease (hereditary dystrophic lipidosis)—rare, corkscrew tortuosity of veins, retinal edema, dilatation of conjunctival vessels
   C. von Hippel-Lindau disease (angiomatosis)—familial in 20% of cases, bilateral in 50%
   D. Racemose (arteriovenous) aneurysm—rare, arteriovenous anastomoses localized to sector of retina
   E. Longfellow-Graether syndrome—rare, intermittent attacks of uniocular blindness associated with grossly dilated retinal veins
   F. Retrolental fibroplasia—veins dilated and tortuous
   G. Ocular fundi in newborns

2. Trauma and inflammation
   A. Carotid-cavernous fistula—fracture of base of skull, progressive exophthalmos, bruit
   B. Cavernous sinus thrombosis—rare, proptosis and orbital edema
   C. Periphlebitis—sheathing of vessels
   D. Anterior uveitis—dilatation of veins, often slight hyperemia of disc
   E. Impending obstruction of the central retinal vein (see p. 406)

3. Cardiovascular disease—dilatation may be present but rarely dominates the fundus picture
   A. Arteriosclerosis
   B. Involutionary sclerosis (later stages)
   C. Secondary to defective arterial flow, such as in:
      (1) Aortic arch syndrome (pulseless disease)
      (2) Congenital heart disease

(3) Stenosis or occlusion of common carotid

(4) Venous stasis (hypotensive retinopathy of Kearns and Hollenhorst)

(5) Temporal arteritis

(6) Cardiac insufficiency

(7) Severe blood loss

(8) Iatrogenic (lowering of blood pressure)

4. Respiratory disease—venous dilatation may occur with purplish hue of whole retina; obstruction of venous return from the head, such as in:

A. Mechanical compression of chest

B. Mediastinal tumor obstructing superior vena cava

C. Emphysema

D. Congenital septal defect (Fallot's tetralogy)

E. Heart failure of any type

5. Diseases of the central nervous system

A. Carotid-cavernous fistula—fractured base of skull; rupture of berry aneurysm, arteriosclerosis; proptosis, diplopia, dilatation of retinal veins and edema of disc may be late signs

B. Hemangioma of posterior fossa—rare, papilledema, often grossly dilated veins

C. Subarachnoid hemorrhage—head injury; subhyloid hemorrhages near disc, dilated veins, sometimes papilledema

D. Papilledema (see p. 482)

E. Optic nerve lesion—rare, secondary to orbital space-occupying lesion

6. Blood diseases

A. Polycythemia rubra vera (primary; Vaquez' disease) —common, males, hemorrhages; papilledema may be marked and venous thrombosis may occur

B. Secondary polycythemia—common; hemorrhages, papilledema and venous thrombosis may occur

C. Macrocytic anemia of all types—common, retinopathy absent unless hemoglobin below 50%; pale fundus, superficial hemorrhages, cotton-wool spots

(1) Pernicious anemia

(2) Steatorrhea

    (3) Celiac disease

    (4) Carcinoma of stomach

D. Sickle cell disease—dilatation of peripheral veins with retinal, subhyaloid and vitreous hemorrhages

E. Lymphatic leukemia

F. Myelogenous leukemia

G. Monocytic leukemia

H. Thrombocytopenic purpura—retinal and subhyaloid hemorrhages near disc, moderate venous dilatation

I. Aplastic anemia—hemorrhages the most striking sign, often spreading and around the disc

J. Macroglobulinemia—rare; veins dilated, tortuous and sometimes beaded; hemorrhages and occasionally microaneurysms

    (1) Primary

    (2) Secondary to leukemia, nephrosis, or cirrhosis

K. Cryoglobulinemia—rare; may occur with multiple myeloma; veins dilated, tortuous, and sometimes beaded

7. Acute febrile illnesses—rare, occasionally dilatation of retinal veins with a few hemorrhages and mild edema of disc

  A. Septicemia

  B. Influenza

  C. Rickettsial infections

  D. Infectious mononucleosis

8. Metabolic diseases

  A. Proliferative diabetic retinopathy—larger veins affected, often beaded

  B. Cystic fibrosis of pancreas—venous congestion, often swelling of disc

9. Collagen diseases

  A. Polyarteritis nodosa—among other fundus lesions, dilated veins may occur

  B. Systemic lupus erythematosus—cotton-wool spots, occasional hemorrhages, and moderate dilatation of veins

10. Toxic conditions, such as methyl alcohol ingestion

de Freitas, J. A. H., and Garcia, F. N.: Ocular Fundus of the Newborn. Rev. Brasil. Oftal. 27:199–255, 1968.

14

Frank, R. N., and Ryan, S. J.: Peripheral Retinal Neovascularization with Chronic Myelogenous Leukemia. Arch. Ophthal. *87*:585–589, 1972.

Madsen, P. H.: Venous Stasis Retinopathy in Insufficiency of Ophthalmic Artery. Acta Ophthal. *44*:940–947, 1966.

Newell, F. W.: Ophthalmology, Principles and Practice. St. Louis, C. V. Mosby Co., 1969, pp. 251, 252, 261.

Perkins, E. S., and Dobree, J. H.: The Differential Diagnosis of Fundus Conditions. St. Louis, C. V. Mosby Co., 1972, pp. 82–89.

Rahman, A. N.: The Ocular Manifestations of Hereditary Dystrophic Lipidosis. Arch. Ophthal. *69*:708, 1963.

Central Retinal Vein Occlusion (characterized by massive hemorrhage into the posterior portion of the eye and dilated retinal veins)

1. External compression of the vein
   A. Atherosclerosis of central retinal artery
   B. Connective tissue strand within the floor of the physiologic excavation
   C. Multiple crossings of the same artery and vein or congenital venous loops or twists in the retinal surface

2. Degenerative or inflammatory venous disease, causing detachment, proliferation, and hydrops
   A. Arterial hypertension
   B. Cardiac decompensation
   C. Diabetes mellitus
   D. Optic nerve inflammation
   E. Systemic granulomatous disease, particularly tuberculosis

3. Thrombosis from venous stagnation
   A. Spasm of corresponding retinal arterioles
   B. Blood dyscrasias
      (1) Polycythemia vera
      (2) Emphysema with secondary erythrocytosis
      (3) Sickle cell disease

      (4) Leukemias

      (5) Multiple myeloma

C. Increased viscosity of the blood

      (1) Macroglobulinemia

      (2) Hyperproteinemia

      (3) Cystic fibrosis of pancreas

      (4) Following peritoneal dialysis

D. Sudden reduction of systemic blood pressure due to cardiac decompensation, surgical or traumatic shock, or therapy for arterial hypertension

E. Glaucoma (pre-existing)

F. Increase in fibrinolytic inhibitors of blood

Archer, D. B., Ernest, J. T., and Newell, F. W.: Classification of Branch Vein Obstruction. Trans. Amer. Acad. Ophthal. Otolaryng. 78:148–165, 1974.

Blankenship, G. W., and Okun, E.: Retinal Tributary Vein Occlusion. Arch. Ophthal. 89:363–368, 1973.

Cogan, D. G.: Neurology of the Visual System, 3rd ed. Springfield, Ill., Charles C Thomas, 1968, p. 50.

Michels, R. G., and Gass, J. D. M.: Natural Course of Retinal Vein Obstruction. Trans. Amer. Acad. Ophthal. Otolaryng. 78:166–177, 1974.

Newell, F. W.: Ophthalmology, Principles and Concepts. St. Louis, C. V. Mosby Co., 1969, pp. 260–261.

Pandolfi, M., Hedner, N., and Nilsson, I. M.: Bilateral Occlusion of the Retinal Veins in a Patient with Inhibition of Fibrinolysis. Ann. Ophthal. 2:481–484, 1970.

Pratt, M. V., and deVenecia, G.: Central Retinal Vein Occlusion Following Peritoneal Dialysis. Amer. J. Ophthal. 70:337–341, 1970.

Rothstein, T.: Bilateral Central Retinal Vein Closure as the Initial Manifestation of Polycythemia. Amer. J. Ophthal. 74:256–260, 1972.

Dilated Retinal Veins and Retinal Hemorrhages

1. Macroglobulinemia
2. Multiple myeloma
3. Cryoglobulinemia

4. Lymphomas

5. Paraproteinemias and dysproteinemias

6. Leukemia

7. Polycythemia vera

8. Diabetes mellitus

9. Sickle cell disease

10. Central retinal vein occlusion (see p. 406)

11. Carotid-cavernous fistula

12. Congenital tortuosity and dilation of the retinal vessels

13. Ophthalmic vein thrombosis

14. Cavernous sinus thrombosis

Boniuk, M.: The Ocular Manifestations of Ophthalmic Vein and Aseptic Cavernous Sinus Thrombosis. Trans. Amer. Acad. Ophthal. Otolaryng. 76:1519–1534, 1972.
Kalina, R. E., and Kaiser, M.: Familial Retinal Hemorrhages. Amer. J. Ophthal. 74:252–255, 1972.
Luxenberg, M. N., and Mansolf, F. A.: Retinal Circulation in the Hyperviscosity Syndrome. Amer. J. Ophthal. 70:588–598, 1970.

Retinal Hemorrhages (bleeding that may be intraretinal or preretinal hemorrhages into the vitreous, or subretinal hemorrhages)

1. Congestion of head and neck, such as in newborns, hanging, or choking

2. Trauma

3. Vascular obstruction, such as thrombosis, papilledema, or subarachnoid hemorrhages

4. Inflammatory conditions, such as perivasculitis

5. Toxic states, such as acute, febrile and infectious illnesses

6. Vascular disease, such as arteriosclerosis; atherosclerosis; the retinopathies, particularly diabetic and hypertensive, and when the circulation through the eye is diminished in hypotensive retinopathy, such as in carotid insufficiency or pulseless disease, and in conditions of extreme cachexia

7. Hemopoietic system, such as the anemias, leukemias, purpuras, polycythemia, and hemophilia; also following blood transfusion with incompatibility of blood groups

8. Vascularized neoplasms, including hereditary hemorrhagic telangiectasia (Rendu-Osler-Weber disease)

9. Drugs, such as anticoagulants and penicillamine

10. Sarcoidosis

11. Fat emboli

Bigger, I. F.: Retinal Hemorrhages during Penicillamine Therapy of Cystinuria. Amer. J. Ophthal. *66*:954–955, 1968.
Duke-Elder, S.: System of Ophthalmology, Vol. X. St. Louis, C. V. Mosby Co., 1967, pp. 137–145.

Large Hemorrhages in the Fundus of an Infant or Young Child (suggestive of increased intracranial pressure and paralysis of cranial nerves)

1. Subdural hematoma

2. Hygroma

3. Subarachnoid hemorrhage

Haessler, F. H.: Eye Signs in General Disease. Springfield, Ill., Charles C Thomas, 1960, pp. 95–96.

Retinovitreal Hemorrhage in a Young Adult

1. Sickle cell anemia
2. Prediabetes or diabetes mellitus
3. Incontinentia pigmenti (Bloch-Sulzberger syndrome)
4. Trauma

Duke-Elder, S.: System of Ophthalmology, Vol. X. St. Louis, C. V. Mosby Co., 1967, pp. 132–145.

Retinal Hemorrhage with Central White Spot

1. Septic retinitis
    A. Subacute bacterial endocarditis
    B. Rheumatic mitral and aortic valvulitis
    C. Syphilitis aortitis
    D. Phlebitis
    E. Viral pneumonia
    F. Kala-azar
    G. *Candida albicans* infection
    H. Rocky Mountain spotted fever

2. Hemopoietic system
    A. Anemias
    B. Leukemia
    C. Multiple myeloma

3. Diabetes mellitus

4. Vascular disease

5. Collagen disease

6. Intracranial hemorrhage (infants)

7. Cyanosis retinae—carcinoma of lung

8. Following heart operation

9. Vascular diseases

Duke-Elder, S.: Diseases of the Retina. System of Ophthalmology, Vol. X. St. Louis, C. V. Mosby Co., 1967, pp. 206–211, 373–400.
Leinfelder, P. J.: Ophthalmoscopy: An Investigative Challenge. Amer. J. Ophthal. 61:1211, 1966.
Leinfelder, P. J.: Ophthalmoscopy: Outline of Differential Diagnosis. In Current Concepts in Ophthalmology, Vol. III. St. Louis, C. V. Mosby Co., 1972, pp. 48–63.
Presley, G. D.: Fundus Changes in Rocky Mountain Spotted Fever. Amer. J. Ophthal. 67:263–267, 1969.

Microaneurysms of Retina (punctate red spots scattered over the region of the posterior pole)

* = Most important

*1. Diabetes mellitus

2. Hypertensive retinopathy

3. Associated with cotton-wool spots (see p. 419)

4. Venous occlusion—occlusion of central retinal vein or one of its branches (see p. 406)

5. Chronic uveitis

6. Macroglobulinemia

7. Sickle cell hemoglobin C disease

8. Hypotensive retinopathy, such as pulseless disease

9. Retinoblastoma

10. Variation of Coats' syndrome—Leber's miliary aneurysms with retinal degeneration

11. Venous stasis retinopathy, such as that secondary to carotid-occlusive disease

12. Leukemias—punctate hemorrhages

13. Aplastic anemia—punctate hemorrhage

14. Subacute bacterial endocarditis

15. Infection with *Loa loa*

16. Choroiditis

17. Eales' disease

18. Polycythemia

19. Component of aging

20. Fabry's disease

21. Osler's hemorrhagic telangiectasia

Duke-Elder, S.: Diseases of the Retina. System of Ophthalmology, Vol. X. St. Louis, C. V. Mosby Co., 1967, pp. 159–163.

Duke, J. R., Wilkinson, C. P., and Sigelman, S.: Retinal Microaneurysms in Leukemia. Brit. J. Ophthal. *52*:368–374, 1968.

Grace, E.: Diffuse Angiokeratosis (Fabry's Disease). Amer. J. Ophthal. *62*:139–145, 1966.

Leinfelder, P. J.: Ophthalmoscopy: An Investigative Challenge. Amer. J. Ophthal. *61*:1211, 1966.

Leinfelder, P. J.: Ophthalmoscopy: Outline of Differential Diagnosis. *In* Current Concepts in Ophthalmology, Vol. III. St. Louis, C. V. Mosby Co., 1972, pp. 48–63.

Macroaneurysms of the Retinal Arteries (found within the first three orders of bifurcation of arterioles; frequently associated with localized hemorrhage and exudation)

1. Hypertension
2. Generalized arteriosclerosis
3. Congenital
4. Idiopathic

Robertson, D. M.: Macroaneurysms of the Retinal Arteries. Trans. Amer. Acad. Ophthal. Otolaryng. 77:OP 55–67, 1973.

Retinitis Proliferans (growth of new vessels into the vitreous; hemorrhage and irritation are needed to stimulate the vessel formation)

1. Diabetes mellitus
2. Eales' disease
3. Retinal detachment with hemorrhage (see p. 408)
4. Hypertension (malignant and essential)
5. Sickle cell disease
6. Anemia and leukemia
7. Lupus erythematosus
8. Macroglobulinemia
9. Central retinal vein occlusion (see p. 406)
10. Trauma
11. Syphilis

Duke-Elder, S.: Diseases of the Retina. System of Ophthalmology, Vol. X. St. Louis, C. V. Mosby Co., 1967, pp. 150–152, 183, 408–445.

Predisposition to Rhegmatogenous (Perforated) Retinal Detachment

1. Aphakia

2. High myopia

3. Chorioretinitis

4. Peripheral retinal degeneration
   A. Vitreous base excavation
   B. Retinal hole
   C. Retinoschisis
   D. Cystic retinal tuft
   E. Zonular traction tuft
   F. Meridional folds
   G. Partial-thickness retinal tear
   H. Full-thickness retinal tear
   I. Lattice degeneration

5. Trauma—blunt and perforating, including operation for strabismus

Everett, W. G., and Katzin, D.: Meridional Distribution of Retinal Breaks in Aphakic Retinal Detachment. Amer. J. Ophthal. 66:928–932, 1968.

Feman, S. S., Hepler, R. S., and Straatsma, B. R.: Rhegmatogenous Retinal Detachment Due to Macular Hole. Arch. Ophthal. 91:371–372, 1974.

Foos, R. Y., Spencer, L. M., and Straatsma, B. R.: Trophic Degenerations of the Peripheral Retina. In Symposium on Retina and Retinal Surgery. Transactions of New Orleans Academy of Ophthalmology. St. Louis, C. V. Mosby, 1969, pp. 90–102.

Gottlieb, F., and Castro, J. L.: Perforation of the Globe During Strabismus Surgery. Arch. Ophthal. 84:151–157, 1970.

Hyams, S., and Neumann, E.: Peripheral Retina in Myopia. Brit. J. Ophthal. 53:300–306, 1969.

Spencer, L. M., Straatsma, B. R., and Foos, R. Y.: Tractional Degeneration of the Peripheral Retina. In Symposium on Retina and Retinal Surgery. Transactions of New Orleans Academy of Ophthalmology. St. Louis, C. V. Mosby, 1969, pp. 103–127.

Retinal Detachment (location and morphologic classification)

1. Equator
   A. Myopic type—equatorial horseshoe tear
   B. Equatorial type associated with lattice degeneration

2. Ora serrata
   A. Aphakic, with multiple small breaks often in nasal periphery
   B. Dialysis in young, lower temporal quadrant, often bilateral
   C. Giant dialysis, often bilateral

3. Posterior pole
   A. Macular breaks, rare
   B. Other breaks at posterior pole, from cellular proliferation in inner retinal surface

Pierce, L. H., Norton, E. W. D., Shafer, D. M., and Machemer, R.: Surgery of Retinal Detachment. Course 61. Amer. Acad. Ophthal., Sept. 1972.

Retinal Detachment (separation of the retina between the neural retina and the pigment epithelium)

1. Exudative
   A. Systemic disease
      (1) Hypertension—grade IV
      (2) Renal disease, including chronic glomerulonephritis or uremia
      (3) Toxemia of pregnancy
      (4) Blood diseases
         a. Sickle cell disease

      b. Dysproteinemias

      c. Leukemia

    (5) Polyarteritis nodosa

    (6) Extreme venous congestion, such as occurs during choking

    (7) Lupus erythematosus

    (8) Regional enteritis

    (9) Atopic dermatitis

 B. Ocular disease

    (1) Sympathetic ophthalmia

    (2) Harada's disease and Vogt-Koyanagi's syndrome

    (3) Scleritis or tenonitis (unusual)

    (4) Postinflammation of the orbit or sinuses, or cyclitis

    (5) Choroidal or retinal tumor

      a. Melanoma

      b. Hemangioma

      c. Retinoblastoma

      d. Metastasis—including that from breast, lung, and stomach

    (6) Uveal effusion syndrome

    (7) Toxocara infection

    (8) Lymphoid hyperplasia of the uveal tract

 C. Associated with retinal or choroidal vascular disease

    (1) von Hippel's disease

    (2) Coats' disease

      a. In juvenile

      b. In adult

    (3) Central serous choroidopathy

    (4) Detached pigment epithelium

    (5) Subpigment epithelial hemorrhage

    (6) Eales' disease

    (7) Postirradiation

2. Traction

 A. Pull of adherent and degenerated vitreous

 B. Organized vitreous band

    (1) Posthemorrhagic retinitis proliferans (see p. 413)

    (2) Sickle cell retinopathy

   (3) Hypertensive retinopathy
   (4) After vitreous hemorrhage
    a. Spontaneous
    b. Traumatic
  C. Postneovascularization of vitreous (see retinitis proliferans, p. 413)
   (1) Proliferative diabetic retinopathy
   (2) Eales' disease
   (3) Retrolental fibroplasia
   (4) Severe uveitis
  D. Congenital deformities, such as retinal dysplasia, coloboma, persistence of fetal vascular system, and pit of optic nerve
  E. Penetrating injury
  F. Postoperative retinal detachment with scar contracture

 3. Perforated (rhegmatogenous)
  A. Retinal degeneration at periphery
   (1) Pre-senile or myopic type
   (2) Lattice and paving-stone types
  B. Vitreous degeneration
  C. Myopia, including staphyloma
  D. Accommodation spasm, including strong miotics
  E. Trauma
   (1) Direct injury—perforating wound and foreign body
   (2) Indirect injury
   (3) Following cataract operation
  F. Equatorial or anterior choroiditis
  G. Retinoschisis—adult or juvenile
  H. Juxtapapillary microholes
  I. Hereditary ocular vitreoretinal degeneration and skeletal abnormality (cleft palate)

Ashrafzadeh, M. T., et al.: Aphakic and Phakic Retinal Detachment. Arch. Ophthal. *89*:476–483, 1973.
Duke-Elder, S.: Diseases of the Retina. System of Ophthalmology, Vol. X. St. Louis, C. V. Mosby Co., 1967, pp. 772–788.
Gass, J. D. M.: Bullous Retinal Detachment: an Unusual Manifestation of Idiopathic Central Serous Choroidopathy. Amer. J. Ophthal. *75*:810–821, 1973.

Jarrett, W. H., Green, W. R., Berlin, A. J., and Brawner, J. N.: Retinal Detachment as the Initial Manifestation of Carcinoma of the Lung. Trans. Amer. Acad. Ophthal. Otolaryng. 74:52–59, 1970.

Kanter, P. J., and Goldberg, M. F.: Bilateral Uveitis with Exudative Retinal Detachment. Arch. Ophthal. 91:13–19, 1974.

Knoblock, W. H., and Layer, J. M.: Clefting Syndromes Associated with Retinal Detachment. Amer. J. Ophthal. 73:517–530, 1972.

Norton, E. W. D.: Differential Diagnosis of Retinal Detachment. In Symposium on Retina and Retinal Surgery. Transactions of New Orleans Academy of Ophthalmology. St. Louis, C. V. Mosby Co., 1969, pp. 52–53.

Regenbagen, L., and Stein, R.: Retinal Detachments Due to Juxtapapillary Microholes. Arch. Ophthal. 80:155–160, 1968.

Wilson, R. S., and Dodson, J.: Giant Tear Dialysis in the Outer Layer of Retinoschisis. Arch. Ophthal. 88:336–340, 1972.

Retinal Folds

1. Proliferative retinal folds—inner layer outstrips outer layer

2. Traction folds
   A. Associated with remnants of hyaloid artery
   B. Secondary to vitreous traction
   C. Stage III—cicatricial form of retrolental fibroplasia

3. Falciform retinal fold (congenital retinal septum)

Duke-Elder, S.: System of Ophthalmology, Vol. III, Part 2. St. Louis, C. V. Mosby Co., 1964, pp. 634–639.

Cotton-Wool Spots (soft exudates) (fluffy, white, superficial deposits in the retina)

1. Untreated malignant hypertension

2. Toxemic retinopathy of pregnancy

3. Collagen diseases
    A. Disseminated lupus erythematosus
    B. Dermatomyositis
    C. Polyarteritis nodosa
    D. Diffuse scleroderma
    E. Scleromalacia perforans due to rheumatoid arthritis or rheumatic fever

4. Diabetic retinopathy

5. Anemic conditions
    A. Ligation of the carotid artery
    B. Severe systemic blood loss
    C. Hypotensive retinopathy
    D. Severe primary and secondary anemias
    E. Traumatic retinopathy due to fat embolism
    F. Gastric ulcer syndrome
    G. Following heart operation
    H. Cirrhosis of the liver

6. Dysproteinemia

7. Hodgkin's disease

8. Infective conditions
    A. Roth's septic retinitis
    B. Pneumonia
    C. Subacute bacterial endocarditis

9. Serum disease

10. Carcinomatous cachexia

11. Microemboli following cardiac operation

12. Carbon monoxide poisoning

13. Purtscher's retinopathy

14. Primary amyloidosis

15. Renal disease

16. Blood disease
    A. Leukemia
    B. Multiple myeloma
    C. Pernicious anemia
    D. Aplastic anemia

Bilchik, R. C., Muller-Beigh, H. A., and Freshman, M. E.: Ischemic Retinopathy Due to Carbon Monoxide Poisoning. Arch. Ophthal. *86*:142–144, 1971.

Duke-Elder, S.: Diseases of the Retina. System of Ophthalmology, Vol. X. St. Louis, C. V. Mosby Co., 1967, pp. 17–24.

Leinfelder, P. J.: Ophthalmoscopy. An Investigative Challenge. Amer. J. Ophthal. *61*:1211, 1966.

Leinfelder, P. J.: Ophthalmoscopy: Outline of Differential Diagnosis. *In* Current Concepts in Ophthalmology, Vol. III. St. Louis, C. V. Mosby Co., 1972, pp. 48–63.

Hard Exudates (yellowish white discrete masses deep in the retina)

1. Diabetes mellitus

2. Hypertensive disease

3. Coats' disease

4. Circinate retinopathy or xanthomatosis

Duke-Elder, S.: Diseases of the Retina. System of Ophthalmology, Vol. X. St. Louis, C. V. Mosby Co., 1967, pp. 30–34.

Retinal Exudate and Hemorrhage

1. von Hippel-Lindau, with absence of visible angioma

2. Coats' disease

3. Eales' disease

4. Multiple retinal aneurysms (Leber)

5. Capillary telangiectasis of retina (Reese)

6. Racemose hemangioma of the retina

Ballantyne, A. J., and Michaelson, I. C.: Textbook of the Fundus of the Eye, 2nd ed. Baltimore, Williams & Wilkins Co., 1972.

Pseudoretinitis Pigmentosa (pigment may be bone-corpuscular dots or heaped-up masses)

1. Retinitis pigmentosa—usually autosomal recessive but may be autosomal dominant or sex-linked
   A. Retinitis pigmentosa alone
   B. Retinitis pigmentosa associated with myopia, keratoconus, and/or glaucoma
   C. Usher's syndrome—retinitis pigmentosa, deaf-mutism
   D. Hallgren's syndrome—retinitis pigmentosa, congenital deafness, vestibulocerebellar ataxia, schizophrenia-like symptoms, mental deficiency
   E. Refsum's syndrome—atypical retinitis pigmentosa, polyneuritis, spinocerebellar ataxia
   F. Cockayne's syndrome—retinitis pigmentosa, dwarfism, deafness
   G. Bassen-Kornzweig syndrome—atypical retinitis pigmentosa, acanthocytosis, Friedreich's ataxia

H. Spielmeyer-Vogt syndrome—retinitis pigmentosa, multiple CNS manifestations

I. Kearns-Sayre syndrome—retinitis pigmentosa, heart block, progressive ophthalmoplegia externa

J. Laurence-Moon-Bardet-Biedl syndrome—retinitis pigmentosa, obesity, hypogenitalism, polydactyly, mental retardation

K. Hurler's syndrome (MPS I)—retinitis pigmentosa, corneal haze, gargoylism

L. Hunter's syndrome (MPS II)

M. Sanfilippo's disease (MPS III)

N. Scheie's disease (MPS V)—coarse features, corneal clouding, claw-hand deformity, short neck

2. Senile changes—degenerative pigmentation

3. Vascular lesion, such as occlusion of arteriole

4. Inflammatory
   A. Rubella (German measles)
   B. Rubeola (measles)
   C. Vaccinia
   D. Cytomegalic inclusion disease
   E. Behçet's disease
   F. Harada's disease
   G. Toxoplasmosis
   H. Onchocerciasis
   I. Syphilis
   J. Typhoid fever
   K. Polyarteritis nodosa
   L. Nematode endophthalmitis
   M. Chickenpox virus
   N. Influenza virus

5. Toxic
   A. Pregl's solution (Septojod)—(formerly used for treatment of puerperal sepsis)
   B. Diaminodiphenoxyalkanes—possible drug for treatment of schistosomiasis
   C. Phenothiazines
      (1) Chlorpromazine
      (2) Thioridazine (Mellaril)

D. Chloroquine and Atabrine

E. Sparsomycin

F. Indomethacin

G. Quinine

H. Accidental intraocular injection of depot corticosteroids

6. Cystinosis—peripheral pigment migration, bilateral, symmetrical

7. Sjögren-Larsson syndrome—congenital ichthyosis, spastic paralysis, mental retardation, degenerative retinitis

8. Lens dislocated into vitreous

9. Trauma, including blunt, penetrating, obstetrical, and radiotherapy

10. Cryogenic "pigmentary fall-out"—following use of cryosurgery for retinal detachment

11. Acute lymphocytic leukemia

12. Myotonic dystrophy

13. Progressive cone-rod degeneration

14. Pellagra

15. Waardenburg's syndrome—pigmentation in sector of hyperchromic iris

16. Leber's congenital amaurosis

17. Rud's syndrome—congenital ichthyosis with infantilism (hypophyseal deficiency) and epilepsy

Bernstein, H. N.: Some Iatrogenic Ocular Diseases from Systemically Administered Drugs. *In* Symposium on Ocular Pharmacology and Therapeutics. Transactions of the New Orleans Academy of Ophthalmology. St. Louis, C. V. Mosby Co., 1970, pp. 143–163.

Berson, E. L., Gouras, P., and Gunkel, R. D.: Progressive Cone-Rod Degeneration. Arch. Ophthal. *80*:68, 1968.

Betten, M. G., Bilchik, R. C., and Smith, M. E.: Pigmentary Retinopathy of Myotonic Dystrophy. Amer. J. Ophthal. *72*:720–723, 1971.

Davidorf, F. H.: Thioridazine Pigmentary Retinopathy. Arch. Ophthal. *90*:251–255, 1973.

Duke-Elder, S.: Diseases of the Retina. System of Ophthalmology, Vol. X. St. Louis, C. V. Mosby Co., 1966, pp. 530–533.

Clayman, H. M., et al.: Retinal Pigment Epithelial Abnormalities in Leukemic Disease. Amer. J. Ophthal. *74*:416–419, 1972.

Francois, J., Hanssens, M., Coppieters, R., and Evans, L.: Cystinosis —a Clinical and Histopathologic Study. Amer. J. Ophthal. *73*: 643–650, 1972.

Gellis, S. S., and Feingold, M.: Atlas of Mental Retardation Syndromes. Washington, D.C., U.S. Government Printing Office, 1968.

Goldberg, M. F.: Waardenburg's Syndrome with Fundus and Other Anomalies. Arch. Ophthal. *76*:797, 1966.

Kenyon, K. R., et al.: The Systemic Mucopolysaccharidoses. Amer. J. Ophthal. *73*:811–833, 1972.

McFalane, J. R., Yanoff, M., and Schiae, H. G.: Toxic Retinopathy Following Sparsomycin Therapy. Arch. Ophthal. *76*:532–540, 1966.

Mathur, S. P.: Maculopathy in Pellagra. Brit. J. Ophthal. *53*:350–351, 1969.

Metz, H. S., and Harkey, M. E.: Pigmentary Retinopathy Following Maternal Measles Infection. Amer. J. Ophthal. *66*:1107, 1968.

Moorman, L. T.: Cryogenic Surgery of the Retina. Trans. Pac. Coast Otoophthalmol. Soc. *48*:155–165, 1967.

Nooh, V. B.: Genetic Counseling in Retinitis Pigmentosa. Med. Col. Va. Qrt. *8*:283–285, 1972.

Schlaegel, T. F., and Wilson, F. M.: Accidental Intraocular Injection of Depot Corticosteroids Trans. Amer. Acad. Ophthal. Otolaryng. In press.

Smith, J. L.: The University of Miami Neuro-Ophthalmology Symposium, Vol. 1. Springfield, Ill., Charles C Thomas, 1964, p. 367.

Sorsby, A.: Ophthalmic Genetics, 2nd ed. New York, Appleton-Century-Crofts, Inc., 1970, pp. 165–176.

Wilson, F. M., Grayson, M., and Pierson, D.: Corneal Changes in Ectodermal Dysplasia: Case Report, Histopathology, and Differential Diagnosis. Amer. J. Ophthal. *75*:17–27, 1973.

Lesions Confused with Retinoblastoma

1. Coats' disease

2. Larval granulomatosis (*Toxocara canis*)

3. Retinal detachment due to choroidal or vitreous hemorrhage

4. Persistent primary vitreous

5. Glioma of the retina

6. Developmental retinal cyst

7. Retrolental fibroplasia

8. Retinal dysplasia (massive retinal fibrosis)

9. Uveitis in secondary retinal detachment

10. Rhegmatogenous and falciform retinal detachment

11. Oligodendroglioma of the retina

12. Norrie's disease

13. Juvenile retinoschisis

14. Retrolental membrane associated with Bloch-Sulzberger syndrome (incontinentia pigmenti)

15. 13-15 Trisomy

16. Metastatic endophthalmitis

17. Toxoplasmosis

18. Fetal rubella

19. Sex-linked microphthalmia

20. Organization of intraocular hemorrhage

21. Tumors other than retinoblastoma

22. Coloboma of choroid and optic disc

23. "White-with-pressure" sign

24. Juvenile xanthogranuloma

25. Anomalous optic disc

26. Cysts in a remnant of the hyaloid artery

27. Congenital corneal opacity

28. Secondary glaucoma

29. Tapetoretinal degeneration

30. Anterior dislocated lens with secondary glaucoma

31. Hematoma under retinal pigment epithelium

32. High myopia with advanced chorioretinal degeneration

33. Medullation of nerve fiber layer

34. Traumatic chorioretinitis

Boniuk, M., and Bishop, D. W.: Oligodendroglioma of the Retina. Survey Ophthal. *13*:284–289, 1969.

Hansen, A. C.: Norrie's Disease. Amer. J. Ophthal. *66*:328–332, 1968.

Howard, G. M.: Erroneous Clinical Diagnoses of Retinoblastoma and Uveal Melanoma. Trans. Amer. Acad. Ophthal. Otolaryng. *73*: 199–203, 1969.

Howard, G. M., and Ellsworth, R. M.: Differential Diagnosis of Retinoblastoma: A Statistical Survey of 500 Children. Amer. J. Ophthal. *60*:610, 1965.

Leelawongs, N., and Regan, C. D. J.: Retinoblastoma. Amer. J. Ophthal. *66*:1050–1060, 1968.

Single White Lesion of Retina

1. Retinoblastoma

2. Astrocytoma of tuberous sclerosis

3. Neurofibroma of von Recklinghausen

4. Glioma of optic nerve

5. Astrocytoma

6. Metastatic or direct extension of a tumor

7. Diktyoma

8. *Toxocara canis*

9. Amelanotic melanoma

10. Degeneration of retinal pigment epithelium

11. Hamartomas of the optic disc of retinitis pigmentosa

Duke-Elder, S.: Diseases of the Retina. System of Ophthalmology, Vol. X. St. Louis, C. V. Mosby Co., 1966, pp. 672, 736, 754, 766.
Robertson, D. M.: Hamartomas of the Optic Disc with Retinitis Pigmentosa. Amer. J. Ophthal. 74:526–531, 1972.

Pale Fundus Lesions

1. Generalized pallor
   A. Albinism—photophobia; defective vision; absence of pigment in iris, retina, and choroid
   B. Chediak-Higashi syndrome—rare, ocular albinism
   C. Waardenburg's syndrome—rare, pale fundus on side with hypochromic iris
   D. Choroideremia—rare; night blindness; contraction of visual fields; degeneration of pigment epithelium in periphery with exposure of choroidal vessels
   E. Myopia—thinning of retina and choroidal crescent at disc
   F. Retinal ischemia
      (1) Occlusion of retinal arteries—sudden onset of loss of vision; narrowing of arteries, sludging of blood column; retinal edema, cherry-red spot at macula
      (2) Spasm of retinal arteries—angiospasm: quinine, lead poisoning, migraine, or Raynaud's disease; sudden onset of loss of vision; narrowing of arteries, sludging of blood column; retinal edema; cherry-red spot at macula
      (3) Anemia—retinal edema, pallor of fundus, hemorrhages common
   G. Vascular retinopathies—hypertension, edema, hemorrhages, swelling of disc

427

H. Leukemia—creamy outlining of retinal vessels, engorgement of veins, hemorrhages with white centers

I. The lipidoses—pale area at posterior pole with cherry-red spot at macula, vessels become attenuated, optic atrophy and blindness
    (1) Congenital, rare
    (2) Infantile (Tay-Sachs disease)
    (3) Late infantile—2 to 4 years of age
    (4) Juvenile—5 to 8 years of age, optic atrophy
    (5) Adult—15 to 25 years of age, eyes may be normal or show some pigmented macular changes

J. Gaucher's disease—lipid deposit in cornea, conjunctiva, and choroid; edema of macula

K. Hereditary dystropic lipidosis (Fabry)

L. Hyperlipemia
    (1) Diabetes—rare, yellowish retinal and choroidal vessels
    (2) Essential hyperlipemic xanthomatosis—rare, yellowish retinal and choroidal vessels

M. Oguchi's disease—hereditary, Japanese, grayish-white fundus reflex

2. Localized pale areas
    A. Opaque nerve fibers—common, fan-shaped, glistening white sheets from optic disc; scotoma over affected region
    B. Retrolental fibroplasia—rare; excessive oxygen administration in treatment of prematurity; peripheral pallor; patches of retinal edema
    C. Localized retinal edema
        (1) Inflammation
        (2) Trauma
        (3) Vascular lesions
    D. Retinal detachment and schisis (see p. 415)
    E. Retinoblastoma
    F. Coats' disease—young males, yellow exudative lesions with vascular abnormalities, crystalline deposits common
    G. Coloboma—common, pale area with some pigment in region of fetal cleft

H. Normal fundus features—pale streaks mark site of ciliary nerves
I. Atrophic areas—diathermy, light coagulation, or cryosurgery
J. Scattered retinal exudates
    (1) Preretinal—severe posterior uveitis; discrete white spots, often most marked along vessels adjacent to a patch of choroiditis
    (2) Retinal
        a. Purtscher's compression syndrome—cotton-wool spots
        b. Fat emboli
        c. Hemangiomatosis—yellow exudates
        d. Hypertensive retinopathy—cotton-wool and hard exudates
        e. Toxemia of pregnancy
        f. Hypotensive retinopathy
        g. Pulseless disease
        h. Arterial occlusion
        i. Blood loss—cotton-wool spots
        j. Anemia (all types)
        k. Leukemia
        l. Purpura
        m. Macroglobulinemia
        n. Hodgkin's disease—soft exudates
        o. Diabetes—cotton-wool and hard exudates
        p. Hypercholesterolemia—lipid deposits
        q. Systemic lupus erythematosus
        r. Dermatomyositis—cotton-wool spots
        s. Polyarteritis nodosa
        t. Scleroderma
        u. Vitamin A deficiency—small white spots along course of retinal vessels, night blindness
        v. Retinal capillarosis—yellowish-white spots in substance of retina
        w. Leber's congenital retinal aplasia—bilateral blindness, multiple white specks
        x. Female carrier of retinitis pigmentosa—brilliant silvery reflex with shining yellow spots deep to retinal vessels

3. Dystrophic conditions
   A. Gyrate atrophy—rare, irregular atrophic areas with visual defects and night blindness
   B. Choroidal sclerosis—rare, diffuse peripapillary or central choroidal atrophy with larger choroidal vessels prominent
   C. Infarction or occlusion of ciliary arteries—rare, embolism (air, fat), injury, atrophic area with prominent choroidal vessels
   D. Pseudoinflammatory macular dystrophy—rare, fourth to sixth decades, central edema, hemorrhage and exudate, bilateral and symmetrical
   E. Helicoid peripapillary chorioretinal atrophy—rare, congenital and adult forms, star-shaped atrophic areas radiating from disc
   F. Retinitis punctata albescens—rare, onset in second and third decades, multiple discrete whitish dots which may appear crystalline, night blindness and field defects in progressive type
   G. Fundus flavimaculatus—rare, onset in second and third decades, yellow flecks deep in the retina
   H. Geographic choroiditis—rare, map-like pigmentary disturbance at posterior pole or more widespread over posterior fundus
   I. Doyne's honeycomb dystrophy—rare; middle age and older; colloidal deposits at posterior pole, with pigmentary or cystoid macular changes
   J. Progressive bifocal chorioretinal atrophy—atrophy temporal to disc, extending later; night blindness in late stage

Perkins, E. S., and Dobree, J. H.: The Differential Diagnosis of Fundus Conditions. St. Louis, C. V. Mosby Co., 1972, pp. 118–141.

Medullated Nerve Fibers (opaque white patch usually adjacent to and may cover disc, localized to one sector of the disc, peripapillary or arcuate with a peripheral, feathered edge)

1. Isolated finding
2. Autosomal recessive or dominant inheritance
3. Associated with:
     A. Myopia
     B. Coloboma of optic nerve or choroid
     C. Conus of disc
     D. Hyaloid remnants
     E. Macular colobomas
     F. Aplasia of macula
     G. Neurofibromatosis
     H. Cranial dysostosis (oxycephaly, dolichocephaly, brachycephaly, and craniofacial dysostosis)

Duke-Elder, S.: System of Ophthalmology, Vol. III, Part 2. St. Louis, C. V. Mosby Co., 1964, pp. 646–651.

Pigmented Lesion of the Fundus (single, dark, fundus lesion)

1. Retina
     A. Retinal detachment (see p. 415)
          (1) Macular, such as in central serous retinopathy
          (2) More extensive
          (3) Associated with uveitis, such as that associated with Vogt-Koyanagi-Harada syndrome
          (4) Hemorrhagic macrocyst

B. Retinoschisis
C. Macular degeneration of Kuhnt-Junius type
D. Chorioretinitis—either active choroiditis, sequela of choroiditis, or active effusive choroiditis with large bullous elevations of the retina
    (1) Peripheral
    (2) Macular
    (3) Peripapillary
E. Lesions of retinal pigment epithelium, such as those in the congenital group of pigmentation of the retina
F. Foreign body
G. Coats' disease
H. Peripheral giant cysts

2. Ciliary body and choroid
    A. Tumors
        (1) Metastatic carcinoma, such as that from the lungs, breast, testis, kidney, prostate gland, bladder
        (2) Hemangioma
        (3) Nevus
        (4) Neurilemomma
        (5) Neurofibroma
        (6) Malignant melanoma
    B. Detachment—serous or hemorrhagic (p. 415)
    C. Lymphoid hyperplasia
    D. Nodular choroidal hemorrhage
    E. Lymphoma and leukemias

3. Vitreous body
    A. Hemorrhage
    B. Abscess

4. Staphyloma of sclera

5. Optic nerve head (melanocytoma)

Ferry, A. P.: Lesions Mistaken for Malignant Melanoma of the Posterior Uvea. Arch. Ophthal. 72:463–469, 1964.
Hogan, M. J.: Clinical Aspects, Management, and Prognosis of Melanomas of the Uvea and Optic Nerve. Ocular and Adnexal Tumors, New and Controversial Aspects. St. Louis, C. V. Mosby Co., 1964, pp. 203–302.

Reese, A. B., and Jones, I. W.: The Differential Diagnosis of Malignant Melanoma of the Choroid. Arch. Ophthal. *58*:477–482, 1957.

Ruiz, R. S.: Hemorrhagic Macrocyst of the Retina. Arch. Ophthal. *83*:588, 1970.

Ryan, S. J., Zimmerman, L. E., and King, F. M.: Reactive Lymphoid Hyperplasia. Trans. Amer. Acad. Ophthal. Otolaryng. *76*:652–671, 1972.

Pigmented Fundus Lesions

1. Diffuse pigmentation
   A. Negroid fundus—accentuation of fundus pigmentation
   B. Melanosis bulbi—rare, pigmentation of external eye and fundus
   C. Nevus of Ota—rare, pigmentation of outer eye and diffuse pigmentation of fundus
   D. Waardenburg's syndrome—rare, patchy increased pigmentation in eyes with bi-colored iris

2. Single pigmented lesions
   A. Flat lesions
      (1) Benign melanoma—flat bluish, gray, or black lesion
      (2) Pigmented scar—flat patch of dense pigment, usually atrophic area in center
      (3) Fuchs' dark spot—dark spot in macular region with other atrophic changes
   B. Raised lesions
      (1) Simple detachment (see p. 415)
      (2) Malignant melanoma—raised pigmented lesion with secondary detachment, abnormal vessels
      (3) Choroidal hemorrhage—trauma, spontaneous in patients with vascular disease, high myopia
      (4) Exudative macular lesion—common, old age, subretinal exudate

        (5) Hemangioma of choroid—rare, raised grayish tumor near disc, secondary detachment later

        (6) Metastatic tumor—flattish tumor with little pigment, primary in breast, lung, etc.

3. Multiple pigmented lesions
   A. Scattered focal lesions
        (1) Congenital melanosis—cat's-paw patches of pigment in one sector of fundus
        (2) Postinflammatory—flat pigment with areas of atrophy
        (3) Hypertensive retinopathy—hypertensive vascular changes with scattered pigmentation
        (4) Siegrist's streaks—rare, chain of pigment spots along sclerosed choroidal vessel
        (5) Paravenous retinochoroidal atrophy—paravenous pigmentation with chorioretinal atrophy
        (6) Incontinentia pigmenti (Bloch-Sulzberger syndrome)—blotchy pigmentation and depigmentation, retrolental mass in some cases
        (7) Retinal detachment from cryosurgery
   B. Widely disseminated pigmentary changes
        (1) Genetic conditions
           a. Typical retinitis pigmentosa—attenuation of retinal vessels, optic atrophy (myopia, posterior polar cataract, keratoconus)
           b. Atypical retinitis pigmentosa—rare, little or no pigment, pigment in clumps
           c. Retinitis pigmentosa syndromes
              1. Laurence-Moon-Biedl—common, obesity, oligophrenia, hypogenitalism, polydactyly
              2. Cockayne's—deafness, dwarfism, progeria oligophrenia
              3. Hallgren's—rare, deafness, ataxia, mental deficiency
              4. Pelizaeus-Merzbacher—rare, retinitis pigmentosa, nystagmus and constant ocular movement, ataxia, dwarfism
              5. Myotonic dystrophy—rare, ptosis, lens changes, retinitis pigmentosa, sometimes with macular changes

6. Kearn's—rare, retinitis pigmentosa and myopathy, external ophthalmoplegia
7. Lignac-Fanconi (cystinosis)—rare, retinitis pigmentosa
8. Leber's congenital retinal aplasia—rare, blindness from birth, retina may appear normal or show pepper-and-salt pigmentation

(2) Infectious conditions—secondary retinitis pigmentosa
   a. Syphilis (congenital)—pepper-and-salt pigmentation, interstitial keratitis
   b. Syphilitic neuroretinitis—rare, retinitis pigmentosa
   c. Rubella—cataract, secondary retinitis pigmentosa (non-progressive)
   d. Vaccinia—rare, retinitis pigmentosa, history of vaccination

(3) Metabolic disturbances
   a. Refsum's syndrome—rare, retinitis pigmentosa with nystagmus, polyneuritis cerebellar ataxia
   b. Bassen-Kornzweig syndrome—rare, retinitis pigmentosa, celiac disease

(4) Toxic conditions, such as chloroquine, phenothiazine derivatives; usually central pigmentation; corneal and lens change

Hilton, G. F.: Subretinal Pigment Migration: Effects of Cryosurgical Retinal Reattachment. Arch. Ophthal. *91*:445–450, 1974.
Perkins, E. S., and Dobree, J. H.: The Differential Diagnosis of Fundus Conditions. St. Louis, C. V. Mosby Co., 1972, pp. 158–171.

Cholesterol Emboli of Retina (Hollenhorst plaques) (bright-orange plaques often observed at the bifurcation of arterioles, indicative of generalized atherosclerosis and should signal ophthalmologist to measure retinal artery pressures and refer patient for general medical evaluation)

1. New or old strokes or transient attacks of cerebral ischemia

2. Coronary heart disease with myocardial infarct or angina

3. Peripheral atherosclerosis obliterans, popliteal or femoral aneurysms

4. Torsion and calcification of aorta (x ray)

5. Bruits in one or both carotid arteries

6. Calcification of internal carotids (x ray)

7. Abdominal aortic aneurysms

8. Retinal arterial occlusions (see p. 395)

9. Arteriography showing occlusions in one or more cervical arteries

10. Congestive heart failure

11. Atrial fibrillation

12. Renal artery occlusions

13. Aortic stenosis

14. Bleeding duodenal or gastric ulcer

15. Vocal cord paralysis (aortic arch aneurysm)

16. Diabetes mellitus

Hollenhorst, R. W.: Vascular Status of Patients Who Have Cholesterol Emboli in the Retina. Amer. J. Ophthal. *61*:1159–1165, 1966.

Pfaffenbach, D. D., and Hollenhorst, R. W.: Morbidity and Survivorship of Patients with Embolic Cholesterol Crystals in the Ocular Fundus. Amer. J. Ophthal. *75*:66–72, 1973.

Wylie, E. J., and Ehrenfeld, W. K.: Extracranial Occlusive Cerebrovascular Disease: Diagnosis and Management. Philadelphia, W. B. Saunders Co., 1970, pp. 64–95.

	Platelet-Fibrin	Cholesterol-Lipid	Calcific or Fibrinoid
Color	White, non-reflective	Orange-yellow, orange or bright metallic gold; variable color	Gray-white, dull and non-reflective
Shape	Long, smooth segments with flat discrete ends; homogeneous	(a) Globular, containing bright crystals with indistinct interface with blood; (b) small, rectangular flakes alone	Ovoid, discrete, and filling arterial lumen
Apparent caliber	Same as blood column	Larger than blood column	Same or slightly larger than proximal blood column
Mobility	Highly mobile; jerks from one bifurcation to the next	Ameboid-gelatinous movement with massage of eye. Move or break up over period of days	Fixed
Location in retinal artery	Usually in motion	At bifurcations of medium and small vessels, unless large and mixed with stable fibrin	In unbranched segments of main or medium-sized retinal arteriole
Ischemic	Transient slowing of blood flow, no infarction	Dilated vein indicating mild hypoxia. Retinal infarction from multiple plaques is variable in density and without clear borders	Usually produce dense, sharply delimited retinal infarct. Small ischemic hemorrhages
Vessel change	No damage seen	Gray-white segmental mural opacity at bifurcation; slow appearance	Segmental mural changes with narrowing, collateral capillary shunt, or both
Source and significance	Mural or "tail" thrombus in carotid occlusion (acute or imminent)	Eroding atheroma in carotid bifurcation; carotid patent and often without stenosis	Calcific valvular disease (apparent in x ray of heart), rheumatic heart disease, myocardial disease

Wylie, E. J., and Ehrenfeld, W. K.: Extracranial Occlusive Cerebrovascular Disease: Diagnosis and Management. Philadelphia, W. B. Saunders Co., 1970, p. 81.

15

Lipemia Retinalis (arterioles and venules are similar in color and appear orange-yellow to white)

1. Primary hyperlipoproteinemia
   A. Type I—familial fat-induced hyperlipoproteinemia (hyperchylomicronemia)
   B. Type III—familial hyper-beta- and hyper-pre-beta-lipoproteinemia (carbohydrate-induced hyperlipemia)
   C. Type IV—familial hyper-pre-beta-lipoproteinemia (carbohydrate-induced hyperlipemia)
   D. Type V—familial hyperchylomicronemia with hyper-pre-beta-lipoproteinemia (mixed hyperlipemia)

2. Diabetes mellitus with hyperlipemia

3. Secondary hyperlipoproteinemia
   A. Insulin-deficient diabetes mellitus
   B. Hypothyroidism
   C. Nephrotic syndrome
   D. Biliary obstruction
   E. Chronic pancreatitis
   F. Glycogen storage disease
   G. Hypergammaglobinemia
   H. Malignant neoplasms
   I. Idiopathic hypercalcemia
   J. Progressive lipodystrophy
   K. Chronic renal failure
   L. Coats' disease in adults

Blodi, F. C., and Yarbrough, J. C.: Ocular Manifestations of Familial Hypercholesterolemia. Amer. J. Ophthal. *55*:714–720, 1963.

Imre, G.: Coats' Disease and Hyperlipemic Retinitis. Amer. J. Ophthal. *64*:726–728, 1967.

Spaeth, G. L.: Ocular Manifestations of the Lipidoses. *In* Tasman, W. (Ed.): Retinal Diseases in Children. New York, Harper & Row, 1971, pp. 127–206.

Hemorrhagic or Serous Exudates Beneath Pigment Epithelium

1. Histoplasmosis

2. Macular drusen

3. Doyne's honeycomb macular degeneration

4. Best's macular degeneration

5. Coats' disease

6. Angioid streaks

7. Solid neoplasms

8. Myopia

9. Trauma

Gitter, K. A., et al.: Traumatic Hemorrhagic Detachment of Retinal Pigment Epithelium. Arch. Ophthal. 79:729–732, 1968.

Retinal Vascular Tumors and Angiomatosis Retinae Syndromes

1. Retinal telangiectasis (Leber's miliary aneurysms)—telangiectasia retinae of Reese

2. Cavernous retinal hemangioma—intraretinal angiomas

3. Racemose angioma—with arteriovenous anomalies of central nervous system (Wyburn-Mason syndrome)

4. Coats' disease

5. Bonnet-Dechaune-Blanc—arteriovenous retinal angiomas, papilledema, reduced corneal sensitivity, anisocoria, strabismus, angiomas in mesencephalon and thalamus, facial angiomas, hydrocephalus, slow speech, hemiplegia, neurologic symptoms

6. von Hippel-Lindau—retinal angiomatosis, vascular proliferation, retinal detachment, secondary glaucoma, cerebral angiomatosis, epilepsy, psychic disturbances, dementia

7. Sturge-Weber—chorioretinal angiomas, vascular proliferation, glioma, retinal detachment, conjunctival telangiectases, glaucoma, "portwine" nevus, cerebral angiomas, hemiparesis, hemiatrophy, mental retardation, epilepsy

8. Associated with pheochromocytoma

Gass, J. D. M.: Cavernous Hemangioma of the Retina. Amer. J. Ophthal. *71*:799–814, 1971.

Geeraets, W. J.: Ocular Syndromes, 2nd ed. Philadelphia, Lea & Febiger, 1969, p. 284.

McDonald, P. R., and Sarin, C. K.: Treatment of Intraretinal Angiomas. Amer. J. Ophthal. *71*:298–302, 1971.

Traumatic Retinopathies

	Purtscher's Retinopathy	Commotio Retinae	Traumatic Asphyxia	Fat Embolism
Type of trauma	Chest compression	Local	Chest	Fractures
Accompanying signs	None	None	Cyanosis	Chest, cerebral, and cutaneous signs
Onset of systemic picture	None	None	Immediate	Symptom-free, 48-hour interval
Initial vision	Variable	20/200	Variable	Occasionally reduced
Duration of loss of vision	Several weeks	Days	Several weeks	Several weeks
Ultimate vision	Normal	Normal	Variable	Normal
External eye	Normal	Contused	Hemorrhage	Normal or petechiae
Fundus picture	Exudates and hemorrhage	Retinal edema	Normal or hemorrhage	Exudates, edema, and hemorrhages
Onset of fundus abnormalities	Within 1 to 2 days	A few hours	Immediate or a few hours	After 1 to 2 days

Marr, W. G., and Marr, E. G.: Some Observations on Purtscher's Disease: Traumatic Retinal Angiopathy. Amer. J. Ophthal. *54*:693, 1962.
 For further information see Kelley, J. S.: Purtscher's Retinopathy Related to Chest Compression by Safety Belts. Amer. J. Ophthal. *74*:278–283, 1972.

Retinal "Sea-Fans" (vasoproliferative lesions with a characteristic fan-shaped appearance; "parachute" lesion)

1. Sickle cell thalassemia

2. Sickle cell disease (SS, SC, and SA)

3. Retrolental fibroplasia (RLF)

4. Diabetes mellitus

5. Chronic myelocytic leukemia

Frank, R. N., and Ryan, S. J.: Peripheral Retinal Neovascularization with Chronic Myelogenous Leukemia. Arch. Ophthal. 87:585–589, 1972.

Goldberg, M. F.: Classification and Pathogenesis of Proliferative Sickle Retinopathy. Amer. J. Ophthal. 71:649, 1971.

L'Esperance, F. A.: Argon Laser Photocoagulation of Diabetic Retinal Neovascularization. Trans. Amer. Acad. Ophthal. Otolaryng. 77:OP6–24, 1973.

Morse, P. H., and McCready, J. L.: Peripheral Retinal Neovascularization in Chronic Myelocytic Leukemia. Amer. J. Ophthal. 72:975–978, 1971.

Welsh, R. B., and Goldberg, M. F.: Sickle-Cell Hemoglobin and Its Relation to Fundus Abnormality. Arch. Ophthal. 75:353, 1966.

Retinal Vessels Displaced Temporally

1. Retrolental fibroplasia (RLF)

2. Sickle cell disease

3. Familial vitreous retinopathy

4. Myopia with lattice-like retinal degeneration

5. Hamartomas

6. Trauma

7. Inflammation

Gass, J. D. M.: Personal communication.

Retinal Vessels Displaced Nasally

1. Trauma

2. Inflammation

3. Glaucoma

4. Axial myopia

Keeney, A. H.: Ocular Examination: Basis and Technique. St. Louis, C. V. Mosby Co., 1970, pp. 165–170.

Peripheral Fundus Lesions

1. Pale raised lesions
    A. Vitreous opacities—white fluffy or discrete opacities, associated with pars planitis or sarcoid uveitis
    B. Retrolental fibroplasia—excessive oxygen administration in treatment of prematurity, retinal edema and dense white lesions with neovascularization
    C. Toxocariasis—young children, close contact with dogs; vitreous opacities with peripheral granuloma
    D. Leprosy—Africa and Asia, peripheral exudates with anterior uveal involvement

E. Vitreoretinal dystrophies—rare, bands in vitreous with retinoschisis or retinal detachment

F. Angiomatosis—rare, retinal tumor with enlarged, feeding vessels

G. Retinoblastoma—rare, raised creamy-white fluffy lesion without inflammatory signs

2. Flat lesions

    A. Coloboma—rare, pale area with pigmented edge in region of fetal cleft

    B. Chorioretinitis

        (1) Disseminated, congenital syphilis—pepper-and-salt or larger confluent lesions

        (2) Toxoplasmosis—pigmented scars of old lesions

        (3) Cytomegalic inclusion disease—infants, localized chorioretinitis or general peripheral infiltration

        (4) Histoplasmosis—peripheral punched-out lesions with or without pigmentation

    C. Peripheral degenerations

        (1) Senile changes—75% of eyes older than 50 years of age, depigmented areas with pigmented margins (cobblestone degeneration)

        (2) Secondary pigmentary degeneration—peripheral pigmentary changes similar to senile type or to retinitis pigmentosa

        (3) Cystoid degeneration—multiple cystic spaces and thin areas in peripheral retina

        (4) Lattice degeneration—lacework of white lines with depigmented and pigmented patches

        (5) Cystinosis—granular rings of pigment in periphery of fundus, similar to cobblestone degeneration

3. Dark raised lesions

    A. Choroidal detachment (see page 456)

        (1) Spontaneous—slowly progressive detachment, no inflammatory signs

        (2) Postoperative—intraocular operation, particularly for cataract and glaucoma; shallow anterior chamber; leaking wound

(3) Exudative
    a. Inflammatory—shallow anterior chamber, myopia and peripheral detachment
    b. Vascular—nephritis, hypertension, toxemia of pregnancy, polyarteritis nodosa, leukemia
    c. Tumors—intraocular tumors; tumors of orbit and lacrimal gland
    d. Traumatic—contusion injuries, perforating wounds, hypotony, anterior chamber may be shallow or deep if perforation occurs posteriorly

B. Exudative retinal detachment (see p. 415)
    (1) Secondary to general disease with retinopathy—hypertension, toxemia of pregnancy, leukemia, dysproteinemia, polyarteritis nodosa, rickettsial arteritis, venous congestion
    (2) Secondary to local disease of the eye—inflammatory signs with exudative detachment, Harada's disease, sympathetic ophthalmitis, scleritis, tenonitis, choroidal tumor

C. Simple detachment—myopia in two thirds of patients, trauma, may follow cataract extraction or discission for congenital cataract

D. Cysts
    (1) Ciliary body—larger cysts usually push iris forward; rarely, cyst extends backward to be seen ophthalmoscopically
    (2) Pars plana—may enlarge and appear as a multilocular reddish-brown cyst

E. Scleral indentation—retinal detachment operation

F. Neoplasms of ciliary body
    (1) Benign epithelioma—brown spot 1 to 5 mm in diameter on surface of ciliary body
    (2) Other tumors—diktyoma, leiomyoma, reticuloses, neurofibroma, malignant melanoma, rare, usually present as a mass protruding through root of iris, may cause glaucoma, dark bulge seen ophthalmoscopically, lens changes adjacent to tumor

G. Neoplasms of choroid
  (1) Congenital melanosis—cat's-paw patches of pigment in one sector of fundus
  (2) Benign melanoma—flat bluish gray or black lesion
  (3) Malignant melanoma—raised pigmented lesion with secondary detachment
  (4) Secondary metastatic—rare, primary lesion in breast, lung, etc.
4. Vascular lesions
  A. Periphlebitis (Eales' disease)—common; young adults; sheathing of peripheral veins; hemorrhages in new vessels and later retinal detachment
  B. Perivasculitis secondary to uveitis—perivascular infiltration, particularly in pars planitis, sarcoidosis, Behçet's disease, and toxoplasmosis
  C. Systemic diseases
    (1) Rickettsiae—engorgement of veins, retinal edema, hemorrhages, and exudates
    (2) Multiple sclerosis—sheathing of veins
    (3) Polyarteritis nodosa—hemorrhages, exudates, and serous detachment of retina
    (4) Tuberculin or BCG inoculation—rare, sheathing of peripheral veins with hemorrhages
    (5) Sickle cell retinopathy—dilatation of peripheral veins, hemorrhages and connective tissue sheets in periphery, new vessel formation

Perkins, E. S., and Dobree, J. H.: The Differential Diagnosis of Fundus Conditions. St. Louis, C. V. Mosby Co., 1972, pp. 172–191.

Retinal Disease Associated with Corneal Problems

1. Syphilis—interstitial keratitis and chorioretinitis
2. Bietti's marginal crystalline dystrophy with retinitis punctata albescens

3. Leber's infantile tapetoretinal degeneration with keratoconus

4. Atopic keratoconus and retinal detachment

5. Refsum's syndrome—band keratopathy and retinitis pigmentosa

6. Hydrotic ectodermal dysplasia—juvenile macular degeneration

7. Behçet's—posterior corneal abscess and retinal vascular changes

8. Rubella—microcornea and pigmentary retinal changes

9. Chloroquine—corneal epithelial pigmentation and macular lesions

10. Phenothiazine—epithelial and endothelial pigmentation and retinal pigmentation

11. Cystinosis—crystals in cornea and pigment in retina

12. Mucopolysaccharidosis—Hurler's (MPS I), Hunter's (MPS II), Sanfilippo's (MPS III), and Scheie's (MPS V)

13. Fabry's disease—whorl-like changes in cornea and vascular changes in retina

14. Cryoglobulinemia—deep corneal opacities and venous stasis

15. Hypercholesterolemia—xanthoma and lipemia retinalis

16. Myotonic dystrophy—keratoconjunctivitis sicca and white streaks on retina

17. Idiopathic hypercalcemia—band keratopathy, optic atrophy, and papilledema

18. Ischemic necrosis—edema of cornea and midperipheral hemorrhages

19. Tuberous sclerosis—corneal deposits and retinal tumors

20. Neurofibromatosis—corneal tumors and retinal tumors

21. Marfan's syndrome—keratoconus and retinitis pigmentosa

22. Ehlers-Danlos—keratoconus and angioid streaks

23. 13-15 Trisomy—malformed cornea and retinal dysplasia

24. Sarcoidosis—corneal opacity and wax-candle lesions

25. Norrie's disease—malformation of sensory cells of retina with deafness, mental retardation, and persistent hyperplastic vitreous associated with corneal nebulae

Grayson, M., and Keates, R. H.: Manual of Diseases of the Cornea. Boston, Little, Brown & Co., 1969, p. 297.

Retinal Lesions Associated with Deafness

1. Rubella (German measles)—cardiac disorders, cataract, salt-and-pepper pigmentation

2. Hunter's syndrome—atypical retinitis pigmentosa

3. Waardenburg's syndrome—pigmentation corresponds to same sector as iris heterochromia

4. Harada's syndrome

5. Alport's syndrome—fundus albi punctatus

6. Cockayne's syndrome—retinal pigmentary degeneration

7. Dialinas-Amalric syndrome—retinal pigmentary degeneration

8. Hollgren's syndrome—retinitis pigmentosa

9. Laurence-Moon-Bardet-Biedl syndrome—retinitis pigmentosa, polydactyly, obesity, and hypogonadism

10. Usher's syndrome—retinitis pigmentosa

11. Refsum's syndrome—retinitis pigmentosa, ataxia, polyneuropathy

12. Syphilis—acquired or congenital

448

13. Norrie's disease—mental retardation, X-linked retinal malformation, and hearing loss

14. Alström's disease—retinitis pigmentosa

15. Retinal vessel changes, muscular dystrophy, mental retardation, and hearing loss

Geeraets, W. J.: Ocular Syndromes. Philadelphia, Lea & Febiger, 1969.

Konigsmark, B. W., et al.: Dominant Congenital Deafness and Progressive Optic Nerve Atrophy. Arch. Ophthal. 91:99–103, 1974.

Roy, F. H., et al.: Ocular Manifestations of Congenital Rubella Syndrome. Arch. Ophthal. 75:601, 1966.

CHOROID

Contents

Angioid Streaks (ruptures of Bruch's membrane characterized ophthalmoscopically by brownish lines surrounding the disc and radiating toward the periphery)

1. Senile (actinic) elastosis of the skin
2. Pseudoxanthoma elasticum (Grönblad-Strandberg syndrome)
3. Fibrodysplasia hyperelastica (Ehlers-Danlos syndrome)
4. Osteitis deformans (Paget's disease)
5. Cardiovascular disease with hypertension
6. Sickle cell disease
7. Diffuse lipomatosis
8. Dwarfism
9. Acromegaly
10. Pituitary tumor
11. Epilepsy
12. Lead poisoning
13. Hyperphosphatemia
14. Thrombocytopenic purpura
15. Facial angiomatosis
16. Previous choroidal detachment
17. Francois' dyscephalic syndrome

Duke-Elder, S., and Perkins, E. S.: Diseases of the Uveal Tract. System of Ophthalmology, Vol. IX. St. Louis, C. V. Mosby Co., 1966, pp. 722–727.

Francois, J., and Pierard, J.: The Francois Dyscephalic Syndrome and Skin Manifestations. Amer. J. Ophthal. 71:1241–1250, 1971.

Gerde, L. S.: Angioid Streaks in Sickle Cell Trait Hemoglobinopathy. Amer. J. Ophthal. 77:462–464, 1974.

Kalina, R. E.: Facial Angiomatosis with Angioid Streaks. Arch. Ophthal. 84:528, 1970.

Krill, A. E., Klien, B., and Archer, D.: Precursors of Angioid Streaks. Amer. J. Ophthal. 76:875–879, 1973.

Paton, D.: The Relation of Angioid Streaks to Systemic Disease. Springfield, Ill., Charles C Thomas, 1972.

Zagora, E.: Eye Injuries. Springfield, Ill., Charles C Thomas, 1970, p. 24.

Choroidal Folds (folds of the posterior pole, at the level of the choroid, with Hruby lens and a pattern of alternating light lines on fluorescein angiography)

1. Idiopathic—no underlying pathologic state

2. High hyperopia

3. Orbital mass

4. Postoperative condition, such as scleral buckle

5. Choroidal tumor, such as a melanoma

6. Primary retinal detachment

7. Posteriorly located choroidal detachment

8. Long-standing orbital inflammation

9. Infection of paranasal sinuses

10. Graves' disease

11. Ocular hypotony

12. Uveitis

13. Papilledema

14. Disciform degeneration

15. Exophthalmos

Hyvarinea, L., and Walsh, F. B.: Benign Chorioretinal Folds. Amer. J. Ophthal. 70:14–17, 1970.

Kroll, A. J., and Norton, E. W. D.: Regression of Choroidal Folds. Trans. Amer. Acad. Ophthal. Otolaryng. 74:515–525, 1970.

Newell, F. W.: Choroidal Folds. Amer. J. Ophthal. 75:930–942, 1973.

Norton, E. W. D.: A Characteristic Fluorescein Angiographic Pattern in Choroidal Folds. Proc. Royal Soc. Med. 62:119–128, 1969.

Pannu, J. S., and Lawson, L. J.: Acute Transient Chorioretinal Folds. Ann. Ophthal. 5:880–882, 1973.

Wolter, J. R.: Parallel Horizontal Choroidal Folds Secondary to an Orbital Tumor. Amer. J. Ophthal. 77:669–673, 1974.

Lesions Confused with Malignant Melanoma

1. Retina
    A. Retinal detachment
        (1) Macular
        (2) More extensive
    B. Retinoschisis
    C. Disciform macular degeneration
    D. Chorioretinitis
    E. Lesions of pigment epithelium
    F. Foreign body
    G. Hemorrhagic macrocyst of retina

2. Ciliary body and choroid
    A. Tumors
        (1) Metastatic carcinoma
        (2) Hemangioma
        (3) Nevus
        (4) Neurilemmoma
        (5) Neurofibroma
        (6) Melanocytoma
    B. Detachment
    C. Lymphoid hyperplasia
    D. Nodular
    E. Choroiditis
    F. Angioid streaks
    G. Leukemia and lymphoma
    H. Uveal effusion
    I. Sclero-uveitis
    J. Coats' disease

3. Vitreous body
    A. Hemorrhages
    B. Abscess

4. Optic nerve head
    A. Melanocytoma
    B. Congenital crater

Berkow, J. W., and Font, R. L.: Disciform Macular Degeneration with Subpigment Epithelial Hematoma. Arch. Ophthal. *82*:51–56, 1969.

Ferry, A. P.: Lesions Mistaken for Malignant Melanoma of the Posterior Uvea. Arch. Ophthal. *72*:463–469, 1964.

Howard, G. M.: Erroneous Clinical Diagnoses of Retinoblastoma and Uveal Melanomas. Trans. Amer. Acad. Ophthal. Otolaryng. *73*:199–203, 1969.

Reese, A. B., and Jones, I. S.: The Differential Diagnosis of Malignant Melanomas of the Choroid. Arch. Ophthal. *58*:477, 1957.

Ruiz, R. S.: Hemorrhagic Macrocyst of the Retina, Mistaken for Malignant Melanoma of the Choroid. Arch. Ophthal. *83*:588–590, 1970.

Ryan, S. J., Zimmerman, L. E., and King, F. M.: Reactive Lymphoid Hyperplasia. Trans. Amer. Acad. Ophthal. Otolaryng. *76*:652–671, 1972.

Shields, J. A., and Font, R. L.: Melanocytoma of the Choroid Clinically Simulating a Malignant Melanoma. Arch. Ophthal. *87*:396–400, 1972.

Shields, J. A., and Zimmerman, L. E.: Lesions Simulating Malignant Melanoma of the Posterior Uvea. Arch. Ophthal. *89*:466–471, 1973.

Susac, J. O., Smith, J. L., and Scelfo, R. J.: The "Tomato-Catsup" Fundus in Sturge-Weber Syndrome. Arch. Ophthal. *92*:69–70, 1974.

Zimmerman, L. E.: Problems in the Diagnosis of Malignant Melanoma of the Choroid and Ciliary Body. Amer. J. Ophthal. *75*:917–929, 1973.

Localized Choroidal Hemorrhage

1. Acute choroiditis
2. Choroidal vascular sclerosis, such as senile macular degeneration with hemorrhage (disciform degeneration of the macula)
3. Myopia—accompanied by choroidal atrophy
4. Papilledema—rare
5. General diseases
   A. Arteriosclerosis
   B. Blood dyscrasias

        (1) Pernicious anemia
        (2) Purpura
        (3) Leukemia
    C. Diabetes mellitus
    D. Paget's disease

Duke-Elder, S., and Perkins, E. S.: Diseases of the Uveal Tract. System of Ophthalmology, Vol. IX. St. Louis, C. V. Mosby Co., 1966, pp. 26–27.
Winslow, R. L., Stevenson, W., and Yanoff, M.: Spontaneous Expulsive Choroidal Hemorrhage. Arch. Ophthal. *92*:33–36, 1974.

Choroidal Detachment (may be differentiated from retinal detachment and tumor by solid appearance, smooth surface, and the appearance of normal retinal vessels with color unchanged and good transillumination)

1. Inflammatory disease
    A. Scleritis and tenonitis
    B. Chronic cyclitis
    C. Harada's disease
    D. Sympathetic ophthalmitis
    E. Acute sinusitis
    F. Orbital abscess

2. Vascular diseases
    A. Hypertension
    B. Toxemia of pregnancy
    C. Diabetes mellitus
    D. Nephritis
    E. Syphilitic vascular disease
    F. Periarteritis nodosa
    G. Leukemia
    H. Multiple myeloma

3. Neoplastic disease
    A. Orbital tumor

B. Leukemia

C. Intraocular tumor, such as metastatic or malignant melanoma

4. Trauma

   A. Contusion of globe without perforation

   B. Following perforation injury including that due to perforating corneal ulcer

   C. In phthisical eye with traction of organized inflammatory tissue

5. Acute ocular hypotony (see p. 279)

   A. Operative or perforating wounds, including those required for surgical treatment of cataract, glaucoma, grafting of cornea, and retinal detachment

   B. Myopia

   C. Severe uveitis with severe visual loss, intense ocular pain, unusually low tension, and extremely deep anterior chamber in women

6. Spontaneous detachment associated with uveal effusion, such as non-rhegmatogenous retinal detachment, shifting subretinal fluid, and peripheral annular choroidal detachment affecting males almost exclusively

Chignell, A. H.: Choroidal Detachment Following Retinal Detachment Surgery without Drainage of Subretinal Fluid. Amer. J. Ophthal. 73:860–862, 1972.

Duke-Elder, S., and Perkins, E. S.: Diseases of the Uveal Tract. System of Ophthalmology, Vol. IX. St. Louis, C. V. Mosby Co., 1966, pp. 949–960.

Gottlieb, F.: Combined Choroidal and Retinal Detachment. Arch. Ophthal. 88:481–486, 1972.

Kreiger, A. E., Meyer, D., Smith, T. R., and Riemer, K.: Metastatic Carcinoma to the Choroid with Choroidal Detachment. Arch. Ophthal. 82:209–213, 1969.

Scheie, H. G., and Morse, P. H.: Shallow Anterior Chamber as a Sign of Non-surgical Choroidal Detachment. Ann. Ophthal. 6:317–322, 1974.

Schepens, C. L., and Brockhurst, R. J.: Uveal Effusion. Arch. Ophthal. 70:189–201, 1963.

Seelenfreund, M. H., et al.: Choroidal Detachment Associated with Primary Retinal Detachment. Arch. Ophthal. 91:254–258, 1974.

Swyers, E. M.: Choroidal Detachment Immediately Following Cataract Extraction. Arch. Ophthal. 88:632–634, 1972.

Conditions Simulating Posterior Uveitis or Choroiditis

1. Jensen's disease (juxtapapillary retinopathy)

2. Ischemic optic neuropathy (vascular pseudopapillitis)

3. Relapsing polychondritis

4. Primary familial amyloidosis

5. Opacities of the macular retina
   A. Lipoid deposits
   B. Inspissated exudates
   C. Glial scars
   D. Cotton-wool patches
   E. Hemorrhage
   F. Hemosiderin
   G. Pigment epithelium
      (1) Simple proliferation
      (2) Proliferation in response to demand for phagocytes
      (3) Proliferation with formation of cuticular masses
      (4) Proliferation with metaplasia
      (5) Pigment epithelium migration
      (6) Pigment epithelium seeds
      (7) Pigment epithelium secretion

6. Macular degeneration

7. Malignant melanoma

8. Drusen due to:
   A. Senility
   B. Disease (vascular, inflammatory, or neoplastic)
   C. Hereditary (primary degeneration)

9. Doyne's homogeneous retinal degeneration

10. Metastatic carcinoma

11. Hemangioma of the choroid

12. Solar burns

13. Circinate retinopathy

14. Congenital macular dysplasia

15. Angioid streaks (see angioid streaks, p. 452)

16. Sorsby's pseudo-inflammatory (hemorrhagic) macular degeneration

17. Central serous retinopathy
    A. Retinal
    B. Chorioretinal
    C. Choroidal
    D. Central serous retinopathy associated with crater-like holes in the optic disc
    E. Central serous retinopathy and exudative chorioretinopathy associated with systemic vasculitis

18. Retinal perforation during surgical treatment for strabismus

19. Sickle cell retinopathy

20. Hemorrhage into the vitreous

21. Idiopathic hyperlipemia

22. Night-blinding retinochoroidopathies
    A. Predominately tapetoretinal heredodegenerations
       (1) Retinitis pigmentosa group
       (2) Retinitis punctata albescens
    B. Predominately choroidal heredodegenerations
       (1) Choroidal sclerosis
       (2) Gyrate atrophy of choroid
       (3) Choroideremia
       (4) Myopic retinopathy and choroidopathy
       (5) Fuchs' spot

23. Drug-induced macular disease
    A. Thioridazine (Mellaril)
    B. Chloroquine (Aralen)
    C. Indomethacin (Indocin)

24. Fundus flavimaculatus

25. Peripheral chorioretinal atrophy

26. Helicoid peripapillary chorioretinal degeneration

27. Pigmentary perivenous-chorioretinal degeneration

28. Ischemic ocular inflammation

29. Chorioretinopathy with hereditary microcephaly

30. Retinal vasculitis
    A. With involvement of central retinal vein (papillophlebitis)
    B. Retinal periphlebitis
    C. Retinal periarteritis

31. Retinoblastoma

Schlaegel, T. F.: Essentials of Uveitis. Boston, Little, Brown & Co., 1969, pp. 277–303.

Choroiditis (Posterior Uveitis) (major types listed in order of frequency)*

1. Histoplasmosis

2. Unknown

3. Toxoplasmosis

4. Syphilis

5. Toxocariasis

6. Sarcoidosis

7. Anterior and posterior uveitis
   A. Toxoplasmosis
   B. Peripheral uveitis (cyclitis)
   C. Unknown
   D. Syphilis

*This section from Schlaegel, T. F.: Essentials of Uveitis. Boston, Little, Brown & Co., 1969, Cols. 2 and 3 of Table 1-1, p. 2.

460

E. Tuberculosis
F. Sarcoidosis
G. Vogt-Koyanagi-Harada syndrome
H. *Coccidioides immitis*

Chandler, J. W., Kalina, R. E., and Milam, D. F.: Coccidioidal Choroiditis Following Renal Transplantation. Amer. J. Ophthal. *74*:1080–1085, 1973.
Schlaegel, T. F.: Histoplasmic Choroiditis. Ann. Ophthal. *6*:237–256, 1974.

Conditions Simulating Posterior Uveitis in Children

1. Massive retinal fibrosis

2. Cockayne's disease

3. Retinopathy of childhood cystinosis

4. Retinoblastoma

5. Coats' syndrome

6. Idiopathic hyperlipemia

7. Hypogammaglobulinemia

Kazdan, J. J., et al.: Uveitis in Children. Canad. Med. Assoc. J. *96*: 385–391, 1967.
Schlaegel, T. F.: Essentials of Uveitis. Boston, Little, Brown & Co., 1969, pp. 71–75.
Stafford, W. R., Yanoff, M., and Parnell, B. L.: Retinoblastomas Initially Misdiagnosed as Primary Ocular Inflammations. Arch. Ophthal. *82*:771–773, 1969.

Choroiditis (Posterior Uveitis) in Children

1. Toxoplasmic retinochoroiditis

2. Chorioretinitis of unknown cause
   A. Juxtapapillary chorioretinitis
   B. Disseminated chorioretinitis

3. Anterior and posterior uveitis
   A. Vogt-Koyanagi-Harada syndrome
   B. Sarcoidosis
   C. Sympathetic ophthalmia

4. Herpes simplex chorioretinitis

5. Nematode (Toxocara) retinochoroiditis

6. Syphilitic retinochoroiditis

7. Neonatal cytomegalic inclusion disease

8. Reticulum cell sarcoma of brain

9. Inability of leukocytes to kill microorganisms

Kazdan, J. J., et al.: Uveitis in Children. Canad. Med. Assoc. J. *96*: 385–391, 1967.

Kimura, S. J., and Hogan, M. J.: Uveitis in Children: Analysis of 274 Cases. Trans. Amer. Ophthal. Soc. *62*:173, 1964.

Lonn, L. I.: Neonatal Cytomegalic Inclusion Disease Chorioretinitis. Arch. Ophthal. *88*:434–438, 1972.

Martyn, L. J., et al.: Chorioretinal Lesions in Familial Chronic Granulomatous Disease of Childhood. Amer. J. Ophthal. *73*:403–418, 1972.

Neault, R. W., et al.: Uveitis Associated with Isolated Reticulum Cell Sarcoma of the Brain. Amer. J. Ophthal. *73*:431–436, 1972.

Witmer, R., et al.: Uveitis in Childhood. Ophthalmologica *152*:272–282, 1966.

Uveitis and Associated Systemic Disease*

1. Arthralgia
   A. Histoplasmosis
   B. Whipple's disease

2. Arthritis
   A. Ankylosing spondylitis
   B. Ulcerative colitis
   C. Whipple's disease
   D. Behçet's syndrome
   E. Gonococcosis
   F. Leprosy
   G. Reiter's syndrome
   H. Sporotrichosis
   I. Sarcoid
   J. Van Metre's peripheral polyarthritis or monoarthritis
   K. Rheumatoid arthritis including Still's disease

3. Diarrhea
   A. Whipple's disease
   B. Ulcerative colitis
   C. Regional enteritis

4. Hepatomegaly
   A. Toxocariasis
   B. Cytomegalic inclusion disease
   C. Toxoplasmosis

5. Influenza-like disease
   A. Leptospirosis
   B. Toxoplasmosis
   C. Histoplasmosis

6. Jaundice
   A. Leptospirosis

*Adapted from Schlaegel, T. F.: Essentials of Uveitis. Boston, Little, Brown & Co., 1969, Table 1–14, p. 28.

7. Like infectious mononucleosis
    A. Toxoplasmosis
    B. Cytomegalic inclusion disease

8. Meningism
    A. Tuberculosis
    B. Sympathetic ophthalmia
    C. Vogt-Koyanagi-Harada syndrome
    D. Leptospirosis
    E. Toxoplasmosis
    F. Behçet's syndrome
    G. Listerellosis
    H. Cryptococcosis
    I. Histoplasmosis
    J. Herpes simplex

9. Nodules in the leg
    A. Histoplasmosis
    B. Sarcoid
    C. Ulcerative colitis

10. Pneumonitis
    A. Cytomegalic inclusion disease
    B. Toxocariasis

11. Prostatitis
    A. Gonococcosis
    B. Whipple's disease

12. Stomatitis
    A. Behçet's syndrome
    B. Herpes simplex
    C. Reiter's syndrome
    D. Ulcerative colitis
    E. Disseminated systemic histoplasmosis—not the ocular form

13. Tonsillitis
    A. Whipple's disease

Specific Types of Uveitis*

1. Exudative detachment
   A. Toxoplasmosis
   B. Vogt-Koyanagi-Harada syndrome

2. Iris neovascularization, such as Knox's ischemic ocular inflammation (see rubeosis iridis, p. 318)

3. Iritis associated with ulcerative colitis

4. Microphthalmia
   A. Toxoplasmosis
   B. Cytomegalic inclusion disease

5. Neovascularization of the disc
   A. Ischemic uveitis of Knox
   B. Papillophlebitis

6. Neuroretinitis
   A. Behçet's syndrome
   B. Influenza
   C. Mumps
   D. Syphilis
   E. Peripheral uveitis (pars planitis)

7. Optic neuritis (see p. 477)
   A. Sarcoid
   B. Toxoplasmosis
   C. Cytomegalic inclusion disease
   D. Syphilis
   E. Brucellosis
   F. Regional enteritis
   G. Sympathetic ophthalmia

8. Papilledema
   A. Sarcoid
   B. Papillophlebitis

*Items 1 through 12 from Schlaegel, T. F.: Essentials of Uveitis. Boston, Little, Brown & Co., 1969, adapted from Table 1–15.

9. Perivascular sheathing
   A. Syphilis
   B. Tuberculosis
   C. Peripheral uveitis (multiple sclerosis)
   D. Candidiasis
   E. Coccidioidomycosis
   F. Sarcoidosis

10. Predilection for choroid
    A. Histoplasmosis
    B. Sympathetic ophthalmia

11. Predilection for retina
    A. Toxoplasmosis
    B. Cytomegalic inclusion disease
    C. Moniliasis

12. Salt-and-pepper fundus (see p. 421)
    A. Cockayne's disease
    B. Cystinosis
    C. Choroideremia in males
    D. Prenatal syphilis
    E. Prenatal influenza
    F. Prenatal rubella

13. Syndromes associated with uveitis
    A. Bing's syndrome: chorioretinitis, glaucoma, ptosis, paralysis of extraocular muscles
    B. Degos' syndrome: choroiditis, atrophic skin of eyelids, conjunctival telangiectasis—white skin lesions, anorexia, gastrointestinal involvement
    C. Fuchs' syndrome: choroiditis, heterochromia, cataract
    D. Harada's syndrome: uveitis, choroiditis, visual loss, retinopathy, retinal detachment—headaches, vomiting, deafness, meningeal irritation
    E. Heerfordt's disease: granulomatous uveitis—parotid gland swelling, lymphadenopathy, slight fever
    F. Laurence-Moon-Bardet-Biedl syndrome: choroiditis, retinitis pigmentosa, optic atrophy, nystagmus, strabismus, visual loss, scotoma, anterior segment involvement—obesity, hypogenitalism, polydactylia, mental retardation

G. Romberg's syndrome: choroiditis, keratitis, iritis, cataract, ptosis, paralysis of ocular muscles—atrophy of soft tissue on one side of face, neuralgia of fifth nerve, seizures

H. Sabin-Feldman syndrome: chorioretinal degenerative changes—cerebral calcifications, convulsions (congenital toxoplasmosis)

I. Schaumann's syndrome: uveitis, keratitis, retinopathy, lymphadenopathy, fatigue

J. Siegrist's syndrome: choroiditis, exophthalmos—hypertension, albuminuria

K. Vogt-Koyanagi syndrome: uveitis, glaucoma, retinal detachment, choroiditis—alopecia, vitiligo, hearing defect

Aaberg, T. M., Cesarz, T. J., and Rytel, M. W.: Correlation of Virology and Clinical Course of Cytomegalovirus Retinitis. Amer. J. Ophthal. *74*:407–415, 1972.

Geeraets, W. J.: Ocular Syndromes, 2nd ed. Philadelphia, Lea & Febiger, 1969, p. 225.

Schlaegel, T. F.: Essentials of Uveitis. Boston, Little, Brown & Co., 1969, p. 29.

Chorioretinitis Juxtapapillaris (large, irregular opaque mass that protrudes 3 to 4 diopters and obscures the retinal vessels is seen near the disc. It may be confused with acute optic neuritis or a tumor)

1. Tuberculosis

2. Syphilis

3. Sarcoid

4. Histoplasmosis

5. Toxoplasmosis

6. *Coccidioides immitis*

Haessler, F. H.: Eye Signs in General Disease. Springfield, Ill., Charles C Thomas, 1960, p. 98.

Rosen, E. S., and Ashworth, B.: Early Diagnosis and Natural History of Juxtapapillary Choroiditis. Amer. J. Ophthal. *69*:105–111, 1970.

Characteristics of Granulomatous and Non-granulomatous Inflammation in Posterior Uvea

Symptomatology	Granulomatous Uveitis	Non-granulomatous Uveitis	
		Due to Acute, Self-limited Insult	Due to Chronic or Oft-Repeated Insult
Anterior ocular changes	Sometimes epithelioid or "mutton-fat" keratotic deposits; often Koeppe's nodules	Usually none	None in early stage; irreversible in terminal stages
Vitreous changes	Usually heavy vitreous blurring; heavy veil-like opacities	Slight to intense general blurring; fine muscae or string-like fibrinous opacities	Slowly increasing blur with heavy opacities in terminal stages
Retinal and subretinal edema	Usually slight or moderate and localized around exudates; intense only when there is a secondary allergic reaction	Marked and generalized, with blurring of neuroretinal vascular bed	Low grade at onset; may become intense in later stages
Choroidal exudates	Heavy massive exudates—edges may be blurred by surrounding retinal and subretinal edema	No heavy massive exudates; occasionally localized areas of deeper infiltration	Great tendency to localized deep ill-defined infiltrates (lymphocytes, etc.)
Secondary retinal involvement	Almost invariable with retinal destruction	None or limited to pigment and neuroepithelium	None in early stage; irreversible in later stages with involvement of neuroepithelium
Residual organic damage in retina and choroid	Heavy glial scars with massive pigment heaping which often surrounds the lesion	No fine granular changes in pigment epithelium but damage to neuroepithelium and occasionally superficial gliosis	Fine granular changes in early stages; superficial gliosis in terminal stages

Choroidal Neovascularization (new vessel formation from the choriocapillaris through defects in Bruch's membrane; suggested by fluorescein angiography)

1. Choroidal neovascular ingrowth through breaks in Bruch's membrane in the macular area
    A. Macular drusen
    *B. Presumed ocular histoplasmosis syndrome
    C. Angioid streaks (see p. 452)
    D. Myopic degeneration
    E. Idiopathic choroidal neovascularization
    F. Choroidal tumors
    G. Trauma
    H. Scars from previous deep macular hemorrhage (see p. 385)
    I. Senile disciform macular degeneration (Kuhnt-Junius disease)

2. Choroidal neovascular ingrowth at the margin of the optic nerve head
    A. Idiopathic choroidal neovascularization
    B. Macular drusen
    *C. Peripapillary choroiditis
    *D. Presumed ocular histoplasmosis syndrome
    E. Hyaline bodies of the optic nerve head
    F. Angioid streaks (see p. 452)

Fuller, B, and Gitter, K. A.: Traumatic Choroidal Rupture with Late Serous Detachment of Macula. Arch. Ophthal. *89*:354–355, 1973.

Gass, J. D. M.: Choroidal Neovascular Membranes—Their Visualization and Treatment. Trans. Amer. Acad. Ophthal. Otolaryng. *77*:310–320, 1973.

Krill, A. E., and Archer, D.: Choroidal Neovascularization in Multifocal (Presumed Histoplasmin) Choroiditis. Arch. Ophthal. *84*: 595–604, 1970.

*These are the diseases in which the choroidal neovascular membrane usually lies beneath the retina rather than beneath the pigment epithelium.

16

Ischemic Infarcts of the Choroid (Elschnig Spots) (when healed, they may show small, disseminated yellowish scars with central pigment deposits. They may be associated with retinal separation when acute.)

1. Malignant hypertension
2. Chronic glomerulonephritis
3. Collagen disease, such as scleroderma
4. Toxemia of pregnancy

Klien, B. A.: Ischemic Infarcts of Choroid (Elschnig Spots). Amer. J. Ophthal. *66*:1069–1074, 1968.

Pars Planitis (Peripheral Uveitis) (inferior exudates in the peripheral retina, ora, pars plana, and peripheral vitreous, vitreous ray and cells, posterior cortical cataract, perivasculitis, partial thrombosis of central retinal vein, glaucoma, peripheral retinal hemorrhages and retinal detachment may be present)

1. Idiopathic
2. Syphilis
3. Toxoplasmosis
4. Sarcoidosis
5. Nematoidosis
6. Streptococcal hypersensitivity
7. Sinus infection

8. Dental infection

9. Rheumatic disease

10. Multiple sclerosis

Giles, C. L.: Peripheral Uveitis in Patients with Multiple Sclerosis. Amer. J. Ophthal. *70*:17–19, 1970.

Gills, J. J.: Combined Medical and Surgical Therapy for Complicated Cases of Peripheral Uveitis. Arch. Ophthal. *79*:723, 1968.

Maumenee, A. E.: Clinical Entities in "Uveitis": An Approach to the Study of Intraocular Inflammation. Trans. Amer. Acad. Ophthal. Otolaryng. *74*:497, 1970.

Welch, R., et al.: Peripheral Posterior Segment Inflammation, Vitreous Opacities, and Edema of the Posterior Pole. Arch. Ophthal. *64*:540, 1960.

Differential Diagnosis of Pars Planitis

	Chronicity	Vitreous Opacities	Retinal Edema	Fluorescein Leakage	Organized Vitreous	Distinguishing Features
Acute non-granulomatous iritis	−	±	±	±	−	Acute red eye
Acute recurrent cyclitis	+	+	+	+	+	Localized area of inflammation in ciliary body
Nematode	+	+	+	+?	+	Nodular focus and dragged retina, one eye
Irvine-Gass syndrome	+	+	+	+	±	Usually postoperative
Behçet's syndrome	+	+	+	+?	+	Retinal vasculitis
Peripheral toxoplasmosis	±	+	±	±	±	Localized area of inflammation
Sarcoidosis	+	+	+	+	+	Other ocular signs of sarcoidosis

Maumenee, A. E.: Clinical Entities in "Uveitis": An Approach to the Study of Intraocular Inflammation. Trans. Amer. Acad. Ophthal. Otolaryng. 74:497, 1970.

OPTIC NERVE

Contents

Blurred Optic Nerve Heads

	Vision	Visual Fields	Retinal Veins	Color of Nerve Head	Retinal Hemor- rhages	Peripap- illary Retinal Edema	Vitreous Cells	Symmetry of Nerve Heads	Comments
Early papilledema	Normal	Normal (except blind spot en- largement)	Slightly dis- tended; early loss of sponta- neous pulsations	Pink	±	±	−	Often asym- metrical	Headaches
Advanced papill- edema	Normal or, at times, some- what reduced	Normal (except blind spot en- largement)	Distended with- out spontane- ous pulsations	Very pink to pale	+	+	−	Often sym- metrical	Sixth nerve pal- sies are addi- tional clue to intracranial pressure
Hyperopia and physiologic variants	Normal	Normal	Normal	Normal	−	−	−	Often sym- metrical	Fundus seen with + lens. Central disc cupping usually present
Optic neuritis	Impaired	Central scotoma ± peripheral loss	Distended ± spontaneous pulsations	Pink	±	±	±	Usually uni- lateral	Precipitous onset; may have pain with ocular motility

Optic nerve tumor	Normal or markedly reduced	Normal or markedly reduced	Normal or distended	May be pigmented if disc contains melanin. Very pink to pale	±	±	—	Usually unilateral	May involve **only** or the orbital or intracranial optic nerve, **and not the intraocular portion.** Primary nerve tumors are **rarely observed on the disc**
Optic nerve avulsion	Blind eye	—	Sludged	Pale	±	—	±	Contralateral eye normal	Contre-coup or direct trauma
Hyaline bodies of nerve head	Normal	Normal or a variety of field cuts	Normal	Normal	— (Very rarely +)	—	—	Often symmetrical; hyaline bodies sometimes seen at disc margins in one eye only	Often familial (examine parents and siblings)
Hypotony of eye (after trauma)	Slightly impaired	Usually normal	Distended	Pink ±	±	Peripheral edema	—	Unilateral	Soft eye; commotio retinae

Paton, D., and Goldberg, M. F.: Injuries of the Eye, the Lids, and the Orbit. Philadelphia, W. B. Saunders Co., 1968, pp. 6 and 7.

Hyperemia of Disc

1. Papilledema

2. Polycythemia

3. Hypermetropia

4. Optic neuritis

5. Neovascularization

6. Central retinal vein thrombosis

7. Hemangioma

8. Hypertensive retinopathy

9. Ischemic optic neuropathy

10. von Hippel-Lindau

Duke-Elder, S., and Scott, G. I.: System of Ophthalmology, Vol. XII. St. Louis, C. V. Mosby Co., 1971.

Pseudo-optic Neuritis (lesions that mimic optic neuritis)

1. Central scotomas produced by expanding lesions of anterior and middle cranial fossa
   A. Meningiomas
   B. Pituitary adenomas
   C. Nasopharyngeal carcinomas
   D. Lymphomas
   E. Hodgkin's disease
   F. Craniopharyngiomas
   G. Metastatic carcinomas

H. Ectopic pinealomas

I. Plasmacytoma

2. Blurring of the disc from drusen or papilledema (see pp. 482 and 493)

3. Ischemic optic neuropathy

4. Retinal lesions that also exhibit metamorphopsia, such as serous or angiospastic retinopathy

5. Tumors of disc, such as metastatic carcinoma, gliomas, neurofibromas, hematomas, and meningiomas

Cogan, D. G.: Neurology of the Visual System, 3rd ed. Springfield, Ill., Charles C Thomas, 1966, pp. 177–178.

Ginsberg, J., Freemand, A. S., and Calhoun, J. B.: Optic Nerve Involvement in Metastatic Tumors. Ann. Ophthal. 2:604–612, 1970.

Huber, A.: Eye Symptoms in Brain Tumors, 2nd ed. St. Louis, C. V. Mosby Co., 1971, pp. 143–150.

Kamin, D. F., and Hepler, R. S.: Solitary Intracranial Plasmacytoma Mistaken for Retrobulbar Neuritis. Amer. J. Ophthal. 73: 584–586, 1972.

Papillitis and Retrobulbar Neuritis

1. Progressive loss of vision and possibly complete amaurosis

2. Pain in or behind eye, especially on lateral movement

3. Marcus Gunn pupillary phenomenon

4. Central and paracentral scotoma

Papillitis—lesions of the disc, manifest by exudate in the vitreous, swelling of the optic disc, obliteration of the physiologic cup, congestion of the vessels, and central scotoma

Retrobulbar neuritis—lesion of the optic nerve that shows no abnormality in the fundus

1. Primary demyelinative and degenerative diseases
   A. Multiple sclerosis
   B. Diffuse sclerosis, such as that associated with Schilder's disease and leukodystrophies
   C. Opticomyelitis (Devic's disease)
   D. Hereditary optic atrophy
      (1) Autosomal dominant hereditary atrophy
      (2) Leber's optic atrophy—sex-linked

2. Vasculitis
   A. Temporal arteritis
   B. Relationship to Raynaud's disease
   C. Trypanosomiasis
   D. Rheumatic fever
   E. Periarteritis nodosa and Still's disease
   F. Syphilis
   G. Drug reaction
   H. Systemic diseases of blood vessels
   I. Idiopathic

3. Secondary inflammatory processes
   A. Spread from sinuses, such as from sphenoid and posterior ethmoidal sinuses
   B. Meningitis—common in first decade of life, due to infection, such as tuberculosis, or bacterial, fungal, or viral infections
   C. Brain inflammation, such as encephalitis
   D. Inflammation of the orbit, such as in herpes zoster, infections of the gasserian ganglion, and orbital abscess
   E. Following measles, chickenpox, mumps, pertussis, equine encephalitis, poliomyelitis, infectious mononucleosis, torula meningitis, Asiatic influenza, smallpox, smallpox vaccination, infectious hepatitis, Q fever, epidemic keratoconjunctivitis, toxoplasmosis, malaria, trypanosomiasis, typhus, bacterial endocarditis, brucellosis, botulism, and relapsing fever
   F. Uveitis and retinitis, including sympathetic ophthalmitis
   G. Behcet's disease and Vogt-Koyanagi syndrome
   H. Nematode, such as Toxocara
   I. Leukemia, lymphoma, and Hodgkin's disease

J. Syphilis

K. Venoms

4. Systemic diseases and poisons
   A. Diabetes mellitus
   B. Dysthyroidism and hyperthyroidism
   C. Chronic glomerulonephritis with secondary renal hypertension or pyelonephritis
   D. Paget's disease
   E. Fibrous dysplasia
   F. Nutritional diseases, such as beriberi, hyperemesis gravidism, pellagra, and carcinomatosis
   G. Megaloblastic (pernicious) anemia, especially in smokers due to lack of vitamin B_{12}, severe hemorrhage, macroglobulinemias, and polycythemias
   H. Fibrocystic disease of pancreas
   I. Hypoparathyroidism
   J. Lactation, pregnancy, and puberty
   K. Porphyria
   L. Amyloidosis and sarcoidosis
   M. Alcohol ingestion and use of tobacco
   N. Emphysema
   O. Toxins
      (1) Thallium salts
      (2) Carbon disulfide
      (3) Chloramphenicol
      (4) Sulfonamides
      (5) Disulfiram (Antabuse)
      (6) Antimony
      (7) Antipyrine
      (8) Apiol
      (9) Arsenicals
      (10) Carbon tetrachloride
      (11) Chlorpropamide
      (12) Emetine
      (13) Ergot
      (14) Ergothioneine
      (15) Ethambutol
      (16) Fava beans
      (17) Lead

(18) Methyl acetate
(19) Methyl bromide
(20) Methyl chloride
(21) Methylene blue
(22) Oil of chenopodium
(23) Penicillamine
(24) Pyridoxine
(25) Tartar emetic
(26) Thioglycolates
(27) Tin and tin alkyl compounds
(28) Trichloroethylene
(29) Tricresyl phosphate
(30) Tryparsamide
(31) Vinylbenzene
(32) Methyl ethyl ketone
(33) Carbon monoxide
(34) Methyl alcohol

5. Laser burn

Barron, G. J., Tepper, L., and Iovine, G.: Ocular Toxicity from Ethambutol. Amer. J. Ophthal. 77:256–260, 1974.
Berg, E. F.: Retrobulbar Neuritis: a Case Report from Presumed Solvent Toxicity. Ann. Ophthal. 3:1349, 1971.
Bilchik, R. C., Muller-Beigh, H. A., and Freshman, M. E.: Ischemic Retinopathy Due to Carbon Monoxide Poisoning. Arch. Ophthal. 86:142–144, 1971.
Bird, A. C., Smith, J. L., and Curtin, V. T.: Nematode Optic Neuritis. Amer. J. Ophthal. 69:72–77, 1970.
Carroll, F. D.: Optic Nerve Complications of Cataract Extraction. Trans. Amer. Acad. Ophthal. Otolaryng. 77:623–629, 1973.
Cogan, D. G.: Neurology of the Visual System, 3rd ed. Springfield, Ill., Charles C Thomas, 1966, pp. 158–177.
Duke-Elder, S., and Scott, G. I.: System of Ophthalmology, Vol. XII. St. Louis, C. V. Mosby Co., 1971, pp. 82–196.
Huber, A.: Eye Symptoms in Brain Tumors, 2nd ed. St. Louis, C. V. Mosby Co., 1971, pp. 130–140, 351.
Walsh, F. B., and Hoyt, W. F.: Clinical Neuro-ophthalmology, 3rd ed. Baltimore, Williams & Wilkins Co., 1969.
Zittle, H. L., and Zweng, H. C.: Complications of Argon Laser Photocoagulation. Trans. Amer. Acad. Ophthal. Otolaryng. In press.

Pseudopapilledema (may be mistaken for swelling of optic nerve)

1. Normal variant

2. Drusens of optic nerve (see p. 493)

3. High hyperopia or astigmatism

4. Optic neuritis or papillitis (see p. 482)

5. Epipapillary membrane and Bergmeister's papilla

6. Cervico-oculo-acusticus syndrome

7. Medullated nerve fibers (opaque nerve fibers)

8. Tortuosity and anomalous early branching of the retinal vessels

9. Arteriovenous aneurysms (racemose aneurysms) of the retina (Wyburn-Mason syndrome)

10. Tumors of disc, such as gliomas, meningiomas, neurinomas, neurofibromas, metastatic tumor, hematoma, and sarcoid

11. Opacities or haziness of the media, especially nuclear sclerosis of the lens

Duke-Elder, S., and Scott, G. I.: System of Ophthalmology, Vol. XII. St. Louis, C. V. Mosby Co., 1971, pp. 76–78.

Howorth, C. H., and Havener, W. H.: Differential Diagnosis of an Edematous Optic Disc. Amer. J. Ophthal. *49*:150, 1959.

Huber, A.: Eye Symptoms in Brain Tumors, 2nd ed. St. Louis, C. V. Mosby Co., 1971, pp. 143–150.

Jampol, L. M., Woodfin, W., and McLean, E. B.: Optic Nerve Sarcoidosis. Arch. Ophthal. *87*:355–360, 1972.

Kirkham, T. H.: Cervico-oculo-acusticus Syndrome with Pseudopapilledema. Arch. Dis. Child. *44*:504–508, 1969.

Leinfelder, P. S.: Pathogenesis of Papilledema. Amer. J. Ophthal. *48*:107, 1959.

Perkins, E. S., and Dobree, J. H.: The Differential Diagnosis of Fundus Conditions. St. Louis, C. V. Mosby Co., 1972, p. 41.

Schlezinger, N. S., Waldman, J., and Alpers, B. J.: Drusen of Optic Nerve Simulating Cerebral Tumor. Arch. Ophthal. *31*:509, 1944.

Papilledema (swelling of optic disc)

1. Ocular cause—usually unilateral
   A. Hypotony (see page 279), including that following cataract extraction
   B. Acute glaucoma
   C. Inflammatory
      (1) Uveitis, particularly chronic cyclitis, and that due to sarcoidosis
      (2) Juxtapapillary choroiditis
      (3) Retinal vasculitis
      (4) Syphilitic neuroretinitis
      (5) Gumma of nerve head
      (6) Tuberculoma of nerve head
      (7) Rocky Mountain spotted fever
   D. Ocular tumors
      (1) Tuberous sclerosis
      (2) Neurofibromatosis (von Recklinghausen's disease)
      (3) Hemangioma
      (4) Melanocytoma
      (5) Glioma
      (6) Melanotic sarcoma
      (7) Secondary carcinoma
   E. Central retinal vein or artery occlusion (see p. 395 or p. 406)
   F. Ocular trauma
   G. Unilateral optic atrophy and contralateral papilledema (Foster Kennedy syndrome)
      (1) Previous unilateral optic nerve atrophy
      (2) Frontal lobe tumors or abscess
      (3) Arteriosclerotic plaques of internal carotid or anterior cerebral arteries
      (4) Chiasmal arachnoiditis secondary to trauma, spinal anesthesia, or syphilis
      (5) Aneurysm of internal carotid, anterior cerebral, or anterior communicating artery

(6) Olfactory groove, sphenoid ridge, and supra-sellar meningioma
(7) Craniopharyngioma with forward extension
(8) Glioma of the intracranial portion of optic nerve
(9) Internal hydrocephalus due to tumor of posterior fossa
H. Unilateral condition that prevents choked disc
   (1) Myopia (over 5 diopters)
   (2) Optic atrophy
   (3) Anomalous disc and/or anomalous optic nerve sheaths

2. Orbital cause—usually unilateral, may have exophthalmos
A. Orbital tumors
   (1) Benign, such as dermoid cyst, cystic angioma, Paget's disease, osteopetrosis (Albers-Schönberg disease), and glioma
   (2) Malignant, such as tumor of lacrimal gland, lymphosarcoma, fibrosarcoma, melanotic sarcoma, osteosarcoma, myosarcoma, secondary metastasis, and extension from nasopharynx or sinuses
B. Aneurysm of the ophthalmic artery
C. Orbital abscess
D. Sinusitis
E. Endocrine exophthalmos—more likely bilateral
F. Optic nerve trauma

3. Intracranial causes—usually bilateral
A. Increased intracranial pressure
   (1) Tumors
      a. Frontal lobe lesion—mental changes (apathy, euphoria, and social behavioral changes); normal visual field if confined to frontal lobe; most likely tumors are medulloblastoma, meningioma, astrocytoma, glioblastoma, or metastasis from lung or breast
      b. Temporal lobe lesions—formed hallucinations, superior homonymous quadrantanopia, or homonymous hemianopia, ipsilateral mydriatic fixed pupil and oculomotor paresis,

and contralateral facial palsy; most likely tumors are medulloblastoma, meningioma, astrocytoma, glioblastoma, or metastasis from lung or breast

c. Parietal lobe lesions—visual agnosia, such as alexia or dyslexia, complete homonymous hemianopia, or inferior homonymous quadrantanopia, disturbances of trigeminal nerve including decreased corneal sensation, and positive (asymmetrical response) optokinetic nystagmus; most likely tumors are medulloblastoma, meningioma, astrocytoma, glioblastoma, or metastasis from lung or breast

d. Occipital lobe lesions—unformed visual hallucinations and homonymous congruous visual field defect; most likely tumors are hemangioma, meningioma, astrocytoma, glioblastoma, or metastasis from lung or breast

e. Third ventricle and sellar lesions—visual field of bitemporal hemianopia or unilateral blindness and contralateral temporal hemianopia; most likely tumors are craniopharyngioma, glioblastoma, medulloblastoma, or astrocytoma

f. Fourth ventricle and cerebellum lesions—ataxia, asynergy, dysmetria, hypotonia, and acquired jerk nystagmus, usually horizontal and more pronounced in lateral gaze; most likely tumors are medulloblastoma, astrocytoma, hemangioblastoma, or metastasis from lung or breast

(2) Hydrocephalus

(3) Abscess

(4) Tuberculomas

(5) Gummas

(6) Aneurysms

(7) Cavernous sinus thrombosis

(8) Meningitis, anterior poliomyelitis, and encephalitis

(9) Cerebral hemorrhage

(10) Trauma, including subdural and subarachnoid bleeding

(11) Parasitic infections, such as cysticercosis and cryptococcus

B. Decreased intracranial capacity, such as in tower skull (oxycephaly), craniofacial dysostosis (Crouzon's disease), hypertelorism, and acrocephalosyndactyly (Apert's disease)

C. Changes in the cerebrospinal fluid (CSF), such as in (Landry) Guillain-Barré syndrome with high CSF protein content and defective absorption

D. Tumors of spinal cord located caudally as far as the cauda equina, more likely higher

E. Pseudotumor cerebri—bilateral papilledema and increased intracranial pressure but negative neurologic and general physical findings

(1) Drugs
   a. Adrenal corticosteroids
   b. Antimicrobials, such as tetracyclines and their derivatives and Nalidixic acid (Neg Gram)
   c. Vitamin A intoxication
   d. Manganese
   e. Oral contraceptives

(2) Menarche

(3) Pregnancy

(4) Addison's disease

(5) Thrombosis of the sagittal or lateral sinus, such as that following otitis media in children

4. Systemic diseases—usually bilateral

A. Blood dyscrasias, including leukemia, pernicious and iron-deficiency anemias, thrombocytopenic purpura, polycythemia vera, macroglobulinemia, and multiple myeloma

B. Hypertension, sometimes benign, usually malignant including lead encephalopathy

C. Cardiopulmonary insufficiency, such as in pulmonary emphysema, cystic fibrosis of lungs, emphysema, chronic bronchitis, types of congenital heart disease, and cystic fibrosis of pancreas

D. Infectious (rare, usually optic neuritis), such as infectious mononucleosis, malaria, sandfly fever, cryptococcosis, and subacute sclerosing panencephalitis (Dawson's disease)

E. Endocrine, such as hyperthyroidism, parathyroid deficiency, Addison's disease, pregnancy, menses, diabetes, and suppression of adrenal function from prolonged use of steroids

F. Sarcoidosis

G. Giant-cell arteritis

H. Muscular dystrophy and Maroteaux-Lamy syndrome (MPS VI)

I. Collagen disorders, such as polyarteritis nodosa and lupus erythematosus

J. Nutritional diseases
   (1) Beriberi
   (2) Pellagra
   (3) Vitamin B_{12} deficiency

K. Drugs—rare and usually optic atrophy
   (1) D-L Penicillamine
   (2) Thioridiazine
   (3) Corticosteroid therapy
   (4) Salicylate intoxication
   (5) Intrathecal injection of methylene blue
   (6) Lead
   (7) Quinine
   (8) Methyl alcohol
   (9) Carbon monoxide

Bigger, J. F.: Retinal Hemorrhages during Penicillamine Therapy of Cystinuria. Amer. J. Ophthal. 66:954–955, 1968.

Bilchik, R. C., Muller-Beigh, H. A., and Freshman, M. E.: Ischemic Retinopathy Due to Carbon Monoxide Poisoning. Arch. Ophthal. 86:142–144, 1971.

Brenner, R. L., et al.: Eye Signs of Hypophosphatasia. Arch. Ophthal. 81:614, 1969.

Chumbley, L. C., and Kearns, T. P.: Retinopathy of Sarcoidosis. Amer. J. Ophthal. 73:123–131, 1972.

Cogan, D. G.: Neurology of the Visual System, 3rd ed. Springfield, Ill., Charles C Thomas, 1968.

Duke-Elder, S., and Scott, G. I.: System of Ophthalmology, Vol. XII. St. Louis, C. V. Mosby Co., 1971, pp. 32–65.

Ellis, W., and Little, H. L.: Leukemic Infiltration of the Optic Nerve Head. Amer. J. Ophthal. *75*:867–871, 1973.

Gass, J. D. M., and Norton, E. W. D.: Cystoid Macular Edema and Papilledema Following Cataract Extraction. Arch. Ophthal. *76*:646–661, 1966.

Goldberg, M. F., Scott, G. I., and McKusick, V. A.: Hydrocephalus and Papilledema in the Maroteaux-Lamy Syndrome (Mucopolysaccharidosis Type VI). Amer. J. Ophthal. *69*:969–974, 1970.

Gonyea, E. F., and Heilman, K. M.: Neuro-ophthalmic Aspects of Central Nervous System Cryptococcosis. Arch. Ophthal. *87*:164–168, 1972.

Grant, W. M.: Toxicology of the Eye, 2nd ed. Springfield, Ill., Charles C Thomas, 1973.

Howorth, C. H., and Havener, W. H.: Differential Diagnosis of an Edematous Optic Disc. Amer. J. Ophthal. *49*:150, 1959.

Huber, A.: Eye Symptoms in Brain Tumors, 2nd ed. St. Louis, C. V. Mosby Co., 1971.

Kirkpatrick, B. V., and David, R. B.: Subacute Sclerosing Panencephalitis. J. Pediat. Ophthal. *10*:74–76, 1973.

Massey, J. Y., Roy, F. H., and Bornhofen, J. H.: Ocular Manifestations of Reye Syndrome. Arch. Ophthal. *91*:441–444, 1974.

Presley, G. D.: Fundus Changes in Rocky Mountain Spotted Fever. Amer. J. Ophthal. *67*:263–267, 1969.

Trujillo, M. H., Desenne, J. J., and Berrain Pinto, H.: Reversible Papilledema in Iron Deficiency Anemia. Ann. Ophthal. *4*:378–380, 1972.

Van Dyk, H. J. L., and Swan, K. C.: Drug-Induced Pseudotumor Cerebri. *In* Leopold, I. H. (Ed.): Symposium on Ocular Therapy, Vol. 4. St. Louis, C. V. Mosby Co., 1969, pp. 71–77.

Walsh, F. B., and Hoyt, W. F.: Clinical Neuro-ophthalmology, 3rd ed. Baltimore, Williams & Wilkins Co., 1969, pp. 567–607.

Optic Atrophy (pallor of optic disc; may follow papilledema or optic neuritis [see pp. 477 and 482])

In children

1. Tumors
   A. Intraorbital—glioma of optic nerve
   B. Intracranial—craniopharyngiomas, gliomas, meningiomas, and ectopic pinealomas
   C. Papilledema, initially of fourth ventricle and cerebellum

2. Developmental cause
   A. Cerebral palsy
   B. Hydrocephalus and anencephaly
   C. Craniostenosis including Crouzon's disease
   D. Cerebellar ataxia

3. Hereditary degenerative disease
   A. Bielschowsky's disease
   B. Tay-Sachs disease and Batten-Mayou disease (Spiel-meyer-Vogt disease)
   C. Metachromatic leukoencephalopathy
   D. Leber's disease—sex-linked
   E. Behr's disease (optic atrophy-ataxia syndrome)—autosomal dominant
   F. Charcot-Marie-Tooth disease (progressive neuritic muscular atrophy)

4. Metabolic disease
   A. Hyperparathyroidism
   B. Osteopetrosis—marble-bone disease or Albers-Schön-berg disease
   C. Generalized gangliosidosis (GM_1-gangliosidosis)
   D. Juvenile diabetes—rare
   E. Cystic fibrosis of the pancreas

5. Toxic
   A. Lead poisoning
   B. Devic's disease (neuromyelitis optica)
   C. Thallium (used for treatment of fungi of the scalp)
   D. Toxic drugs (sulfonamides, isoniazid, streptomycin, chloramphenicol)
   E. Chronic cyanide intoxication, such as from eating cassava

6. Congenital optic atrophy

7. Associated syndromes and diseases
   A. Chondrodystrophia calcificans congenita (Conradi's syndrome)
   B. Cri du chat syndrome (crying cat syndrome)
   C. Congenital cytomegalic inclusion disease

D. Happy puppet syndrome
E. Congenital syphilis
F. Osteogenesis imperfecta
G. Osteopetrosis (Albers-Schönberg disease)
H. Chromosome 18 deletion—pallor only, not atrophy
I. De Lange's syndrome—pallor only, not atrophy
J. Apert's syndrome (acrocephalosyndactylism syndrome)
K. Bloch-Sulzberger disease (incontinentia pigmenti)
L. Cockayne's syndrome (dwarfism with retinal atrophy and deafness)
M. Greig's syndrome (ocular hypertelorism syndrome)
N. Hallgren's syndrome (retinitis-pigmentosa-deafness-ataxia syndrome)
O. Systemic mucopolysaccharidosis
    (1) Hurler's disease (MPS I)
    (2) Hunter's disease (MPS II)
    (3) Sanfilippo's disease (MPS III)
    (4) Morquio's disease (MPS IV)
    (5) Scheie's disease (MPS V)
    (6) Maroteaux-Lamy disease (MPS VI)
P. Krabbe's disease—rigidity, convulsions, deafness, and blindness
Q. Kloepfer's syndrome—autosomal recessive trait with 100% penetrance
R. Oculo-oro-genital syndrome—vitamin B_1 deficiency
S. Pelizaeus-Merzbacher disease (aplasia axialis extracorticalis congenita)
T. Rieger's syndrome (hypodontia and iris dysgenesis)
U. Menkes' disease (kinky hair disease)
V. Refsum's syndrome (ophthalmoplegia, ataxia, deafness, and polyneuritis)
W. Diencephalic syndrome (emaciation, locomotor overactivity, euphoria, skin pallor)
X. Leigh's disease (subacute necrotizing encephalomyelopathy)

8. Infections, such as basal meningitis, infectious encephalomeningitis (especially measles, chickenpox, smallpox, vaccinia, epidemic parotitis), congenital neurosyphilis (rare before 2 years of age), and toxoplasmosis

In adults

1. Inflammatory (see optic neuritis, p. 477) with secondary atrophy
   A. Multiple sclerosis
   B. Temporal arteritis

2. Non-inflammatory swelling (see papilledema, p. 482) with secondary atrophy

3. Trauma, evulsion of optic nerve, and ocular contusion

4. Glaucoma

5. Arachnoidal adhesions, including tabes

6. Compressive lesions
   A. Meningiomas
   B. Pituitary adenoma
   C. Craniopharyngioma
   D. Nasopharyngeal carcinomas

7. Aneurysm of internal carotid artery

8. Vascular accident

9. Central nervous system deficiency—bitemporal pallor due to deficient diet in prisoners

10. Orbital operation, such as following orbital floor fracture, reduction of malar fractures, and Kronlein lateral orbitotomy

11. Carbon monoxide

12. Drusen of optic nerve

Bilchik, R. C., Muller-Beigh, H. A., and Freshman, M. E.: Ischemic Retinopathy Due to Carbon Monoxide Poisoning. Arch. Ophthal. 86:142–144, 1971.

Cogan, D. G.: Neurology of the Visual System, 3rd ed. Springfield, Ill., Charles C Thomas, 1968, pp. 133–137.

Davis, W. H., Nevins, R. C., and Elliott, J. H.: Optic Atrophy after Contusion. Amer. J. Ophthal. 73:278–280, 1972.

Duke-Elder, S., and Scott, G. I.: System of Ophthalmology, Vol. XII. St. Louis, C. V. Mosby Co., 1971, pp. 213–229.

Emery, J. M., Green, W. R., and Huff, D. S.: Krabbe's Disease. Amer. J. Ophthal. 74:400–406, 1972.

Geeraets, W. J.: Ocular Syndromes, 2nd ed. Philadelphia, Lea & Febiger, 1969.

Gellis, S. S., and Feingold, M.: Atlas of Mental Retardation. Washington, D.C., U.S. Government Printing Office, 1968.

Howard, R. O., and Albert, D. H.: Ocular Manifestations of Subacute Necrotizing Encephalomyelopathy (Leigh's Disease). Arch. Ophthal. 74:386–393, 1972.

Jampol, L. M., Woodfin, W., and McLean, E. B.: Optic Nerve Sarcoidosis. Arch. Ophthal. 87:355–360, 1972.

Kamin, D. F., Hepler, R. S., and Foos, R. Y.: Optic Nerve Drusen. Arch. Ophthal. 89:359–362, 1973.

Kenyon, K. R., et al.: The Systemic Mucopolysaccharidoses. Amer. J. Ophthal. 73:811–833, 1972.

Layden, W. E., and Edwards, W. C.: Ocular Manifestations of the Diencephalic Syndrome. Amer. J. Ophthal. 73:78–82, 1972.

Massey, J. Y., and Roy, F. H.: Ocular Manifestations of the Happy Puppet Syndrome. J. Pediat. Ophthal. 10:282–284, 1973.

Osuntokun, B. O., and Osuntokun, W.: Tropical Amblyopia in Nigerians. Amer. J. Ophthal. 72:708–715, 1971.

Park, J. H., et al.: Evulsion of the Optic Nerve. Amer. J. Ophthal. 72:969–971, 1971.

Seelenfreund, M. H., Gartner, S., and Vinger, P. F.: The Ocular Pathology of Menkes Disease. Arch. Ophthal. 80:718–720, 1968.

Spaeth, G. L.: Ocular Manifestations of the Lipidoses. In Tasman, W. (Ed.): Retinal Diseases in Children. New York, Harper & Row, Inc., 1971, pp. 181–187.

Shapiro, L. R., et al.: Hereditary Optic Atrophy: an Autosomal Dominant with Incomplete Penetrance. Arch. Ophthal. 81:359–362, 1969.

Sorsby, A.: Ophthalmic Genetics, 2nd ed. New York, Appleton-Century-Crofts, Inc., 1970, pp. 177–182.

Pseudoglaucomatous Atrophy of the Optic Disc (cupping of the nerve head with optic atrophy and field defects simulating true glaucoma, but without ocular hypertension)

1. Tumors arising near the chiasm (rare)

2. Congenital anomalies of the optic disc
   A. Oblique insertion of the optic nerve

    B. Branching of vessels behind the lamina, so that the individual branches appear at the disc margins

    C. Congenital coloboma of the disc

    D. Coloboma within the nerve sheath

    E. Traction of the disc with bowing of the scleral crescent

3. Syphilitic optic atrophy

4. Sclerosis or calcification of the internal carotid arteries with pressure on optic nerves or arteriosclerosis of the nutrient vessels of the optic nerve

5. True low tension glaucoma

6. Open-angle glaucoma with low scleral rigidity (following intraocular operation, association with myopia, and in patients receiving miotic therapy) with low pressure reading with Schiotz tonometry; applanation intraocular pressure high

7. Glaucoma, usually secondary, that causes permanent changes, then subsides spontaneously

8. Open-angle glaucoma with hyposecretion of aqueous as well as decreased facility of outflow; diagnosed by tonography

9. Hypersecretion glaucoma—diurnal variation with intermittent pressure rises; tonography gives diagnosis with normal outflow

10. Large diurnal fluctuations of intraocular pressure

11. Previous damage to optic nerve with normal intraocular pressure (IOP) now as with prior corticosteroid glaucoma, secondary glaucoma, spontaneously "cured" open-angle glaucoma, or intermittent angle closure glaucoma

12. "Weak" optic disc that atrophies at normal pressures, or reduced blood pressure to optic nerve, such as from severe blood loss, gastrointestinal bleeding, acute hypotension, myocardial infarction, carotid insufficiency, or pernicious anemia

13. Schnobel's cavernous atrophy

14. Patients using digitalis

15. Transitory glaucoma due to intraocular inflammation, such as synechiae in the pupil or angle and old pigmented inflammatory deposits

Bedrossian, E. H.: The Eye. Springfield, Ill., Charles C Thomas, 1958, pp. 268–269.

Deutsch, A. R.: Differential Characteristics of Low Tension Glaucoma. J. Tenn. Med. Assoc. *54*:84–89, 1961.

Drance, S. M., et al.: Studies of Factors Involved in the Production of Low Tension Glaucoma. Arch. Ophthal. *90*:457, 1973.

Hiatt, R. L., Deutsch, A. R., and Ringer, C.: Low Tension Glaucoma. Ann. Ophthal. *3*:85–92, 1971.

Kolker, A. E., and Hetherington, J.: Becker-Schaffer's Diagnosis and Therapy of the Glaucomas, 3rd ed. St. Louis, C. V. Mosby, Co., 1970, pp. 223–225.

McDonald, T. J.: Problems of Low Tension Glaucoma. Trans. Ophthal. Soc. U.K. *87*:873–892, 1967.

Vaughan, D., Asbury, T., and Cook, R.: General Ophthalmology, 6th ed. Los Altos, Calif, Lange Medical Publications, 1971, p. 200.

Drusen of the Optic Nerve (white or yellow conglomerate translucent bodies on optic nerve; may cause field defects)

1. Idiopathic

2. Hereditary—autosomal dominant

3. Retinitis pigmentosa

4. Tuberous sclerosis

5. Angioid streaks (see p. 452)

6. Meningioma (unusual)

7. Pituitary tumor (unusual)

8. Nonspecific optic atrophy

9. High hypermetropia and optic disc elevation

10. Pseudoxanthoma elasticum

11. Associated with corneal dystrophy, juvenile diabetes, Friedreich's ataxia, status dysraphicus, Wilson's disease, glaucoma, and syphilis

Cogan, D. G.: Neurology of the Visual System, 3rd ed. Springfield, Ill., Charles C Thomas, 1968, pp. 151–152.

Chamlin, M., and Davidoff, L. M.: Drusen of the Optic Nervehead; Ophthalmoscopic and Histopathologic Study. Amer. J. Ophthal. *35*: 1599, 1952.

Lorentzen, S. E.: Drusen of the Optic Disc: A Clinical and Genetic Study. Acta Ophthal. (Suppl. 90). Copenhagen, Ejnar Munksgaard, 1966.

Newell, F. W.: Ophthalmology, Principles and Concepts. St. Louis, C. V. Mosby Co., 1969, p. 281.

Reese, A. B.: Relation of Drusen of the Optic Nerve to Tuberous Sclerosis. Arch. Ophthal. *24*:187, 1940.

Walsh, F. B., and Hoyt, W. F.: Clinical Neuro-ophthalmology, 3rd ed. Baltimore, Williams & Wilkins Co., 1969, pp. 675–679.

Wise, G. N., Henkind, P., and Alterman, M.: Optic Nerve Drusen and Subretinal Hemorrhage. Trans. Amer. Acad. Ophthal. Otolaryng. *78*:212–219, 1974.

Pigmented Tumors of Optic Disc

1. Malignant melanoma

2. Drusen

3. Giant drusen—family history or presence of tuberous sclerosis

4. Melanocytomas—small, pigmented tumors spilling into adjacent retina (usually lower temporal) with no loss of vision, no growth, and a normal visual field

5. Metastases from remote sites

6. Hemangioma of the disc with hemorrhage and secondary pigmentation

Hogan, M. J.: "Clinical Aspects, Management and Prognosis of Melanomas of the Uvea and Optic Nerve." Ocular and Adnexal Tumors, New and Controversial Aspects. St. Louis, C. V. Mosby Co., 1964, p. 292.

Linear Hemorrhage on Optic Disc

1. Low tension glaucoma
2. Ischemic optic neuropathy
   A. Altitudinal field loss
   B. Dense arcuate field loss
   C. Sector-shaped field loss
3. Drusen of optic nerve

Begg, I. S., Drance, S. M., and Sweeney, V. P.: Haemorrhage on the Disc: A Sign of Acute Ischemic Optic Neuropathy in Chronic Simple Glaucoma. Canad. J. Ophthal. 5:321–330, 1970.

Drance, S. M., et al.: Studies of Factors Involved in the Production of Low Tension Glaucoma. Arch. Ophthal. 90:457, 1973.

Duke-Elder, S., and Scott, G. I.: System of Ophthalmology, Vol. XII. St. Louis, C. V. Mosby Co., 1971, pp. 198–205.

Temporally Displaced Disc (dragged disc)

1. Temporally displaced vessels (see p. 442)

2. Ectopic macula

3. Abnormal tortuous retinal vessels temporally

Gow, J., and Oliver, G. L.: Familial Exudative Vitreoretinopathy. Arch. Ophthal. 86:150–155, 1971.

Optic Nerve Atrophy and Deafness

1. Sylvester's disease—optic atrophy, ataxia, and hearing loss, moderate and slowly progressive

2. Rosenberg-Chutorian syndrome—optic atrophy, polyneuropathy, and neural hearing loss—recessive inheritance

3. Juvenile diabetes mellitus—progressive optic atrophy, progressive neural hearing loss, juvenile diabetes mellitus

4. Turnbridge-Paley disease—recessive inheritance, optic atrophy, deafness

5. Opticocochleodentate degeneration (van Bogaert-Nyssen syndrome)—recessive inheritance, infantile onset of progressive spastic quadraparesis, progressive hearing loss, and mental retardation

6. Dominant inheritance—congenital deafness and progressive optic nerve atrophy

7. Cockayne's syndrome—dwarfism with retinal atrophy and deafness

8. Hollgren's syndrome—retinitis pigmentosa, deafness, and ataxia

9. Krabbe's disease—rigidity, convulsions, and deafness

10. Refsum's syndrome—ophthalmoplegia, ataxia, deafness, and polyneuritis

Emery, J. M., Green, W. R., and Huff, D. S.: Krabbe's Disease. Amer. J. Ophthal. 74:400–406, 1972.

Konigsmark, B. W., Knox, D. L., Hussels, I. E., and Moses, H.: Dominant Congenital Deafness and Progressive Optic Nerve Atrophy. Arch. Ophthal. 91:99–103, 1974.

VISUAL FIELD DEFECTS

Contents

Pseudo-field Defect

1. Facial contour
   A. Prominent nose
   B. Bushy projecting eyebrows
   C. High cheekbones
   D. Ptosis or blepharochalasis

2. Corneal opacities

3. Lenticular opacities, especially if miotics are used to depress fields and exaggerate existing scotomas

4. Aphakia without lens or with convex lens; little distortion with contact lens or intraocular acrylic lens

5. Dull patient—patient may be mentally defective, have toxemia, arteriosclerosis, cerebral tumor, brain abscess, or increased intracranial pressure

6. Pupillary size
   A. Decrease in miotic field, especially with opacities of ocular media
   B. Drooping of upper lid over pupillary aperture decreases field

7. Uncorrected refractive errors—correct presbyopia for distance testing

8. Head tilting—when the head is tilted toward the left shoulder the right blind spot is elevated; when the head is tilted toward the right shoulder the right blind spot is lowered

9. Environmental artifacts
   A. Reduction in illumination of screen and test objects magnifies field defect
   B. Variation in size of test object changes field defect
   C. Standard distance of patient from screen
   D. Attention of patient
   E. Technique of examiner

10. Psychologic artifacts
    A. Patient's misunderstanding of test
    B. Tiring of patient by prolonged testing
    C. Malingering—isopters at different distances are inconsistent
    D. Hysteria—spiral field defects may be found

11. Frames of glasses and segments of multifocal lenses

Kolker, A. E., and Hetherington, J.: Becker-Shaffer's Diagnosis and Therapy of the Glaucomas, 3rd ed. St. Louis, C. V. Mosby Co., 1970, pp. 156–159.

Reed, H.: The Essentials of Perimetry. New York, Oxford University Press, 1960, pp. 37, 66–69.

Bilateral Central Scotomas (bilateral macular defects with decreased visual acuity; the scotomas may be central or centrocecal)

1. Bilateral macular lesions such as cysts or those due to hemorrhage, edema, degeneration, detachment, hole, or infection

2. Bilateral optic nerve lesions
    A. Papillitis (see p. 477)
    B. Retrobulbar neuritis (see p. 477)
    C. Papilledema with macular edema (see p. 482)

3. Toxic agents
    A. Tobacco
    B. Ethyl alcohol
    C. Methyl alcohol
    D. Carbon disulfide
    E. Halogenated hydrocarbons—methyl chloride, methyl bromide, iodoform, trichloroethylene
    F. Aromatic amino- and nitro- compounds—aniline, nitrobenzene, trinitrotoluene

G. Drugs
   (1) Sedatives—barbiturates, ethchlorvynol, pheni-
       prazine, Disulfiram, opium, morphine
   (2) Anti-infection drugs—sulfanilamide, isoniazid,
       chloramphenicol
   (3) Miscellaneous drugs—digoxin, stramonium, thy-
       roxin, ricin, apiol, nicotinic acid
H. Metals—lead, thallium (inorganic), arsenic

4. Familial optic atrophies (see p. 477)

5. Migraine—forerunner of visual aurae

6. Nutritional deficiency, such as thiamine or vitamin B_{12} deficiency

7. Pernicious anemia

8. Diabetes mellitus

9. Occipital cortex lesions

Cocke, J. G.: Chloramphenicol Optic Neuritis. Amer. J. Dis. Child.
   114:424–426, 1967.
Duke-Elder, S., and Scott, G. I.: System of Ophthalmology, Vol. XII.
   St. Louis, C. V. Mosby Co., 1971, pp. 145–166.
Friedman, B.: Migraine: with Special Reference to Scintillating
   Scotoma. Eye Ear Nose Throat Monthly *50*:52–58, 1971.
Harrington, D. O.: The Visual Fields, 3rd ed. St. Louis, C. V. Mosby
   Co., 1971.

Enlargement of the Blind Spot

1. Papilledema (see p. 482)

2. Papillitis (see p. 477)

3. Glaucoma

4. Progressive myopia with a temporal crescent

5. Medullated nerve fibers

6. Drusen of the optic nerve (see p. 493)

7. Coloboma of the optic nerve

8. Senility—senile halo

9. Early manifestation of other defect, such as centrocecal scotoma or arcuate defect

10. Inferior conus

11. Juxtapapillary choroiditis

12. Inverted disc or nasally directed scleral canal

O'Brien, C. S.: Ophthalmology, Notes for Students. Iowa City, Athens Press, 1930, p. 347.
Reed, H.: The Essentials of Perimetry. New York, Oxford University Press, 1960, pp. 69–70.
Zuckerman, J.: Perimetry. Philadelphia, J. B. Lippincott Company, 1954.

Arcuate (Cuneate) Scotoma (the scotoma follows the lines of the nerve fibers in the retina with the narrow end at the blind spot and broad end at horizontal raphe)

1. Glaucoma

2. Vascular accident affecting the optic nerve

3. Acute bleeding episode

4. Drusen of optic nerve

5. Chorioretinitis juxtapapillaris

6. High myopia

7. Coloboma of the disc

17

8. Inferior conus

9. Supratraction

Drance, S. M.: The Glaucomatous Visual Field. Invest. Ophthal. *11*:85–97, 1972.

Harrington, D. O.: The Visual Fields, 3rd ed. St. Louis, C. V. Mosby Co., 1971.

Reed, H.: The Essentials of Perimetry. New York, Oxford University Press, 1960, p. 85.

Unilateral Sector-Shaped Defects (narrow end of scotoma characteristically touches the physiologic blind spot)

1. Optic disc involvement
   A. Secondary optic atrophy after choked disc (more on nasal side)
   B. Papillitis
   C. Glaucoma (early stages primarily on nasal side)

2. Retina
   A. Juxtapapillary chorioretinitis
   B. Branch embolism of the central retinal artery

3. Optic nerve—between disc and chiasm
   A. Tumor
   B. Aneurysm
   C. Drusen

Huber, A.: Eye Symptoms in Brain Tumors, 2nd ed. St. Louis, C. V. Mosby Co., 1971, p. 83.

Knight, C. L., and Hoyt, W. F.: Monocular Blindness from Drusen of the Optic Disc. Amer. J. Ophthal. *73*:890–892, 1972.

Peripheral Field Contraction (central vision present; patient may complain of poor night vision [see p. 545])

1. Optic atrophy (see p. 478)

2. Retinitis pigmentosa

3. Papillitis (see p. 477)

4. Glaucoma

5. Hysteria and malingering

6. Retinitis—periphery of fundus

7. Choroiditis—periphery of fundus

8. Poisons
   A. Quinine
   B. Chloroquine
   C. Arsenic
   D. Salicylates
   E. Optochin (ethylhydrocuprenic poisoning—in the past Optochin was used in the treatment of pneumococcal infection)
   F. Filax mas—drug used in the past in the treatment of worm infestation
   G. Carbon monoxide
   H. Thioridazine
   I. Oxygen poisoning
   J. Carbon tetrachloride
   K. Methyl iodide
   L. Acridine derivatives
   M. Ergot
   N. Aspidium and other vegetable derivatives

9. Many conditions in which night blindness occurs (see p. 545)

10. Drusen of optic disc

11. Double homonymous hemianopia (if the macular sparing in one homonymous hemianopia is larger than that in the other homonymous hemianopia, the spared central portion of the field has small vertical steps, above and below fixaation, where the two areas of macular sparing do not quite coincide)
    A. Stroke or infarction of occipital lobe
    B. Cortical blindness with damage to occipital lobe and macular recovery
        (1) Trauma
        (2) Anoxia
        (3) Carbon monoxide poisoning
        (4) Cerebral angiography
        (5) Cardiac arrest
        (6) Exsanguination

12. Frontal lobe tumors

13. General apathy in a lackadaisical subject

14. Chronic atrophic papilledema

15. Unilateral concentric constriction excluding diseased retina or glaucoma suggests lesion of optic nerve and chiasm
    A. Tumor of optic nerve
    B. Meningioma of tuberculum sellae, sphenoid ridge, or the olfactory groove

Duke-Elder, S., and Scott, G. I.: System of Ophthalmology, Vol. XII. St. Louis, C. V. Mosby Co., 1971, pp. 145–166.

Harrington, D. O.: The Visual Fields, 3rd ed. St. Louis, C. V. Mosby Co., 1971, pp. 125–126.

Huber, A.: Eye Symptoms in Brain Tumors, 2nd ed. St. Louis, C. V. Mosby Co., 1971, pp. 81–82.

Knight, C. L., and Hoyt, W. F.: Monocular Blindness from Drusen of the Optic Disc. Amer. J. Ophthal. 73:890–892, 1972.

O'Brien, C. S.: Ophthalmology, Notes for Students. Iowa City, Athens Press, 1930, p. 347.

Altitudinal Hemianopia (defective vision or blindness in the upper or lower horizontal half of the visual field; may be unilateral or bilateral; the unilateral field defect is prechiasmal)

1. Superior or inferior retinal artery obstruction—unilateral

2. Glaucomatous cupping—usually greatest in lower portion of optic nerve, giving superior altitudinal hemianopia; associated especially with low tension glaucoma

3. Optic nerve lesions, such as papilledema and atrophy (see pp. 482 and 487)

4. Injury to the optic nerve—due to torsion, edema, or shearing of the small vessels supplying the optic nerve

5. Coloboma of optic nerve

6. Sclerotic plaques of internal carotid artery or anterior cerebral arteries—pressure of plaques on optic nerve results in inferior altitudinal hemianopia

7. Fusiform aneurysms (arteriosclerotic or congenital)—may produce inferior altitudinal hemianopia by pressure against the lateral halves of the optic chiasm or nerve

8. Lesion that presses the chiasm upward against the superior margin of the optic foramen

9. Olfactory groove meningioma extending postero-inferior to compress the intracranial portion of the optic nerve

10. Trauma to or vascular insufficiency of occipital lobe—inferior altitudinal hemianopia results when the upper lips of both calcarine fissures are damaged; when the lower lips of both calcarine fissures are damaged, superior altitudinal hemianopia is produced

11. Anemia—produces bilateral inferior altitudinal hemianopia

12. Exsanguination

Cogan, D. G.: Neurology of the Visual System, 3rd ed. Springfield, Ill., Charles C Thomas, 1966, pp. 31, 137, 185, 188, 224.

Harrington, D. O.: The Visual Fields, 3rd ed. St. Louis, C. V. Mosby Co., 1971.

McLean, J. M., and Roy, B. S.: Soft Glaucoma and Calcification of the Internal Carotid Arteries. Arch. Ophthal. *38*:154, 1947.

Walker, C. B., and Cushing, H.: Studies of Optic Nerve Atrophy in Association with Chiasmal Lesions. Arch. Ophthal. *45*:407, 1916.

Binasal Hemianopia (defects in nasal half of visual fields; usually incomplete; due to lateral involvement of the chiasm; presupposes bilateral lesions)

1. Chiasmic arachnoiditis, postneuritic optic atrophy, and bilateral retrobulbar neuritis of multiple sclerosis

2. Drusen of optic nerve (see p. 493)

3. Fusiform aneurysms—arteriosclerotic or congenital—of internal carotid artery

4. Sclerotic plaques of internal carotid artery or anterior cerebral arteries

5. Pituitary tumor with third ventricle dilatation pushing laterally

6. Symmetrical lesions in the temporal halves of both retinas, such as severe retinal edema associated with diabetic retinopathy

7. Nasal quadrant peripheral depression of glaucoma—bilateral and reasonably symmetrical

8. Bilateral occipital lesion (thrombosis)

9. Trauma

10. Severe exsanguination

506

Cogan, D. G.: Neurology of the Visual System, 3rd ed. Springfield, Ill., Charles C Thomas, 1966, pp. 150, 188, 210, 217, 224.

Duke-Elder, S., and Scott, G. I.: System of Ophthalmology, Vol. XII. St. Louis, C. V. Mosby Co., 1971, pp. 292–293.

Harrington, D. O.: The Visual Fields, 3rd ed. St. Louis, C. V. Mosby Co., 1971, pp. 123–124.

Bitemporal Hemianopia (defects in temporal half of visual field; usually incomplete; due to pressure on the optic chiasm)

* = Most important

1. Chiasmal lesions
    A. Vascular lesions
        (1) Arteriosclerosis
        (2) Arterial compression
        (3) Thrombosis of the carotid artery
        *(4) Intracranial aneurysms, such as congenital, endocardial emboli, traumatic, atheromatic, or syphilitic, especially intrasellar aneurysms
    B. Inflammatory lesions
        (1) Chiasmal neuritis
        *(2) Basal meningitis, including chronic chiasmal arachnoiditis, syphilitic, tuberculous, actinomycotic, and cysticercal
    C. Tumors of the chiasma
        *(1) Primary tumors including gliomas in childhood
        *(2) Secondary tumors (rare) including meningiomas, retinoblastoma, pinealoma, and ependymoma

2. Pituitary lesions
    A. Pituitary hyperplasia
    B. Pituitary tumors

    (1) Adenoma
        a. Chromophobe adenoma—varies from no endocrine symptoms to panhypopituitarism; most common type of pituitary tumor
        b. Acidophilic adenoma—varies from gigantism to acromegaly
        c. Basophilic adenoma—hyperadrenalism (Cushing's disease), rare
    (2) Adenocarcinoma (rare)
    (3) Metastatic tumors as from breast (rare)

3. Perisellar lesions
    A. Suprasellar tumors
      *(1) Craniopharyngioma—manifestations may include diabetes insipidus, infantilism, and calcification of hypophyseal-pituitary region
      *(2) Suprasellar meningioma
      (3) Chordoma
      (4) Cholesteatoma
      (5) Epidermoids
      (6) Teratoma
      (7) Pinealoma
      (8) Lymphoblastoma
      (9) Tumors of the frontal lobe including porencephaly (cystic cavity in brain substance) and glioma
      (10) Tumors of the third ventricle and internal hydrocephalus, such as glioma and epidymoma
    B. Presellar tumors
      *(1) Meningioma of the olfactory groove
      (2) Neuroblastoma of the olfactory groove
    C. Parasellar tumors
      *(1) Meningioma of the sphenoid ridge
      (2) Tumors of the sphenoid bone including osteochondroma, sarcoma, anaplastic carcinoma
      (3) Tumors of the basal meninges
      (4) Injuries to the chiasmal pathway, such as from trauma
      (5) Migraine
      (6) Sudden onset without apparent cause
        a. Disseminated sclerosis

b. Arteriosclerotic or giant-cell arteritic occlusion of nutrient vessels of the chiasm in elderly patients

Cogan, D. G.: Neurology of the Visual System, 3rd ed. Springfield, Ill., Charles C Thomas, 1966, pp. 217, 222, 224, 228, 233, 239.
Duke-Elder, S., and Scott, G. I.: System of Ophthalmology, Vol. XII. St. Louis, C. V. Mosby Co., 1971, pp. 299–395.
Finn, J. E., and Mount, L. A.: Meningioma of the Tuberculum Sellae and Planum Sphenoidale. Arch. Ophthal. 92:23–27, 1974.
Walsh, F. B., and Hoyt, W. F.: Clinical Neuro-ophthalmology, 3rd ed. Baltimore, Williams & Wilkins Co., 1969, pp. 69–75, 730, 1674.

Homonymous Quadrantanopia (one quadrant involved in upper or lower and right or left visual fields)

1. Superior homonymous quadrantanopia
   A. Temporal lobe—incongruous
   B. Inferior lip of the calcarine fissure—congruous

2. Inferior homonymous quadrantanopia
   A. Superior radiation in parietal lobe—incongruous
   B. Upper lip of the calcarine fissure in the occipital lobe —congruous

Harrington, D. O.: The Visual Fields, 3rd ed. St. Louis, C. V. Mosby Co., 1971, pp. 121–123.

Crossed Quadrantanopia (upper quadrant of one visual field is lost along with the lower quadrant of the opposite visual field)

1. Chiasm compression from lesion below compressing it against contiguous arterial structure

2. Glaucoma

3. Inflammatory lesion, such as choroiditis juxtapapillaris

4. Asymmetrical homonymous hemianopia, such as vascular lesion of the upper lip of the calcarine area on one side and the lower lip of the opposite calcarine cortex

Harrington, D. O.: The Visual Fields, 3rd ed. St. Louis, C. V. Mosby Co., 1971, p. 124.

Homonymous Hemianopia (hemianopia affecting the right or left halves of the visual fields; the lesion is posterior to the optic chiasm)

1. Optic tract lesions—visual conduction system posterior to optic chiasm and anterior to lateral geniculate body; lesion demonstrates incongruous field defect on side opposite to defect, often with decreased vision
   A. Saccular aneurysms of internal carotid or posterior communicating artery
   B. Pituitary adenomas and craniopharyngiomas (most common); nasopharyngeal carcinomas, chordomas, infundibulomas, and gliomas (less common)
   C. Demyelinative disease—retrobulbar, multiple sclerosis, and Schilder's disease
   D. Trauma
   E. Migraine

2. Temporoparietal lesions—temporal lobe lesions are manifest initially in the upper visual fields, whereas lesions of the parietal lobe are first manifest in the lower visual fields
   A. Vascular lesions—sudden onset
      (1) Thrombosis—premonitory symptoms include unilateral blackouts in one eye
      (2) Embolism—may be associated with rheumatic or arteriosclerotic heart disease, bacterial endocarditis, myocardial infarction, or septic focus in lungs
      (3) Occlusion—middle cerebral occlusion affects primarily the arm and face; anterior cerebral occlusion affects primarily the leg
      (4) Subdural hematoma—spontaneous or following trauma
   B. Tumor—gradual onset of symptoms—lesions include intrinsic astrocytoma and glioblastoma, extrinsic meningioma, and lung metastasis
   C. Diffuse demyelinative diseases
      (1) Schilder's type
      (2) Pelizaeus-Merzbacher type
      (3) Krabbe's type
      (4) Metachromatic leukoencephalopathy
      (5) Progressive multifocal leukoencephalopathy
      (6) Spongy degeneration of the brain
   D. Migraine
3. Occipital lesions—congruous field defect and macular sparing most likely
   A. Vascular lesions—sudden onset
      (1) Occlusion of posterior cerebral artery—thrombotic or embolic
      (2) Arteriovenous anomalies
      (3) Aneurysms (rare)
      (4) Subclavian steal syndrome, with reversal of blood flow through the vertebral artery
   B. Tumors—gradual onset of symptoms—lesions include intrinsic astrocytoma and glioblastoma, extrinsic meningioma, and lung metastasis
   C. Demyelinative disease
      (1) Schilder's type

        (2) Pelizaeus-Merzbacher type

        (3) Krabbe's type

        (4) Metachromatic leukoencephalopathy

        (5) Progressive multifocal leukoencephalopathy

        (6) Spongy degeneration of the brain

D. Trauma

        (1) Direct—penetrating missiles and depressed bone fragments

        (2) Indirect—general concussion syndrome

E. Poisons, such as carbon monoxide, digitalis, mescal, opium, LSD

F. Migraine

Cogan, D. G.: Neurology of the Visual System, 3rd ed. Springfield, Ill., Charles C Thomas, 1966, pp. 249, 256, 262, 290, 296.

Friedman, B.: Migraine: with Special Reference to Scintillating Scotoma. Eye Ear Nose Throat Monthly 50:52–58, 1971.

Harrington, D. O.: The Visual Fields, 3rd ed. St. Louis, C. V. Mosby Co., 1971.

Smith, J. L.: Homonymous Hemianopsia: a Review of 100 Cases. Amer. J. Ophthal. 54:616, 1962.

Trobe, J. D., Lorber, M. L., and Schlezinger, N. S.: Isolated Homonymous Hemianopia. Arch. Ophthal. 89:377–381, 1973.

GENERAL
SIGNS AND SYMPTOMS

VISUAL DISTURBANCE

Contents

Acquired Myopia (error of refraction, in which parallel rays of light focus in front of the retina usually producing blurred distant vision and clear near vision [see Spasm of Accommodation, p. 353])

1. Conditions such as diabetes mellitus or nuclear cataract in which there is increased index of refraction of lens

2. Increased curvature of the refracting surfaces due to:
   A. Ciliary muscle spasm
      (1) Functional—adolescence, hysteria
      (2) Medication—miotics, such as pilocarpine; cholinesterase inhibitors, such as Eserine or Phospholine Iodide
      (3) Trauma—ocular contusion or anterior dislocation of the lens
      (4) Mushroom (*Amanita muscaria*) poisoning
   B. Lens hydration changes—diabetes mellitus, dysentery, or toxemia of pregnancy
   C. Drug reaction—probably due to ciliary body edema
      (1) Sulfa drugs, including some carbonic anhydrase inhibitors such as acetazolamide and ethoxzolamide
      (2) Phenothiazides such as hydrochlorothiazide
      (3) Organic arsenicals such as arsphenamine and neoarsphenamine
   D. Paralysis of accommodation for distance (sympathetic paralysis)—young patient with unilateral Horner's syndrome or migraine
   E. Retrolental fibroplasia

3. Syndromes associated with myopia:
   A. Homocystinuria—subluxation of lens, malar flush, osteoporosis
   B. Kenny's syndrome—short stature, slim medullary cavity, transient hypocalcemia
   C. Marfan's syndrome—arachnodactyly with hyperextensibility, lens subluxation, aortic dilatation, bluish sclerae

D. Marshall's syndrome—cataract, thick lips, partial deafness, low nasal bridge with short depressed nose
E. Schwartz's syndrome—myotonia, blepharophimosis, joint limitation, low-set ears
F. Stickler's syndrome—joint pain and stiffness, myopia, deafness
G. Weil-Marchesani syndrome—brachydactylia, small spherical lens, short stature, malformed and malaligned teeth
H. Cornelia De Lange's syndrome—synophrys of eyebrows, thin down-turning upper lip, micromelia, mental retardation
I. Ehlers-Danlos syndrome—hyperextensibility of joints, hyperextensibility of skin, poor wound healing with thin scar, narrow maxilla
J. XXXXY syndrome—hypogenitalism, limited elbow pronation, low dermal ridge count on fingertips, short neck, wide-set eyes
K. Myasthenia gravis—blepharoptosis, external ophthalmoplegia, internal ophthalmoplegia
L. Noonan's syndrome (male Turner's syndrome)—antimongoloid slant, hypertelorism, epicanthal folds, exophthalmos, keratoconus, posterior embryotoxon, strabismus
M. Alport's syndrome

Grant, W. M.: Toxicology of the Eye, 2nd ed. Springfield, Ill., Charles C Thomas, 1973.
Milot, J., and Denoy, F.: Ocular Anomalies in DeLange Syndrome. Arch. Ophthal. *74*:394–399, 1972.
Romano, P. E., and Stark, W. J.: Pseudomyopia as a Presenting Sign in Ocular Myasthenia Gravis. Amer. J. Ophthal. *75*:872–875, 1973.
Schatz, H.: Alport's Syndrome in a Negro Kindred. Amer. J. Ophthal. *71*:1236–1240, 1971.
Schwartz, D. E.: Noonan's Syndrome Associated with Ocular Abnormalities. Amer. J. Ophthal. *73*:955–960, 1972.
Smith, D. W.: Recognizable Patterns of Human Malformation. Philadelphia, W. B. Saunders Co., 1970, pp. 280, 260, 214, 258, 180, 100, 84, 240, 62, 262, 36.

Tasman, W.: Retrolental Fibroplasia. *In* Tasman, W. (Ed.): Retinal Diseases in Children. New York, Harper & Row, Inc., 1971, pp. 105–120.

Walsh, F. B., and Hoyt, W. F.: Clinical Neuro-ophthalmology, Vol. I, 3rd ed. Baltimore, Williams & Wilkins Co., 1969, pp. 550–551.

Acquired Hyperopia (farsightedness, error of refraction, in which parallel rays of light focus behind the retina usually producing clear distant vision and blurred near vision, see Paresis of Accommodation, p. 354)

1. Drugs
   A. Chloroquine
   B. Phenothiazides
   C. Meprobamate
   D. Antihistamines such as diphenhydramine (Benadryl) and prophenpyridamine (Trimeton)
   E. Systemic parasympatholytic drugs such as atropine sulfate and tincture of belladonna
   F. Topical parasympatholytic drugs such as atropine sulfate, cyclopenolate hydrochloride (Cyclogyl), tropicamide (Mydriacyl)
   G. Cannabis (marihuana)
   H. Imipramine (Tofranil)
   I. Systemic ganglionic blocking agents such as pentolinum tartrate (Ansolysen)

2. Toxin of *Clostridium botulinum*

3. Trauma to the eye with posterior dislocation of the lens, macular edema, or ciliary body contusion

4. Orbital tumor with extraocular globe pressure and retinal striae

5. Adie's syndrome

6. Presbyopia—after the age of about forty-five years

7. Lesions causing internal ophthalmoplegia with paralysis of accommodation (see p. 337)

8. Flat cornea

9. Hyperopia—refractive or axial

10. Aphakia

11. Short eyeball—congenital

12. Microphthalmos

Grant, W. M.: Toxicology of the Eye, 2nd ed. Springfield, Ill., Charles C Thomas, 1973.

Marmor, M. F.: Transient Accommodative Paralysis and Hyperopia in Diabetes. Arch. Ophthal. *89*:419–421, 1973.

Newell, F. W.: Ophthalmology, Principles and Concepts. St. Louis, C. V. Mosby Co., 1969.

O'Brien, C. S.: Ophthalmology, Notes for Students. Iowa City, Athens Press, 1930, p. 346.

Reinecke, R. D., and Herm, R. J.: Refraction, a Programmed Text. New York, Appleton-Century-Crofts, Inc., 1965, p. 184.

Metamorphopsia (visual disturbance in which the shape of objects is distorted; objects may appear smaller [micropsia] or larger [macropsia] than they are)

1. Ocular
   A. Astigmatism
   B. Macular lesions, including orbital tumor and macular striae, macular edema, or macular inflammation
   C. Retinal detachment
   D. Posterior vitreous separation and residual vitreoretinal macular traction
   E. Subnormal accommodation—micropsia
   F. Spasm of accommodation—macropsia

2. Cerebral
   A. Epilepsy
   B. Schizophrenia
   C. Drug intoxications
   D. Focal lesions such as thrombosis of right middle cerebral artery
   E. Migraine
   F. Parietal lobe lesion including tumor and vascular lesion

3. Paget's disease

4. Hysteria

Cogan, D. G.: Neurology of the Visual System, 3rd ed. Springfield, Ill., Charles C Thomas, 1966, p. 268.

Klee, A., and Willanger, R.: Disturbances of Visual Perception in Migraine. Acta Neurol. Scand. *42*:400–411, 1966.

Walsh, F. B., and Hoyt, W. F.: Clinical Neuro-ophthalmology, Vol. I, 3rd ed. Baltimore, Williams & Wilkins Co., 1969, pp. 115–116, 544–545, 1660.

Amaurosis Fugax (transient monocular blackout of vision)

1. Functional—hysteria, neurasthenia

2. Cerebrovascular insufficiency
   A. Unilateral occlusive carotid disease
   B. Fibromuscular hyperplasia
   C. Takayasu's syndrome
   D. Congenital or acquired arteriovenous malformations
   E. Arterial aneurysms
   F. Post-traumatic acute and chronic arterial occlusion

3. Hypotension of fundus
   A. Cardiac arrhythmia
   B. Papilledema—lasts for 15 to 30 seconds (see p. 482)
   C. Increased intracranial pressure, such as from intracranial tumors that interfere with vascular supply to the optic nerve

D. Orbital vascular insufficiency with giant-cell arteritis

E. Negative G-force in pilots—circular maneuver with head toward the center of the circle

F. Impending vascular occlusion, such as spasm of the central retinal artery

G. Increased venous pressure

    (1) Impending central retinal vein occlusion

    (2) Intermittent elevation of intraocular pressure (glaucoma)

4. Uniocular variety of ophthalmic migraine

5. Raynaud's disease

6. Hematologic causes

    A. Polycythemia

    B. Severe anemia

    C. Sickle cell disease

    D. Idiopathic thrombocytosis

    E. Emboli

        (1) Infective, such as subacute bacterial endocarditis

        (2) Gas in dysbarism

    F. Multiple myeloma

7. Arteriosclerosis, hypertension, and hypertensive crisis

8. Uremic amaurosis—with eclampsia

9. Quinine poisoning

10. Large vitreous floater

11. Wasp sting

12. Multiple sclerosis—induced or aggravated by physical exertion (Uhthoff's symptom)

Cogan, D. G.: Neurology of the Visual System, 3rd ed. Springfield, Ill., Charles C Thomas, 1966, pp. 38–40, 188.

Hollenhorst, R. W.: Ophthalmodynamometry and Intracranial Disease. Med. Clin. N. Amer. *42*:951, 1958.

Sandok, B. A., et al.: Clinical Angiographic Correlations in Amaurosis Fugax. Amer. J. Ophthal. *78*:137–142, 1974.

Walter, J. R., and Burchfield, W. J.: Ocular Migraine in a Young Man Resulting in Unilateral Transient Blindness and Retinal Edema. J. Pediat. Ophthal. *8*:173–176, 1971.

Wylie, E. J., and Ehrenfeld, W. K.: Extracranial Occlusive Cerebrovascular Disease: Diagnosis and Management. Philadelphia, W. B. Saunders Co., 1970, pp. 65–72.

Sudden Loss of Visual Acuity

1. Temporal arteritis

2. Occlusion of central retinal artery

3. Optic neuritis, papillitis, retrobulbar neuritis

4. Vitreous or retinal hemorrhage

5. Acute congestive glaucoma

6. Fracture of the lesser wing of the sphenoid bone

7. Quinine poisoning

8. Wood alcohol poisoning (methyl)

9. Injury to the optic nerve

10. Retinal detachment

11. Brain injury

12. Brain stem arteriovenous malformations

13. Following orbital operation

Lessell, S., et al.: Brain Stem Arteriovenous Malformations. Arch. Ophthal. *86*:255–259, 1971.

Long, J. C., and Ellis, P. P.: Total Unilateral Visual Loss Following Orbital Surgery. Amer. J. Ophthal. *71*:218–220, 1971.

O'Brien, C. S.: Ophthalmology, Notes for Students. Iowa City, Athens Press, 1930, pp. 345–346.

Smith, J. L.: The University of Miami Neuro-Ophthalmology Symposium, Vol. 1. Springfield, Ill., Charles C Thomas, 1964, pp. 34–56.

Smith, J. L.: Blindness in Early Syphilis. Arch. Ophthal. *90*:256–258, 1973.

Post-traumatic Loss of Vision

1. Lid swelling, blood or foreign material covering cornea, corneal damage

2. Hyphema, vitreous hemorrhage

3. Traumatic cataract, luxation of the lens

4. Central retinal artery or vein occlusion (from markedly increased orbital pressure or embolus)

5. Traumatic retinal edema and hemorrhages of retina from direct or contre-coup blows

6. Retinal detachment

7. Avulsion of optic nerve by lateral orbital wall trauma or contre-coup blow to head

8. Indirect trauma to optic nerves and/or chiasm

9. Intracranial interruption of visual pathways (hemorrhage, foreign body)

10. Cortical blindness from hematoma, ischemia, or anoxia (patient may be unaware of blindness) (see p. 531)

11. Acute congestive (angle closure) glaucoma precipitated by emotional trauma of recent accident or from intumescent lens or other causes

12. Hysteria

13. Malingering

Paton, D., and Goldberg, M. F.: Injuries of the Eye, the Lids, and the Orbit. Philadelphia, W. B. Saunders Co., 1968, p. 5.

Blindness in Infants

1. Cortical blindness (see p. 531)

2. Congenital or infantile affections of the optic nerve
   A. Retarded myelinization or maturation
   B. Hereditary atrophy of the optic nerve
   C. Secondary atrophy of the optic nerve (see optic atrophy in children, p. 487)
      (1) Hydrocephalus
      (2) Crouzon's craniofacial dysostosis
      (3) Oxycephaly
      (4) Osteopetrosis
      (5) Asphyxia at birth
      (6) Infections such as meningitis and encephalomyelitis
      (7) Accidents such as fractures of the skull; subdural hematoma; and cerebral hemorrhage
      (8) Tumors such as astrocytoma, craniopharyngioma, glioblastoma, angioma, and Burkitt's lymphoma
      (9) Meningioma
      (10) Vascular and inflammatory disease such as tuberculosis or meningitis
      (11) Associated with widespread disease such as mental deficiency, cerebral palsy, epilepsy, deafness, and obesity
      (12) Cavernous sinus thrombosis
      (13) Encephalitis
   D. Aplasia of optic nerve

3. Congenital or infantile affection of the retina
   A. Leber's congenital tapetoretinal heredodegeneration
   B. Reese's retinal dysplasia
   C. Early chorioretinal heredodegenerations including Stargardt's disease, and pigmentary retinopathy (see pseudoretinitis pigmentosa, p. 421)
   D. Myopia with or without detachment
   E. Albinism
   F. Achromatopsia

  G. Retinoschisis
  H. Retrolental fibroplasia
  I. Retinoblastoma
  J. Coats' disease
  K. Infections and embryopathies (toxoplasmosis, rubella, syphilis)

4. Persistence of the primary vitreous

5. Congenital cataracts (see syndromes associated with cataracts, p. 343)

6. Affections and inflammations of the uvea
  A. Fetal or infantile uveitis (pseudoglioma, infective endophthalmitis, posterior uveitis, Still's disease)
  B. Colobomatous affections

7. Congenital glaucoma (see congenital glaucoma, p. 266)

8. Corneal dystrophies

9. Syndromes associated with amaurosis or blindness
  A. Marfan's syndrome
  B. Bardet-Biedl syndrome
  C. Malformative syndrome with cryptophthalmos

10. Porencephaly

11. Niemann-Pick disease

12. Metachromatic leukodystrophy

13. Davidoff's single ventricle

14. Schilder's disease

15. Keratitis
  A. Measles
  B. Smallpox
  C. Ophthalmia neonatorum
  D. Pemphigus

Francois, J.: Diagnosis of Blindness in the Infant. Ann. Ophthal. 2:533–554, 1970.

Fraser, G. R., and Friedmann, A. I.: The Causes of Blindness in Childhood. Baltimore, The Johns Hopkins Press, 1967.

Olurin, O.: Etiology of Blindness in Nigerian Children. Amer. J. Ophthal. 70:533–540, 1970.

Walsh, T. J., Smith, J. L., and Shipley, T.: Blindness in Infants. Amer. J. Ophthal. 62:546–556, 1966.

Binocular Diplopia (double vision using both eyes)*

1. Paralysis of one or more extraocular muscles
    A. Fourth nerve palsy (rare) (p. 137)
    B. Third nerve palsy—with isolated muscle paralysis, one must suspect a nuclear lesion (hemorrhage, syphilis, multiple sclerosis), or myasthenia gravis (p. 134)
    C. Sixth nerve palsy—has no localizing value (p. 139)

2. Intractable postoperative diplopia
    A. Anomalous retinal correspondence with or without amblyopia (common); this is called paradoxical diplopia
    B. "Horror fusonis" (rare)—congenital or developmental deficiency of fusion, i.e., absence of sensory correspondence between two eyes (this is not the same as abnormal retinal correspondence, since visual directions are normal in these cases)
    C. Cyclotropia due to oblique muscle operation
    D. Large surgical overcorrection
    E. Following surgical treatment of retinal detachment due to symblepharon or limitation of extraocular movement

3. Other
    A. Aniseikonia
    B. Psychogenic causes
    C. Physiologic diplopia
    D. Heterophoria—due to lesions such as orbital tumor and cellulitis

Norton, E. W. D.: Complications of Retinal Detachment Surgery. Symposium on Retina and Retinal Surgery. Transactions of New Orleans Academy Ophthalmology. St. Louis, C. V. Mosby Co., 1969, pp. 222–223.

*1 and 2 modified from Bedrossian, E. H.: The Eye. Springfield, Ill., Charles C Thomas, 1958, pp. 252, 254.

Binocular Triplopia (uniocular diplopia)*

1. Optical causes external to the eye
   A. Looking through the edge of a bifocal or margin of lens
   B. Improper correction of a high astigmatism
   C. Double or single prism placed in center of pupil before one eye

2. Optical causes in the eye
   A. High myopia, probably due to irregular astigmatism
   B. Irregular astigmatism such as pressure on the globe
   C. Double pupil
   D. Dislocation of the lens or misalignment of corneal and lenticular optical axis
   E. Lens abnormalities such as fluid clefts or incipient cataract
   F. Air bubbles or transparent foreign bodies in aqueous or vitreous
   G. Retinal detachment
   H. Irregular spasm of the ciliary muscle
   I. Complete or partial contraction of the eyelids, in which the eyelids impinge on the cornea (De Schweintz)
   J. Migration of filtering bleb onto the cornea
   K. Keratoconus
   L. Megalocornea
   M. Spherophakia

3. Abnormal retinal correspondence with single image given two associations of direction, such that the abnormal retinal point is brought into consciousness at the same time as the macula image

4. Malingering, hysteria, or psychogenic causes

5. Central uniocular diplopia (rare)—systemic or neurologic causes include cerebral aneurysm, abscess or gross degener-

---

*1 and 2 modified from Bedrossian, E. H.: The Eye. Springfield, Ill., Charles C Thomas, 1958, pp. 252–253.

ative lesions, encephalitis lethargica, postencephalitis, multiple sclerosis, basal meningitis, cerebellar tumor, and vertebrobasilar insufficiency

Rubin, M. L.: The Woman Who Saw Too Much. Surv. Ophthal. *16*:382–383, 1972.
Sugar, H. S.: Complications, Repair, and Reoperation of Antiglaucoma Filtering Blebs. Amer. J. Ophthal. *63*:825, 1967.

Diplopia Following Head Trauma

1. Orbital fracture (particularly blow-out fracture of the floor, causing restricted function of inferior rectus and inferior oblique muscles)

2. Hematoma in the orbit and/or the ocular muscles

3. Third, fourth, and/or sixth cranial nerve palsies (orbital or intracranial)

4. Avulsion, contusion, or transection of extraocular muscles

5. Avulsion of the pulley of the superior oblique

6. Subluxation of the lens (monocular diplopia)

7. Edema or detachment of the macula (monocular diplopia)

8. Decompensation of a preexisting ocular phoria, becoming a tropia

9. "Whiplash" injury and other diplopias of obscure origin

Paton, D., and Goldberg, M. F.: Injuries of the Eye, the Lids, and the Orbit. Philadelphia, W. B. Saunders Co., 1968, p. 4.

Eccentric Vision (vision is best when the individual is not looking directly at the object of regard)

1. Central scotoma

2. Homonymous hemianopia with macular involvement

3. Glaucoma—late with only eccentric field remaining

4. Eccentric fixation with amblyopia

5. Ectopic macula such as macula displaced by retinal scarring or fibrous strands, often a result of retrolental fibroplasia

6. Craniopharyngioma

Huber, A.: Eye Symptoms in Brain Tumors, 2nd ed. St. Louis, C. V. Mosby Co., 1971, pp. 212–213.

O'Brien, C. S.: Ophthalmology, Notes for Students. Iowa City, Athens Press, 1930, p. 347.

Von Noorden, G. K., and Maumenee, A. E.: Atlas of Strabismus, 2nd ed. St. Louis, C. V. Mosby Co., 1973, p. 38.

Decreased Visual Acuity

1. Amblyopia or anopsia—disuse
   A. Strabismus—esotropia, exotropia, or hypertropia
   B. Monocular occlusion
   C. Anisometropia—difference in refractive error between the eyes

2. Optic neuritis—retrobulbar and papillitis including toxic causes such as those due to tobacco, alcohol, and quinine, see page 477

3. Macular pathology (see pp. 380–387)

4. Achromatopsia

5. Hysterical

6. Malingering

7. Nystagmus

8. Anomalous elevation of optic disc with hyperplastic glial tissue and anomalous retinal vessels

9. Opacities of cornea, lens, or vitreous precluding good vision

10. Myotonic dystrophy—exertional vision loss

11. Sphenoid sinus mucocele

Knight, C. L., Hoyt, W. F., and Wilson, C. B.: Syndrome of Incipient Prechiasmal Optic Nerve Compression. Arch. Ophthal. 87:1–11, 1972.

McCarthy, W. L., Frenkel, M., and Busse, B. J.: Visual Loss as the Only Symptom of Sphenoid Sinus Mucocele. Amer. J. Ophthal. 74:1134–1140, 1972.

Walsh, F. B., and Hoyt, W. F.: Clinical Neuro-ophthalmology, Vol. I, 3rd ed. Baltimore, Williams & Wilkins Co., 1969.

Bilateral Blurring of Vision

1. Vertebrobasilar insufficiency

2. Intracranial hypertension and advanced papilledema

3. Severe systemic hypertension

4. Systemic hypotension

5. Retinal "blackout" experienced by pilots

6. Migraine—attacks last 15 to 20 minutes

7. Drug-induced (see paresis of accommodation, p. 354)

Wylie, E. J., and Ehrenfeld, W. K.: Extracranial Occlusive Cerebrovascular Disease: Diagnosis and Management. Philadelphia, W. B. Saunders Co., 1970, p. 88.

Cortical Blindness (Cerebral Blindness) (complete loss of all visual sensation including all appreciation of light and dark—loss of reflex lid closure to bright illumination and to threatening gestures; retention of pupil constriction to light and accommodation; normal ophthalmoscopic examination; normal motility; may be associated with hemiplegia, sensory disorders, aphasia and disorientation)

1. Trauma
    A. To occipital region
    B. Birth trauma including heart dysfunction, postictal and vertebral artery injury
    C. Chiropractic manipulation of the neck and odontoic subluxation
    D. Ventriculography and ventriculoatrial shunt operation

2. Space-taking lesions, such as tumors, gummas, abscesses, and cysts

3. Inflammatory lesions
    A. Encephalitis (including that due to measles and to pertussis) and subacute sclerosing panencephalitis
    B. Syphilitic meningitis
    C. Meningococcal and pneumococcal meningitis
    D. Influenza and meningitis due to *Haemophilus influenzae*

4. Vascular lesions
    A. Basilar artery thrombosis
    B. Bilateral posterior cerebral artery occlusion
    C. Following cerebral or vertebral angiography
    D. Cerebral hemorrhages
    E. Subarachnoid hemorrhage
    F. Angioma of occipital region
    G. "Subclavian steal syndrome" with reversal of blood flow through the vertebral artery
    H. Anoxia from high altitude
    I. Cardiac arrest

J. Blood transfusion reaction

K. Blood loss syndrome

L. Angiospastic lesions, including hypertension, nephritis, eclampsia, uremia, and chronic lead poisoning (saturnism)

M. Anoxia from chronic respiratory insufficiency

N. Obstruction of the local venous sinus, such as from septic thrombosis of superior longitudinal sinus

O. Air embolism

P. Herniation of hippocampal gyrus associated with subdural hematoma

Q. Thrombotic thrombocytopenic purpura

R. Malaria

S. Following burns and sunstrokes

T. Periarteritis nodosa

U. Electroshock

V. Hydrocephalus and microcephaly

5. Toxic conditions

A. Intoxications, such as from carbon monoxide, carbon dioxide, and nitrous oxide

B. Chronic lead poisoning

C. Corticotropin therapy

D. With use of hexamethonium chloride, tansy poisoning, acute ethyl alcohol poisoning, and nitroglycerin poisoning

6. Degenerative conditions

A. Alper's progressive gray matter

B. Creutzfeldt-Jakob disease (corticostriatospinal degeneration)

C. Pompe's disease (generalized glycogenesis)

D. Scholz' subacute cerebral sclerosis

E. Schilder's disease

7. Common causes of cortical blindness in infants

A. Hydrocephalus

B. Hemorrhages in spastic palsy

C. Meningo-encephalitis

D. Cerebral dysgenesis associated with dementia

E. Subdural hematoma and cerebral edema due to trauma

F. Degenerations

(1) Galactosemia
(2) Phenylpyruvic oligophrenia
(3) Tay-Sachs disease
(4) Porencephaly
(5) Spongy degeneration of the brain
(6) Infantile neuroaxonal dystrophy
(7) Toxoplasmosis (rare)
(8) Cytomegalic inclusion disease (rare)

Altrocchi, P. A., Reinhardt, P. H., and Eckman, P. B.: Blindness and Meningeal Carcinomatosis. Arch. Ophthal. 88:508–512, 1972.
Davis, L. E., Harms, A. C., and Chin, T. D.: Transient Cortical Blindness and Cerebellar Ataxia Associated with Mumps. Arch. Ophthal. 85:366–368, 1971.
Duke-Elder, S., and Scott, G. I.: System of Ophthalmology, Vol. XII. St. Louis, C. V. Mosby Co., 1971, pp. 489–501.
Massey, J. Y., Roy, F. H., and Bornhofen, J. H.: Ocular Manifestations of Reye Syndrome. Arch. Ophthal. 91:441–444, 1974.
Walsh, F. B., and Hoyt, W. F.: Clinical Neuro-ophthalmology. 3rd ed. Baltimore, Williams & Wilkins Co., 1969.

VISUAL COMPLAINT

Contents

Photopsia (sparks or flashes of light before the eyes)

1. Oculodigital phenomenon
2. Moore's lightning streak—traction of a partially liquefied vitreous on the retina
3. Impending retinal detachment
4. Retinitis
5. Phosphene of quick eye motion (Flick phosphene)
6. Focal lesions of occipital region
7. Glaucoma
8. Migraine and epilepsy
9. Brain concussion
10. Idiopathic thrombocytosis
11. Retinal microembolization
12. Associated with arteriovenous aneurysm
13. Clomiphene citrate (Clomid)

Bernstein, H. N.: Some Iatrogenic Ocular Diseases from Systemically Administered Drugs. *In* Symposium on Ocular Pharmacology and Therapeutics. Transactions of New Orleans Academy of Ophthalmology. St. Louis, C. V. Mosby Co., 1970, pp. 143–163.

Cogan, D. G.: Neurology of the Visual System, 3rd ed. Springfield, Ill., Charles C Thomas, 1966, pp. 268, 313.

Levine, J., and Swanson, P. D.: Idiopathic Thrombocytosis: A Treatable Cause of Transient Ischemic Attacks. Neurology *18*:711–713, 1968.

Moore, R. F.: Subjective Lightning Streaks. Brit. J. Ophthal. *19*: 545, 1935.

Morse, P. H., Scheie, H. G., and Aminlari, A.: Light Flashes as a Clue to Retinal Disease. Arch. Ophthal. *91*:179–180, 1974.

Nebel, B.: The Phosphene of Quick Eye Motion. Arch. Ophthal. *58*:235, 1957.

Roy, F. H.: Ocular Autostimulation. Amer. J. Ophthal. *63*:1776, 1967.

Walsh, F. B., and Hoyt, W. F.: Clinical Neuro-ophthalmology, 3rd ed. Baltimore, Williams & Wilkins Co., 1969, p. 1661.

Wylie, E. J., and Ehrenfeld, W. K.: Extracranial Occlusive Cerebrovascular Disease: Diagnosis and Management. Philadelphia, W. B. Saunders Co., 1970, p. 67.

Hallucinations (formed images)

1. Blind persons

2. Bilateral eye covering—such as may be required after an eye operation, especially in elderly patients

3. Diffuse irritative lesion of parietotemporal area including uncinate seizures of the temporal lobe and stimulation of superior colliculus, optic radiation, and hippocampus

4. Psychoses

5. Poisoning
   A. Mushroom (*Amanita muscaria*) and psilocin poisoning
   B. Bromide (usually potassium or sodium) poisoning
   C. Use of cannabis (marihuana), hashish, and hemp
   D. Acute and chronic ethyl alcoholism—most often associated with delirium tremens
   E. Use of lysergic acid diethylamide (LSD)
   F. Intoxication due to mescaline from peyote, the flowering head of a cactus
   G. Myristica (nutmeg) poisoning
   H. Paraldehyde addiction withdrawal
   I. Trihexyphenidyl (Artane) treatment
   J. Topical or systemic use of atropine sulfate or scopolamine, homotropine, and cyclopentolate
   K. Phenergan
   L. Chloral hydrate delirium
   M. Amphetamines including Benzedrine Sulfate, amphetamine phosphate, and Dexedrine
   N. Camphor—camphorated oil, paregoric, liniments, and moth repellents
   O. Chlorpromazine (Thorazine)
   P. Cocaine
   Q. Dimethylacetamine
   R. Dimethyltryptamine (DMT)
   S. Ditran—synthetic psychotomimetic
   T. Ethchlorvynol (Placidyl)
   U. Gasoline

V. Imipramine (Tofranil)

W. Metrazol

X. Mullet poisoning (Hawaiian fish)

Y. Ololiuqui (morning glory seeds)

Z. Pargyline

A^1. Penicillin and probenecid-penicillin

B^1. Sernyl

C^1. Stramonium (Jimson weed)

D^1. Mysoline (primidone)

E^1. Epanutin (phenytoin)

F^1. Mepacrine

G^1. Digitalis

6. Chronic mountain sickness

7. Associated with blind visual fields

8. Retinal hemorrhage, glaucoma, tabetic optic atrophy, myxedema

9. Associated with measles, encephalitis, pellagra, and epidemic encephalitis

10. Vertebrobasilar insufficiency

11. Pituitary and hypophyseal duct tumor

12. Lesion of hippocampus

13. Papilledema

Adams, J. E., and Rutkin, B. B.: Visual Response to Subcortical Stimulation in the Visual and Limbic Systems. Confin. Neurol. 32:158–164, 1970.

Cogan, D. G.: Neurology of the Visual System, 3rd ed. Springfield, Ill., Charles C Thomas, 1966, pp. 268, 313.

Freund, M., and Mein, S.: Toxic Effects of Scopolamine Eye Drops. Amer. J. Ophthal. 70:637–638, 1970.

Grant, W. M.: Toxicology of the Eye, 2nd ed. Springfield, Ill., Charles C Thomas, 1973.

Green, H., and Spencer, J.: Drugs with Possible Ocular Side-Effects. New York, St. Martin's Press, 1969, pp. 187–192.

Huber, A.: Eye Symptoms of Brain Tumors, 2nd ed. St. Louis, C. V. Mosby Co., 1971, p. 103.

Lissner, W., et al.: Localization of Tritiated Digoxin in the Rat Eye. Amer. J. Ophthal. 72:608–614, 1971.

Nashold, B. S., Jr.: Phosphores Resulting from Stimulation of the Midbrain in Man. Arch. Ophthal. *84*:433–435, 1970.

Walsh, F. B., and Hoyt, W. F.: Clinical Neuro-ophthalmology, 3rd ed. Baltimore, Williams & Wilkins Co., 1969, pp. 2617–2630, 116–119.

"Spots" before Eyes (dots or filaments that move with movement of the eyes)

1. Vitreous opacitics—muscae volitantes; associated with pre-retinal hemorrhage, myopia, or intraocular inflammations (see p. 365)

2. Scotomatous defects
   A. Retinal lesions
   B. Myopia

3. Corneal foreign-body reflection

4. Carbon tetrachloride poisoning

Grant, W. M.: Toxicology of the Eye, 2nd ed. Springfield, Ill., Charles C Thomas, 1973.

Vaughn, D., Cook, R., and Asbury, T.: General Ophthalmology, 6th ed. Los Altos, Calif., Lange Medical Publications, 1971.

Colored Halos around Lights (blue and violet are next to the stimulating light with red outermost)

1. Glaucoma
   A. Acute-angle closure with stretching of corneal lamellae or corneal edema
   B. Open-angle glaucoma—halo noted upon awakening (intraocular pressure is highest in the morning)

2. Mucus on the cornea

3. Corneal scar

4. Krukenberg's spindle

5. Lens opacities

6. Vitreous opacities

7. Any haze of the ocular media

8. Drugs—probably affecting corneal epithelium
   A. Chlorine dioxide
   B. Ethylenediamine
   C. Nitronaphthalene
   D. Quinacrine (Atabrin, Atebrin)
   E. Sterile water can cause transient edema of the epithelium

9. Physiologic halos—most common when lens acts as diffracting gradient

10. Too intense exposure to light as in snow blindness

Adler, F. H.: Physiology of the Eye, 2nd ed. St. Louis, C. V. Mosby Co., 1972.

Grant, W. M.: Toxicology of the Eye, 2nd ed. Springfield, Ill., Charles C Thomas, 1973.

Kolker, A. E., and Hetherington, J.: Becker-Shaffer's Diagnosis and Therapy of the Glaucomas, 3rd ed. St. Louis, C. V. Mosby Co., 1970, p. 181.

Photophobia (painful intolerance of the eyes to light)

1. Conjunctivitis-keratitis

2. Iritis

3. Iridocyclitis

4. Uveitis

5. Albinism

6. Total color blindness (achromatopsia)

7. Corneal, lenticular, and vitreous opacities

8. Patients with corneal lesions having diseases characterized by photosensitization (xeroderma pigmentosa, hydroa vacciniforme, and smallpox)

9. Normal ocular findings with photophobia
    A. Trigeminal neuralgia
    B. Migraine
    C. Neurasthenia
    D. Meningitis
    E. Subarachnoid hemorrhage
    F. Acromegaly
    G. Associated with hypophyseal tumor, and craniopharyngioma
    H. During and following retrobulbar neuritis
    I. Acrodynia
    J. Following severe head injury
    K. Hypoparathyroidism
    L. Lesion of gasserian ganglion
    M. Tumors of ophthalmic branch of the trigeminal nerve, such as neuroma, middle fossa tumor, and posterior fossa tumor, such as meningioma or acoustic neuroma
    N. Increased intracranial pressure including subdural hematomas

10. Botulism

11. Chediak-Higashi syndrome

12. Cystinosis

13. Erythropoietic porphyria

14. Hypoparathyroidism

15. Rabies

16. Psittacosis

17. Schistosomiasis

18. Toxic causes to include isoniazid, Stelazine, Steladex, Plaquenil, and mercury poisoning

Green, H., and Spencer, J.: Drugs with Possible Ocular Side-Effects. New York, St. Martin's Press, 1969, pp. 187–192.

Huber, A.: Eye Symptoms in Brain Tumors, 2nd ed. St. Louis, C. V. Mosby Co., 1971, pp. 11–12.

Smith, J. L.: The University of Miami Neuro-Ophthalmology Symposium, Vol. I. Springfield, Ill., Charles C Thomas, 1964, pp. 24–56.

Walsh, F. B., and Hoyt, W. F.: Clinical Neuro-ophthalmology, 3rd ed. Baltimore, Williams & Wilkins, 1969, pp. 413–416.

Asthenopia (uncomfortable ocular sensation)

1. Uncorrected refractive errors

2. Phoria or tropia

3. Spasm from muscles held too long in a restricted position

4. Passive congestion

5. Neurasthenia or hysteria

6. Weak accommodation

7. Unknown

Pine, R. H., and Hultin, G. L.: Treatment of Asthenopia—Non-pathologic and Non-refractive in Origin. Arch. Ophthal. 27:520, 1944.

Eye Ache

1. Hyperopia

2. Astigmatism

3. Iritis

4. Iridocyclitis

5. Retrobulbar neuritis

6. Glaucoma

7. Sinus disease

8. Unknown

O'Brien, C. S.: Ophthalmology, Notes for Students. Iowa City, Athens Press, 1930, p. 284.

Dazzling or Glare Discomfort

1. Corneal scars or foreign bodies

2. Lenticular changes

3. Altered pupillary response

4. Emotional disorders

5. Drugs, such as chloroquine, acetazolamide, or trimethadione (Tridione)

6. Idiopathic

Grant, W. M.: Toxicology of the Eye, 2nd ed. Springfield, Ill., Charles C Thomas, 1973.
Vaughn, D., Cook, R., and Asbury, T.: General Ophthalmology, 6th ed. Los Altos, Calif., Lange Medical Publications, 1971.

Chromatopsia (colored vision, a condition in which objects are abnormally colored, examples, yellow [xanthopsia], red [erythropsia], blue [cyanopsia], or green [chloropsia])

1. Chorioretinal lesion

2. Lenticular change

3. Jaundice—yellow vision

4. Digitalis—yellow, blue, or green vision

5. Barbiturates—yellow or green vision

6. Bromides (usually potassium or sodium)

7. Cannabis (marihuana, Indian hemp, hashish)—ianthinopsia or violet vision

8. Pentylene tetrazol (Metrazol)—yellow vision

9. Picric acid—yellow vision

10. Quinacrine (Atabrin, Atebrin)—yellow, green, blue vision

11. Following cataract extraction—blue, red or yellow vision

12. Vitreous or retinal hemorrhage—red vision

13. After iridectomy—red vision

14. Snow blindness or blindness following electric shock—red vision

15. Tabetic optic atrophy—blue and red vision

16. Leber's hereditary optic atrophy

17. Santonin—yellow or green vision

18. Streptomycin—yellow vision

19. Sulfonamides—yellow vision

20. Amyl nitrite—yellow vision

21. DDT or carbon disulfide poisoning—yellow vision

22. Hysteria—red or yellow vision

23. Aspidium (*Felix mas*)—yellow vision

24. Chromic acid—yellow vision

25. Chlorothiazide (Diuril)—yellow vision

26. Griseofulvin—green vision

27. Methyl salicylate (oil of wintergreen)—yellow vision

28. Post-traumatic intracavernous aneurysm

29. Acetophenetidin (Phenocetin)—yellow vision

30. Fluorescein—topical or intravenous

31. Aconite—yellow vision

32. Doyne's honeycomb dystrophy

Grant, W. M.: Toxicology of the Eye, 2nd ed. Springfield, Ill., Charles C Thomas, 1973.

Keane, J. R., and Talalla, A.: Post-traumatic Intracavernous Aneurysms. Arch. Ophthal. 87:701–705, 1972.

Perkins, E. S., and Dobree, J. H.: The Differential Diagnosis of Fundus Conditions. St. Louis, C. V. Mosby Co., 1972, p. 140–141.

Vaughn, D., Cook, R., and Asbury, T.: General Ophthalmology, 6th ed. Los Altos, Calif., Lange Medical Publications, 1971.

Walsh, F. B., and Hoyt, W. F.: Clinical Neuro-ophthalmology, Vol. I, 3rd ed. Baltimore, Williams & Wilkins Co., 1969, p. 870.

Nyctalopia (night blindness)

1. Vitamin A deficiency
   A. Dietary deficiencies including malnutrition and cystic fibrosis
   B. Pregnancy

C. Liver disease such as chronic cirrhosis
D. Thyroid gland disorder such as hyperthyroidism
E. Digestive tract disturbance
  (1) In stomach—achlorhydria, chronic gastritis or diarrhea, peptic ulcer
  (2) In pancreas—such as chronic pancreatitis
  (3) Colitis and enteritis
F. Skin disorders such as pityriasis rubra pilaris
G. Pulmonary tuberculosis
H. Malaria

2. Psychologic causes—malingering or psychoses

3. Glaucoma—especially open-angle and angle-closure glaucoma

4. Tapetoretinal degenerations
   A. Retinitis pigmentosa
   B. Retinitis punctata albescens
   C. Choroideremia
   D. Gyrate atrophy
   E. General choroidal sclerosis
   F. Congenital night blindness
     (1) Dominant form
     (2) Recessive form
     (3) Recessive, sex-linked
   G. Oguchi's disease—may be abnormal
   H. Detachment of retina
   I. Miners' nystagmus
   J. Fleck retina—non-progressive, congenital, rare
   K. Fundus flavimaculatus—minimal
   L. Drusen (familial)—minimal
   M. Toxic, such as from indomethacin and chloroquine

5. Vitreotapetoretinal degeneration—sex-linked recessive and autosomal recessive

6. Congenital high myopia

7. Refsum's syndrome—ophthalmoplegia, ataxia, deafness, and polyneuritis

Carr, R. E., and Siegel, I. M.: The Vitreo-tapeto-retinal Degenerations. Arch. Ophthal. *84*:436–445, 1970.

Henkes, H. E., von Lith, G. H. M., and Canta, L. R.: Indomethacin Retinopathy. Amer. J. Ophthal. *73*:846–856, 1972.

Hill, D. A., Arbel, K. F., and Berson, E. L.: Cone Electroretinograms in Congenital Nyctalopia with Myopia. Amer. J. Ophthal. *78*:127–136, 1974.

Jayle, G. E., Ourgand, A. G., Baisinger, L. F., and Holmes, W. J.: Night Vision. Springfield, Ill., Charles C Thomas, 1959, pp. 174–300.

Kandari, F., Tamoi, A., Kurimoto, S., and Fukunoga, K.: Fleck Retina. Amer. J. Ophthal. *73*:673–685, 1972.

Merin, S., Rowe, E., Auerbach, E., and Landon, J.: Syndrome of Congenital High Myopia with Nyctalopia. Amer. J. Ophthal. *70*: 541–547, 1970.

Regenbogen, L., Godel, V., and Stein, R.: Retinoschisis and Night Blindness in a Case of Abortive Retrolental Fibroplasia. J. Pediat. Ophthal. *8*:185–187, 1971.

Spaeth, G. L.: Ocular Manifestations of the Lipidoses. *In* Tasman, W. (Ed.): Retinal Diseases in Children. New York, Harper & Row, Inc., 1971, pp. 181–187.

Hemeralopia (day blindness—inability to see as distinctly in a bright light as in a dim one)

1. Congenital—autosomal recessive trait usually associated with amblyopia and color deficiency
2. Partial occlusion of the central retinal artery
3. Intraocular iron
4. Central opacities of the lens—nuclear or perinuclear cataracts
5. Central scotoma
6. Hereditary retinoschisis
7. Refsum's syndrome—ophthalmoplegia, ataxia, deafness, and polyneuritis

Duke-Elder, S.: System of Ophthalmology, Vol. III, Part 2. St. Louis, C. V. Mosby Co., 1963, pp. 660–661.

Grant, W. M.: Toxicology of the Eye, 2nd ed. Springfield, Ill., Charles C Thomas, 1973.

MacVicar, J. E., and Wilbrandt, H. R.: Hereditary Retinoschisis and Early Hemeralopia. Arch. Ophthal. *83*:629–636, 1970.

O'Brien, C. S.: Ophthalmology, Notes for Students. Iowa City, Athens Press, 1930, p. 347.

Spaeth, G. L.: Ocular Manifestations of the Lipidoses. *In* Tasman, W. (Ed.): Retinal Diseases in Children. New York, Harper & Row Inc., 1971, pp. 181–187.

Oscillopsia (illusionary movement of the environment; may be unilateral or bilateral; usually due to acquired nystagmus)

1. Involvement of medial longitudinal fasciculus affecting ipsilateral medial rectus in internuclear ophthalmoplegia (see p. 147)—monocular oscillopsia

2. Following vestibular function loss—occurs during movement of the head or body
   A. Sectioning of vestibular (VIII) nerve for vertigo
   B. Streptomycin toxicity
   C. Spontaneous loss

3. Fixation and voluntary nystagmus

4. Opsoclonus and ocular flutter

5. Intermittent exotropia

Bender, M. B.: Oscillopsia. Arch. Neurol. *13*:204–213, 1965.

Bridkner, R. M.: Oscillopsia, A New Symptom Commonly Occurring in Multiple Sclerosis. Arch. Neurol. Psychiat. *36*:586, 1936.

Cogan, D. G.: Opsoclonus, Body Tremulousness, and Benign Encephalitis. Arch. Ophthal. *79*:545, 1968.

Cogan, D. G.: Down Beat Nystagmus. Arch. Ophthal. *80*:757–768, 1968.

Hoyt, W. F., and Keane, J. R.: Superior Oblique Myokymia. Report and Discussion on Five Cases of Benign Intermittent Unilocular Microtremor. Arch. Ophthal. *84*:461–467, 1970.

Keeney, A. H., and Roseman, E.: Acquired, Vertical Illusory Movement. Amer. J. Ophthal. *51*:1188–1191, 1966.

Kroll, M.: Acquired Idiopathic Nystagmus and Oscillopsia. Amer. J. Ophthal. *67*:139–144, 1969.

Reinecke, R. D.: Translated Myokymia of the Lower Eyelid Causing Uniocular Vertical Pseudonystagmus. Amer. J. Ophthal. *75*:150–151, 1973.

Rosenblum, J. A., and Shafer, N.: Voluntary Nystagmus Associated with Oscillopsia. Arch. Neurol. *15*:560–562, 1966.

Color Blindness

1. Inherited—stable defect, affecting both eyes
    A. Klinefelter's syndrome (XXY or XXYYO)
    B. Turner's syndrome (XO)
    C. Hemophilia
    D. Glucose-6-phosphate dehydrogenase deficiency (G6PD)
    E. Duane's retraction syndrome
    F. Duchenne's muscular dystrophy
    G. "Intrinsic" defect
        (1) Trichromat—three colors mixed to see white
            a. Protanomaly—red anomaly
            b. Deuteranomaly—green anomaly
            c. Tritanomaly—blue anomaly
        (2) Dichromat—two colors mixed to see white
            a. Protanope—red deficiency
            b. Deuteranope—green deficiency
            c. Tritanope—blue deficiency
        (3) Monochromat—one color mixed to see white
            a. Cone deficient
            b. Rod deficient

2. Acquired—defect can increase or decrease; may affect only one eye; impairment of other visual function; often characterized by chromatopsia; hue discrimination primarily affected; yellow-blue defects more common in retinal disease; red-green defects in optic nerve disease

19

A. Peripheral chorioretinal degeneration
B. Chorioretinitis
C. Retinitis pigmentosa
D. Retinal detachment (see p. 416)
E. Diabetic retinitis
F. Macular lesions including juvenile degeneration, senile degeneration dystrophy, and edema (see pp. 380 to 387)
G. Occlusion of retinal vessels (see pp. 395 and 406)
H. Glaucoma including narrow and open angle
I. Papillitis (see p. 477)
J. Night blindness (see p. 545)
K. Snow blindness
L. Optic atrophy (see p. 487)
M. Retrobulbar optic neuritis (see p. 477)
N. Optic pathways including brain tumor
O. Advanced hypertensive retinopathy
P. Oguchi's disease
Q. Drugs and chemical substances causing optic neuropathy (see p. 487)
R. Friedreich's ataxia
S. Color anomia—inability to name colors; may be associated with homonymous hemianopia due to infarct of posterior parietal and corpus callosum
T. Dominantly inherited juvenile optic atrophy
U. Amblyopia
V. Albinism
W. Hepatic cirrhosis

Cruz-Coke, R.: Color Blindness. Springfield, Ill., Charles C Thomas, 1970.

Krill, A. E., and Fishman, G. A.: Acquired Color Vision Defects. Trans. Amer. Acad. Ophthal. Otolaryng. 75:1095–1111, 1971.

Rothstein, T. B., et al.: Dyschromatopsia with Hepatic Cirrhosis: Relation to Serum B_{12} and Folic Acid. Amer. J. Ophthal. 75:889–895, 1973.

Sakuma, Y.: Studies on Color Vision Anomalies in Subjects with Alcoholism. Ann. Ophthal. 5:1277–1296, 1973.

Smith, D. P., Coke, B. L., and Isaacs, J.: Congenital Tritanopia with Neuroretinal Disease. Invest. Ophthal. 12:608–617, 1973.

Walsh, F. B., and Hoyt, W. F.: Clinical Neuro-ophthalmology, Vol. I, 3rd ed. Baltimore, Williams & Wilkins Co., 1969.

Palinopsia (persistence or recurrence of visual images after the exciting stimulus object has been removed; patient has a hemianopic field defect)

1. Parietal-occipital region lesion
    A. Vascular
    B. Degenerative
    C. Neoplastic
    D. Traumatic

2. Encephalitis

3. Epilepsy

4. Acute migraine

5. Intoxications, such as mescal delirium

Bender, M. B., Feldman, M., and Sobin, A. J.: Palinopsia. Brain 91:321–338, 1968.

Duke-Elder, S., and Scott, G. I.: System of Ophthalmology, Vol. XII. St. Louis, C. V. Mosby Co., 1971, p. 569.

Vertical Reading (patient reads from above downwards)

1. Homonymous hemianopia

2. Astigmatism—high error of refraction

O'Brien, C. S.: Ophthalmology, Notes for Students. Iowa City, Athens Press, 1930, p. 350.

HEAD POSITION

Contents

Head Turn (face turn)

1. Head turned toward right
    A. Right lateral rectus muscle palsy
    B. Left medial rectus muscle palsy
    C. Left superior oblique muscle palsy
    D. Left inferior oblique muscle palsy
    E. Right superior rectus muscle palsy
    F. Right inferior rectus muscle palsy
    G. Right supranuclear gaze paresis

2. Head turned toward left
    A. Left lateral rectus muscle palsy
    B. Right medial rectus muscle palsy
    C. Right superior oblique muscle palsy
    D. Right inferior oblique muscle palsy
    E. Left superior rectus muscle palsy
    F. Left inferior rectus muscle palsy
    G. Left supranuclear gaze paresis

3. Head turned toward either left or right
    A. Congenital nystagmus—turned toward field with least amplitude of nystagmus
    B. Hearing defect
    C. Progressive intracranial arterial occlusion syndrome

Walsh, F. B., and Hoyt, W. F.: Clinical Neuro-ophthalmology, 3rd ed. Baltimore, Williams & Wilkins Co., 1969, p. 151.
Zappia, R. J., et al.: Progressive Intracranial Arterial Occlusion Syndrome. Arch. Ophthal. *86*:455–458, 1971.

Head Tilt (head tilted toward either shoulder or around an anteroposterior axis)

1. Head tilted toward right
   A. Left superior oblique muscle palsy
   B. Right inferior oblique muscle palsy
   C. Left superior rectus muscle palsy
   D. Right inferior rectus muscle palsy

2. Head tilted toward left
   A. Right superior oblique muscle palsy
   B. Left inferior oblique muscle palsy
   C. Right superior rectus muscle palsy
   D. Left inferior rectus muscle palsy

3. Head tilted toward either right or left
   A. Non-ocular torticollis—patching of eyes does not eliminate; x ray may help
      (1) Spasm of sternocleidomastoid or contracture of sternocleidomastoid muscle on side of head tilt
      (2) Paralysis or absent muscles on opposite side of head tilt
      (3) Vertibulbar defect
         a. Labyrinthitis
         b. Otitis media
         c. Acoustic neuroma
      (4) Pain from infection
         a. Adenitis
         b. Mastoiditis
         c. Arthritis
         d. Synovitis
      (5) Congenital malformation of fracture of cervical spine or vertebral processes
      (6) Functional habit and hysteria
      (7) Sandifer's syndrome (torticollis associated with hiatal hernia)
   B. Nystagmus—turned toward field with least amplitude of nystagmus
   C. Astigmatism

O'Donnell, J. J., and Howard, R. O.: Torticollis Associated with Hiatus Hernia (Sandifer's Syndrome). Amer. J. Ophthal. *71*:1134–1137, 1971.

Von Noorden, G. K., and Maumenee, A. E.: Atlas of Strabismus, 2nd ed. St. Louis, C. V. Mosby Co., 1973.

Walsh, F. B., and Hoyt, W. F.: Clinical Neuro-ophthalmology, 3rd ed. Baltimore, Williams & Wilkins Co., 1969, p. 151.

Chin Elevation

1. Inferior oblique muscle palsy

2. Superior rectus muscle palsy

3. Incomplete bilateral ptosis

4. A esotropia with fusion in downward gaze

5. V exotropia with fusion in downward gaze

6. Adaptive symptom of contact lens wearer

Von Noorden, G. K., and Maumenee, A. E.: Atlas of Strabismus, 2nd ed. St. Louis, C. V. Mosby Co., 1973.

Chin Depression

1. Superior oblique muscle palsy

2. Inferior rectus muscle palsy

3. V esotropia with fusion in upward gaze

4. A exotropia with fusion in upward gaze

Von Noorden, G. K., and Maumenee, A. E.: Atlas of Strabismus, 2nd ed. St. Louis, C. V. Mosby Co., 1973.

Head Nodding

1. Bobble head (doll syndrome)—(to and fro bobbing of the head and trunk, at 2- to 3-second intervals, due to cyst of third ventricle)

2. Benign or familial tremor

3. Habit spasm

4. Extrapyramidal dysfunction, such as paralysis agitans

5. Spasms nutans—quick head movement

Benton, J. W., et al.: Report of a Unique Truncal Tremor Associated with Third Ventricle Cyst and Hydrocephalus in Children. Neurology 16:725–729, 1966.

Wyber, K.: Disorders of Ocular Motility in Brain Stem Lesions in Children. Ann. Ophthal. 3:645–662, 1971.

INDEX

Albright's disease (hereditary osteodystrophy; pseudohypoparathyroidism), 8, 112, 211, 346, 351
Albers-Schönberg disease (osteopetrosis; marble bone disease), 26, 343, 483, 487-488
Alcohol, 54, 120, 121, 126, 135, 143, 175, 301, 478, 529
Allergic conjunctivitis, 159, 169, 174, 353
Alligator tears, 89
Alpers' progressive gray matter degeneration, 532
Alport's syndrome, 240, 343, 349, 448, 517
Alstöm's disease, 449
Altitudinal hemianopia, 448, 505, 506
Amanita muscaria (mushroom), 516, 537
Amaurosis fugax, 520
Amblyopia, 124, 529
Amebiasis, 135, 332
Aminopterin-induced syndrome, 23, 28, 72
Amniotic fluid embolization, 395
Amodiaquin, 222
Amphetamine phosphate, 537
Amyl nitrite, 544
Amyloidosis, 227, 264, 365
Amyoplasia congenita (arthrogryposis), 17
Amyotrophic lateral sclerosis, 55, 93
Ancylostomiasis, 333
Anemia, 21, 35, 82, 146, 180, 221, 279, 283, 285, 354, 363, 410, 412, 415, 419, 420, 455, 478, 505, 520
Anencephaly, 203, 487
Anesthesia, corneal, 218
Aneurysm(s), arteriovenous, 6, 20, 37
  carotid artery, 15, 139, 142
  conjunctival, varicosities and tortuosities of, 176
  retina, 255, 318, 411
Aneurysmal dilatation of retinal vessels, 393
Angioid streaks, 385, 390, 452, 454, 459, 469, 493
Angiomatosis of retina, 198, 311, 363, 403
Angiomatosis retinae (von-Hippel-Lindau disease), 6, 267, 363, 380, 416
Angle width of anterior chamber, 287
Angular conjunctivitis, 77
Anhidrotic ectodermal dysplasia, 41, 225
Aniline, 499
Aniridia, 119, 253, 266, 271, 297, 316, 350
Anisocoria, 295
Ankylosing spondylitis, 330
Anophthalmia, clinical, 44, 70, 203, 204
Antabuse, 479
Anterior chamber cleavage syndrome, 194, 266
  abnormalities of, 216
  angle width, 287

560

Dellen of cornea, 207, 239, 247
Demodex folliculorum, 232
Dengue fever (bone-break fever), 22, 134, 135, 150, 257, 355
Depigmentation of the lids, 73
Dermachalasis, 44
Dermatitis, atopic, 253, 340, 345
Dermatomyositis, 363, 419
Dermoid, cornea and epibulbar, 6, 10, 12, 184, 200, 255
Descemet's membrane, folds of, 252
  tears of, 252
Detachment, anterior vitreous, 360
  choroidal, 456-457
  retinal, 415-418
Deutman's syndrome (retinal pigment dystrophy), 377
Deuteranomaly, 549
Deuteranope, 549
Devic's disease (opticomyelitis), 477, 487
Dexedrine, 537
Diabetic coma, 201, 279
Diabetes insipidus, 310
Diabetes mellitus, 65, 121, 125, 134, 135, 137, 139, 145, 176, 180,
  214, 218, 221, 236, 238, 252, 259, 270, 283, 284, 291, 301, 303, 310,
  318, 319, 322, 340, 342, 352, 363, 380, 393, 403, 406, 408, 410,
  411, 415, 419, 420, 438, 455, 456, 478, 549
Dialinas-Amalric syndrome, 448
Dichloroacetylene, 140, 143
Dichromat, 549
Diencephalic syndrome, 130, 489
Diffuse catarrhal conjunctivitis, 162, 163, 232
Digitalis, 511, 544
Diktyomas (embryonal medulloepitheliomas), 7, 198, 264, 310, 327,
  426
Dilantin, 120, 140
Dilated retinal veins, 403, 407-408
Dimethylacetamine, 537
Dinitrophenol cataract, 135, 342
Diphenhydramine (Benadryl), 518
Diphtheria, 92, 135, 143, 145, 181, 232, 356
Diplopia, binocular, 526
  following head trauma, 515
  uniocular, 527
Diptera larvae, 332
Disc, hyperemia of, 476
  temporally displaced, 495
Disease, Addison's (idiopathic hypoparathyroidism), 49, 187, 486
  Albers-Schönberg (osteopetrosis; marble bone disease), 26, 346,
    483, 487-488
  Albright's (hereditary osteodystrophy; pseudohypoparathyroidism),
    8, 112, 211, 346, 351

Disease—*(Continued)*

Dystrophy—*(Continued)*
    oculovertebral, 192, 203
    Reis-Buckler, 242
    retinal pigment, 377
    vortex, 242

Eales' disease, 318, 363, 392, 411, 415, 417, 446
Eaton-Lambert syndrome, 51
Eccentric vision, 529
Echinococcosis, 369
Echothiophate iodine (phospholine iodide), 340
Eclampsia (toxemia of pregnancy), 54, 92, 236, 344, 531
Ectodermal dysplasia, 33, 81, 92, 170, 236, 260, 344
Ectopic pupils, 192
Ectropion of lids, 69, 89, 92, 162, 231
Edema, conjunctival, 178, 247
    corneal, 219
    macular, 380-381, 519
Ehlers-Danlos syndrome (fibrodysplasia elastica generalisata), 27, 49, 71, 112, 181, 211, 225, 253, 261, 447
Eighteen (18) deletion chromosome syndrome, 198, 349, 452, 488, 517
Elevated intraocular pressure with normal optic disc, 271
Elephantiasis, 44
Elschnig spots, 470
Ellis-van Crefeld syndrome (chondroectodermal dysplasia), 112, 253, 316, 317, 349, 452, 517
Embolism, 395
Embryonal medulloepitheliomas (diktyoma), 7, 198, 264, 310, 327, 426
Embryotoxon, anterior, 216, 240
Emetine, 352
Emphysema of orbit, 21
Encephalitis, 120, 126, 133, 134, 142, 145, 146, 152, 154, 301, 532, 538
Encephalitis periaxialis diffusa (Schilder's disease), 130, 477, 510, 525, 531
Encephalocele, 13, 34
Encephalomyelitis, acute disseminated, 142
Encephalopathy, Wernicke's, 51, 134, 139, 143, 145, 152
Encephalotrigeminal angiomatosis (Sturge-Weber syndrome), 6, 194, 267, 271
Endophthalmitis, 196-197, 202, 282, 310, 329, 424, 525
Endothelioma, 327
Enlargement of blind spot, 500
Enophthalmos, 17-19, 44, 70, 100, 128
Engelmann's disease (hereditary diaphyseal dysplasia), 35
Entropion, 70, 89, 100, 231
Eosinophilic cellular reaction, 159

Eosinophilic granuloma, 76
Epanutin (phenytoin), 538
Ependymomas, 124
Epiblepharon, 70
Epicanthus, 70-73
Epidemic encephalitis, 125, 538
Epidemic keratoconjunctivitis (type 8 adenovirus), 159, 164, 168, 170
Epidermoid cyst, 33
Epidermolysis bullosa, 92, 170
Epilepsy, 519, 536
Epinephrine, 184, 279, 380
Episclera, dilated vessels of, 213
  pigment spots of, 212
Episcleritis, 206, 210, 247
Episkopi (dystrophy of cornea), 229
Equine encephalitis, 477
Erb-Goldflam syndrome (myasthenia gravis), 6, 48, 49, 112, 137, 143, 147, 354, 526
Ergot, 143, 478, 499
Ergothioneine, 478
Erysipelas, 13, 53, 86
Erythema elevantum diutinum, 206
Erythema multiforme (Stevens-Johnson syndrome), 91, 92, 164, 170, 172, 231, 232, 234, 236, 239
Erythema nodosum, 207
Erythroderma ichthyosiforme, 170
Erythropoietic porphyria, 541
Eserine, 274, 301
Esidrix, 380
Esotropia A, 100
Esotropia V, 100
E syndrome (trisomy 18), 23, 42, 51, 78, 268, 316, 344
Ethambutol, 478
Ethchlorvynol (Placidyl), 537
Ethmocephalus, 30
Ethoxzolamide, 516
Ethyl alcohol, 499, 532
Ethylenediamine, 540
Ethylhydrocupreine (Optochin), 503
Euryblepharon, 79-80
Excessive tears, 89
Exfoliation of lens capsule, 351
Exfoliative dermatitis, 170
Exo-, 103, 151
Exophthalmos, 5-17, 102, 151, 231
  bilateral, 14
  pseudoproptosis, 5
  pulsating, 14

Glaucoma—*(Continued)*
neovascular, 291
phacolytic, 273
pigmentary, 221, 286, 326
secondary, 5, 194, 266, 271, 318, 425
unilateral, 273
Glaucomatocyclitic crisis (Posner-Schlossman syndrome), 273, 297, 320
Glioma, chiasmal, 122, 507
of optic nerve, 7, 10, 12-14, 36, 487
Glioblastomas, 141, 147, 510
Globe, 192-204
Glomerulonephritis, 67, 416
Glucose-6-phosphate dehydrogenase deficiency (G6PD), 549
Glycogen disease (von Gierke's), 265
Gold (chrysiasis), 82, 140, 187, 244
Goldberg's disease, 374
Goldmann-Fayre dystrophy, 129, 374
Goldenhar's syndrome (oculoauriculovertebral dysplasia), 24, 31, 43, 80, 192, 203, 218, 255, 316
Goltz' syndrome, 88, 193, 317
Gonadal dysgenesis syndrome (Turner's), 9, 42, 51, 70, 113, 211, 268, 346, 549
Gonococcus, 283, 285, 463, 464
Gougerot-Sjögren syndrome (Sjögren's), 89, 92, 94, 170, 174, 206, 232, 234, 248, 343
Gout, 174, 207, 217, 229, 249, 256, 331
Gradenigo's syndrome (temporal), 139, 141, 218
Graefe's sign, 59, 61
Granulomatous uveitis, 332, 333, 451
Graves' disease, 89, 105, 478
Greig's syndrome (ocular hypertelorism), 17, 25
Griseofulvin, 545
Gronblad-Strandberg syndrome (pseudoxanthoma elastica), 452, 493
Guillain-Barré syndrome, 117, 145, 355, 482, 485
Gustolacrimal reflex, 89
Gyrate atrophy, 545

Hallerman-Streiff syndrome (oculomandibulodyscephaly), 27, 43, 112, 129, 192, 203, 211, 225, 268, 343
Hallgren's syndrome (retinitis pigmentosa-deafness-ataxia), 434, 448, 488, 496
Hallucinations, 537, 538
Hand-Schüller-Christian disease, 7, 8, 10, 14
Happy puppet syndrome, 488
Harada's disease, 416, 421, 448, 456, 466
Hard exudates of retina, 420
Harlequin orbit, 5

Hashish (cannabis; marihuana), 296, 518, 537, 544
Head nodding, 553, 557
Head tilt, 553, 554
Head turn, 553, 554
Heerfort's disease, 68, 80, 198, 345
Hemangioma, of choroid, 380, 431
  of orbit, 6, 10, 11, 12, 14, 35, 47, 74, 87, 141, 152, 267
Hemangioblastomas of cerebellum, 118, 141
Hemifacial microsomia syndrome (otomandibular dysostosis), 143, 225, 316, 317
Hemeralopia (day blindness), 547
Hemianopia, altitudinal, 505
  binasal, 506
  bitemporal, 507-509
  homonymous, 118, 127, 510
Hemophilia, 13, 87, 283, 284, 363, 549
Hemorrhagic polioencephalitis superior syndrome (Wernicke's), 51, 139, 143, 145, 146, 152
Hemp (hashish), 296, 518, 537, 544
Hennebert's syndrome (luetic otitic nystagmus), 129
Hepatitis, 135
Hereditary dystrophic lipidosis, 403, 428
Hereditary fleck dystrophy, 219
Hereditary hemorrhagic telangiectasis (Rendu-Osler-Weber disease), 87, 174, 236, 392
Hereditary oculo-dento-osseous dysplasia (oculodentodigital syndrome), 30, 70, 78, 192, 194, 225
Hereditary osteo-onychodysplasia, 321
Herpes simplex, 159, 160, 164, 167, 168, 186, 207, 218, 228, 231, 232, 233, 234, 235, 237, 250, 252, 283
Herpes zoster, 53, 93, 134, 137, 139, 143, 160, 207, 218, 231, 232, 233, 235, 236, 250, 273, 296, 322, 329, 330, 333
Heterochromia of iris, 65, 102, 135, 168, 201, 243, 268, 280, 355
Heterochromic iridocyclitis (Fuch's heterochromia syndrome), 320, 325, 328, 330, 331, 466
High AC/A ratio, 100, 101
High-energy microwave radiation, 342
Hippus, 295
Histoplasmosis, 332, 385, 460, 463, 464, 466, 467, 469
Hodgkin's disease, 13, 15, 56, 67, 86, 93, 134, 185, 244, 419, 476, 478, 482
Holes of macula, 396
Hollenhorst plaques of retina, 436
Homocystinuria, 267, 316, 346, 348, 349, 516
Homonymous hemianopia, 504, 510, 511
Homatropine, 537
Hood (hereditary osteo-onychodysplasia), 321
Horizontal gaze palsy, 116, 138
Horizontal nystagmus, 119

Hypogammaglobulinemia, 461
Hypoglycemia, infantile, 347
Hypoparathyroidism (Addison's disease), 51, 187, 341, 478, 482, 541
Hypophosphatasia, 5, 23, 58, 211, 229, 482
Hypopyon, 196, 197, 282
Hypopyon ulcer, 250, 282
Hypotelorism, 100
Hypotension, 395, 411, 419, 530
Hypothyroidism, 28, 67, 82, 131, 174
Hypotonia-obesity syndrome (Praeder-Willi), 113
Hypotony, 44, 279, 288, 319, 380, 453, 456, 486

Ichthyosis, 220, 229, 257
Imipramine (Tofranil), 518, 537
Inclusion bodies of cells, 160
Inclusion conjunctivitis, 159, 160-168, 232, 233, 245
Incontinentia pigmenti (Bloch-Sulzberger disease), 8, 112, 128, 198, 244, 256, 312, 410, 434
Indomethacin (Indocin), 217
Infantile cortical hyperostosis, 35
Infantile gigantism, 26
Infantile hypoglycemia, 269
Infantile poikiloderma, 344
Infantile polyarthritis (Still's disease), 229, 330, 463, 525
Infectious mononucleosis, 86, 243, 477, 482
Influenza, 86, 142, 168, 181, 234, 256, 354, 421, 465, 466, 477
Infranuclear ophthalmoplegia, 142
Infundibulomas, 510
Intermittent exophthalmos, 13, 14
Internal ophthalmoplegia, 315, 354, 356, 518
Internuclear ophthalmoplegia, 104, 128, 147
Interstitial keratitis, 221, 229, 242, 244, 252
Intraepithelial epithelioma, 182, 185
Intraocular adipose tissue, 200
Intraocular calcification, 199
Intraocular cartilage, 198
Intraocular infection, 196, 197
Intraocular pressure, elevated, with normal disc, 271
Intraorbital calcification, 19, 20
Inversus epicanthus, 70
Iodoform, 499
Iridescent crystalline deposits in lens, 337, 352
Ischemic uveitis of Knox, 465
Isoniazid, 140, 542
Iridocyclitis, 342, 354, 543
Iridodialysis, 271, 283
Iridodonesis, 323
Iris, atrophy of, 266, 271, 320, 322
  coloboma of, 316

20

Keratitis—*(Continued)*
  genitourinary disease and, 234
  interstitial, 221, 229, 242, 244, 252
  lid disease and, 231
  limbal conditions and, 233
  neuroparalytic, 217, 220, 231, 235
  non-syphilitic interstitial, 62, 244
  nummular, 243
  punctate epithelial, 231, 236, 237
  respiratory disease and, 234
  sicca, 238
  skin disease and, 231
Keratoacanthoma, 15
Keratoconjunctivitis, 159, 164, 168, 169, 170, 187, 206, 216, 232, 236, 245
  phlyctenular, 248
Keratoconjunctivitis sicca, 89, 232, 234, 235, 239
Keratoconus (conical cornea), 220, 236, 253, 254, 264, 527
Keratoectasia, 264
Keratomalacia, 187
Keratopathy, band-shaped, 229, 230
  bullous, 242
Keratosis follicularis spinalosa decalvans, 221, 246
Kinky hair disease (Menkes'), 488
Kleeblattschadel syndrome (cloverleaf skull), 8, 25, 43
Klein-Waardenburg syndrome, 330
Klinefelter's syndrome, 27, 41, 47, 71, 549
Klippel-Feil syndrome (synostosis of cervical vertebrae), 26, 121
Kloepfer's syndrome, 488
Knox's ischemic uveitis, 465
Koeber-Solus-Elschnig syndrome (sylvian aqueduct), 58, 123, 129, 130
Klumpke's paralysis, 55
Koeppe nodules, 326
Krabbe's demyelinative disease, 496, 510
Krukenberg's spindle, 221, 286, 540
Kuhnt-Junius disease, 311
Kwashiorkor, 73
Kyrle's disease, 223, 343

Labrador keratopathy, 229
Lacrimal gland, 7, 12, 86, 87
Lacrimal sac infection, 95
Lactobacillus, 161
Lactosyl ceramidosis, 374
Lagophthalmos, 61, 247
Landry's ascending paralysis, 143
Large hemorrhages in the fundus of an infant or young child, 409
Larsen's syndrome, 26

584

Macula—*(Continued)*
    heterotopia of, 382
    holes in, 386
    pucker of, 382
    star or stellate retinopathy of, 382
    wisps and foveolar splinter of, 391
Macular anatomic classification of diseases, 371
Macular corneal dystrophy, 218
Madarosis, 82
Malaria, 142, 181, 218, 355, 532
Malattia leventinese, 377
Male Turner's syndrome (Noonan's), 29, 43, 50, 70, 82, 115, 254, 346, 517
Malignant atrophic papulosis (Degos' syndrome), 176, 466
Malignant melanoma of choroid, 7, 47, 87, 188, 202, 206, 212, 221, 286, 320, 325, 328, 336, 431, 454, 456
Mandibulofacial dysostosis (Treacher-Collins and Franceschetti-Klein syndromes), 42, 69, 80, 192, 346
Manganese, 118, 486
Mannitol, 279
Map-dot fingerprint, 242
Maple syrup urine disease, 18, 29, 52, 115, 132, 134
Marble bone disease (osteopetrosis; Albers-Schönberg disease), 9, 26, 346, 487, 488
Marchesani's syndrome (mesodermal dysmorphodystrophy), 28, 31, 43, 226, 349
Marcus Gunn sign (pupillary escape), 297
Marcus Gunn syndrome (jaw winking and inverse jaw winking), 46, 50, 59, 297
Marfan's syndrome (dystrophica mesodermalis congenita), 27, 31, 32, 113, 130, 208, 211, 226, 253, 267, 303, 348, 349, 447, 516, 525
Marginal corneal ulcers, 256
Marihuana (cannabis), 296, 518, 537, 544
Marinesco-Sjögren syndrome (oligophrenia with cerebellar ataxia and cataracts), 130, 343
Maroteaux-Lamy syndrome (mucopolysaccharidosis VI [MPS VI]), 228, 265, 482, 486, 489
Marshall's syndrome, 516
Massive retinal fibrosis, 310
Maxillofacial dysostosis, 43
Measles (rubeola), 86, 142, 160, 181, 354, 355, 421, 477, 525, 532, 538
Mecholyl test, 295
Meckles's syndrome, 193, 204, 347
Median cleft face syndrome (lip), 25, 30
Medullary tegmental paralysis (Babinski-Nageotte syndrome), 17, 49, 128
Medullated nerve fibers, 431
Medulloblastomas, 106, 118 141, 147
Meesmann's dystrophy, 242

Megaloblepharon, 69
Megalocornea, 226, 264, 266, 349
Meibomian gland carcinoma, 74
Melanocytoma, 432
Melanoma, malignant, 7, 12, 48, 87, 131, 188, 202, 212, 221, 233, 286, 318, 320, 325, 328, 431, 454
Melanophoric nevus syndrome (Naegeli's) 113, 130
Melanosis oculi, 187, 268
Melkersson-Rosenthal syndrome, 68, 92
Mellaril, 217
Membranous conjunctivitis, 164
Meniere's syndrome, 130
Meningism, 463
Meningitis, 52, 53, 64, 67, 134, 155, 541
Meningocele, 13, 14, 40
Meningioma, 7, 10, 11, 12, 13, 14, 35, 36, 59, 68, 121, 126, 134, 135, 141, 416, 476, 482, 487, 505
Menkes' disease (kinky hair), 488
Mepacrine, 538
Meprobamate, 518
MER-29, 31, 342
Mercury, 229, 542
Mesantoin, 168
Mescal, 511
Mesodermal dysmorphodystrophy (Marchesani's syndrome), 30, 31, 43, 226, 349
Metaphyseal dysostosis (Jansen's disease), 9, 27
Metachromatic leukodystrophy, 374, 383, 525
Metachromatic leukoencephalopathy, 487, 510
Metastatic lesions, 7, 10, 12, 14, 15
Metastatic tumors of lid, 74
Metamorphopsia, 519
Methyl acetate, 478
Methyl alcohol, 478, 522
Methyl bromide, 478
Methyl chloride, 480
Methyl salicylate (oil of wintergreen), 545
Methylene blue, 480
Metrazol, 537, 545
Meyer-Schwickerath and Weyers syndrome, 30, 70, 78, 192, 194, 225, 268
Meyer's phenomenon, 298
Michel's freckles, 326
Microaneurysms of retina, 411, 413
Microblepharon, 69
Microcephaly, 30, 532
Microcornea, 225, 266, 320
Microphakia, 348
Microphthalmos, 70, 78, 192, 266, 316, 518

Migraine, 56, 499, 510, 511, 516, 519, 530, 536, 541
Mikulicz's syndrome, 6, 65, 86, 93, 236
Milk-alkali syndrome, 229
Millard-Gubler syndrome, 64, 113, 139
Miosis, 301, 303
Misdirected third nerve syndrome, 46
Mobiüs' sign, 151
Mobiüs' syndrome (congenital facial paralysis), 8, 50, 71
Mohr's syndrome, 78
Molluscum contagiosum, 74, 160, 169, 231, 233, 245
Mongolism (trisomy 21) (Down's syndrome), 17, 30, 41, 70, 78, 112, 120, 129, 253, 268, 344
Mongoloid obliquity of lid, 41
Moniliasis, 245
Monochromatism, 119, 549
Monocular limitation of elevation of adducted eye, 109
Monocular nystagmus, 124-125
Mononuclear cellular reaction, 159
Mooren's ulcer, 248
Morphine, 120, 301, 353
Morquio-Brailsford syndrome (mucopolysaccharidosis IV [MPS IV]), 89, 228, 264, 265, 347, 489
Morquio-Ullrich syndrome, 26
Moskowskij's sign, 298
MPS I (Hurler's disease), 25, 32, 50, 70, 264, 267, 383, 423, 488
MPS II (Hunter's syndrome), 380, 423, 488
MPS IV (Morquio-Brailsford syndrome), 89, 264
MPS V (Scheie's syndrome), 264
MPS VI (Maroteaux-Lamy syndrome), 482
Mucocele, 10, 12, 13, 14, 19, 34, 37, 48
Mucolipidosis I, 374
Mucopolysaccharidosis type I (MPS I) (Hurler's syndrome), 25, 32, 50, 70, 113, 264, 267, 316, 322, 383, 423, 488
Mucopolysaccharidosis type II (MPS II) (Hunter's syndrome), 380, 423, 488
Mucopolysaccharidosis type IV (MPS IV) (Morquio-Brailsford syndrome), 89, 264
Mucopolysaccharidosis type V (MPS V) (Scheie's syndrome), 83, 264
Mucopolysaccharidosis type VI (MPS VI) (Maroteaux-Lamy syndrome), 322
Mucopurulent conjunctivitis, acute, 162
    chronic, 163
Mucormycosis, 6, 254, 321
Mullet, 538
Multiple basal cell nevi syndrome (Garlin-Goltz), 346
Multiple lentigenes syndrome, 27
Multiple myeloma, 177, 217, 363, 406, 407, 411, 456, 520
Multiple sclerosis, 47, 53, 58, 120, 121, 123, 124, 125, 126, 133, 134, 137, 145, 147, 150, 152, 301, 309, 356, 401, 446, 466, 471, 477, 488, 506, 507, 510, 521, 526, 527

Mumps, 86, 134, 135, 142, 207, 234, 244, 355, 356, 465, 477
Muscular dystrophy, 630
Mushroom poisoning, 516, 537
Mustard gas, 222
Myasthenia gravis (Erb Goldflam syndrome), 6, 47, 49, 63, 69, 90, 111, 112, 135, 137, 142, 145, 147, 309, 354, 356, 517, 526
Myoclonic encephalopathy, 117
Myoclonic syndrome, 383
Mycoplasma, 166
Mycosis fungoides, 244
Mydriacyl, 296
Mydriasis, 296, 298, 300
Myokymia, superior oblique, 122, 124
Myleran, 342
Myologenous leukemia, 401
Myopia, 5, 13, 58, 119, 201, 208, 214, 221, 252, 270, 442, 443, 455, 456, 460, 500, 501, 516, 517, 524, 527, 539
Myositis, 14, 22, 106, 148, 150
Myositis ossificans, 19
Myotonia atrophica, 36, 63
Myotonic dystrophy, 61, 146, 151, 193, 201, 259, 260, 303, 318, 340, 343, 344. 352, 355, 377, 434, 447, 530
Myotonic periodic paralysis, 61
Myristica (nutmeg), 537
Mysoline (primidone), 538

Naegeli's syndrome (melanophoric nevus), 113, 130
Naffziger's syndrome (scalenus anticus), 50
Naphthalene, 340
Narcolepsy, 151
Narrow-angle glaucoma, 218, 225, 274, 296, 342, 522, 540, 545, 549
Nasal nerve syndrome (Charlin's), 22
Nasopharyngeal carcinomas, 7, 134, 148, 476, 490, 510
Negative angle kappa, 100
Nematodes, 332, 380, 421, 462
Neoarsphenamine, 516
Neovascularization of anterior chamber, 291-292
   of choroid, 469
Nephritis, 180, 456
Nephrosis, 67
Nerve(s), corneal, increased visibility of, 220
   fourth (trochlear), 137, 138
   sixth (abducens), 139, 140, 141
   third (oculomotor), 134, 136
Neuritis, 476, 477, 478, 522, 550
   papillitis, 475, 477
   pseudo-optic, 476
   retrobulbar, 477, 478

594

Syndrome(s)—*(Continued)*

De Lange's, 42, 51, 82, 114, 129, 211, 488

diencephalic, 129, 489

dorsolateral medullary (Wallenberg's), 18, 51, 131

doll, 557

Down's (mongolism, trisomy 21), 17, 30, 41, 70, 78, 112, 120, 129, 253, 268, 228

Duane's retraction, 44, 59, 110, 138, 140, 155, 156, 255, 549

Eaton-Lambert, 51

Ehlers-Danlos (fibrodysplasia elastica generalisata), 27, 28, 49, 71, 112, 181, 211, 225, 261, 377

Ellis-van Crefeld (chondroectodermal dysplasia), 112, 253, 316, 317, 349, 452, 517

Erb-Goldflam (myasthenia gravis), 6, 47, 49, 112, 137, 142, 145, 147, 354, 526

familial dysautonomia (Riley-Day), 47, 92, 218, 264, 392

Fanconi's (cystinosis), 217, 229, 264, 461, 466, 541

Felty's (rheumatoid arthritis with hypersplenism), 180, 207

Fisher's (polyradiculoneuronitis), 145

focal dermal hypoplasia, 88, 193, 317

Foville's, 64, 139

Franceschetti-Klein (mandibulofacial dysostosis), 42, 69, 80, 192, 346

Francois' dyscephalic, 31, 114, 132, 193, 347

Freeman-Sheldon, 43, 52, 78, 115

Frenkel's (ocular contusion), 349

Fuch's (heterochromic cyclitis), 320, 325, 328, 330, 331, 466

Gansslen's, 225

Garlin-Goltz (multiple basal cell nevi), 346

Goldenhar's (oculo-auriculo-vertebral dysplasia), 24, 31, 43, 80, 192, 203, 218, 255, 316

Goltz's, 88, 193

Gougerot-Sjögren (Sjögren's), 89, 92, 94, 170, 174, 206, 232, 248, 343

Gradenigo's (temporal), 139, 141, 218

Greig's (ocular hypertelorism), 17, 25, 488

Groeblad-Strandberg (pseudoxanthoma elastica), 377, 452, 493

Guillain-Barré, 117, 145, 355, 482, 485

Hallerman-Streiff (oculomandibulodyscephaly), 27, 43, 112, 129, 192, 203, 211, 225, 268, 343

Hallgren's (retinitis-pigmentosa-deafness-ataxia), 434, 448, 488, 496

Happy puppet, 489

Harada's, 448

Hemifacial microsomia (otomandibular dysotosis), 113, 225, 317

Hemorrhagic polioencephalitis superior (Wernicke's), 51, 139, 143, 145, 146, 152

Hennebert's (luetic otitic nystagmus), 129

Horner's (cervical sympathetic paralysis), 5, 7, 47, 55-56, 58, 89, 90, 301, 303, 307, 320, 516

Syndrome(s)—*(Continued)*

Hunter's (mucopolysaccharidosis II [MPS II]), 29, 83, 228, 260, 316, 380, 423, 448, 488, 489

Hurler's (mucopolysaccharidosis I [MPS I]), 25, 32, 50, 70, 83, 260, 264, 316, 322, 383, 390, 488, 489

Hutchinson's, 7, 8, 10, 14, 15, 68, 117, 141, 347

Hutchinson-Gilford, 9, 347

Hypotonia-obesity (Praeder-Willi), 113

Irvine-Gass, 375

Jadassohn-Lewandowski, 346

Johnson's adherence, 110

Kearns-Sayre, 51, 146, 435

Kenny's, 516

Kleeblattschadel (cloverleaf skull), 9, 25, 43

Klein-Waardenburg, 330

Klinefelter (XXXXY), 27, 41, 47, 71, 549

Klippel-Feil (synostosis of cervical vertebrae), 26, 121

Kloepfer's, 488

Koeber-Solus-Elschnig (sylvian aqueduct), 58, 123, 129, 130

Kwashiorkor, 73

Larsen's, 26

lateral bulbar (Wallenberg's), 17, 51, 55, 131

Laurence-Moon-Biedl (Bardet-Biedl), 12, 26, 41, 113, 119, 129, 225, 346, 421, 434, 448, 466, 525

Lenoble-Aubineau, 129

Leopard, 27

Leri's (pleonostenosis), 41

Leroy's, 71

Linear sebaceous nevi, 42, 316

Louis-Bar (ataxia telangiectasia), 129, 176

Lowe's (oculocerebrorenal), 25, 31, 71, 129, 194, 226, 228, 267, 343, 348

luetic otitic nystagmus (Hennebert's), 129

male Turner's (Noonan's), 29, 43, 50, 70, 82, 115, 254, 346, 517

mandibulofacial dysostosis (Franceschetti and Treacher Collins), 42, 69, 80, 192, 346

Marchesani's (mesodermal dysmorphodystrophy), 30, 32, 43, 226, 349, 517

Marcus Gunn (jaw winking and inverse jaw winking), 46, 50, 59, 297

Marfan's (dystrophica mesodermalis congenita), 26, 28, 31, 113, 130, 132, 208, 211, 253, 267, 292, 303, 348, 349, 516, 525

Marinesco-Sjögren (oligophrenia with cerebellar ataxia and cataracts), 130, 343

Maroteaux-Lamy (mucopolysaccharidosis VI [MPS VI]), 228, 482, 486

Marshall's, 517

median cleft face, 25, 30

melanophoric nevus (Naegeli's), 113, 130

Syndrome(s)—*(Continued)*
  Meckel's, 193, 204, 347
  Melkersson-Rosenthal, 65, 68, 92
  Meniere's, 130
  Meyer-Schwickerath-Weyers (oculodentodigital dysplasia), 30, 70, 78, 192, 194, 225, 268
  Mikulicz's, 6, 65, 86, 93, 236
  Milk-alkali, 229
  Millard-Gubler, 64, 113, 139
  misdirected third nerve, 46
  Möbius' (congenital facial paralysis), 8, 50, 71
  Mohr's, 79
  Morquio-Brailsford (mucopolysaccharidosis IV [MPS IV]), 89, 90, 228, 264, 347
  Morquio-Ulrich, 26
  multiple basal cell nevi (Garlin-Goltz), 346
  multiple lentigenes, 27
  myoclonic, 383
  Naegeli's (melanophoric nevus), 113, 130
  Naffziger's (scalenus anticus), 50
  nasal nerve (Charlin's), 22
  nevoid basal cell carcinoma (basal cell nevus carcinoma), 26, 28, 32, 71, 113, 316
  neurocutaneous, 170, 256
  Noonan's (male Turner's), 29, 43, 50, 70, 82, 115, 254, 346, 517
  Nothnagel's, 300
  ocular hypertelorism (Greig's), 17, 25, 488
  oculoauriculovertebral dysplasia (Goldenhar's), 43, 80, 192, 203, 218, 255
  oculocerebrorenal (Lowe's), 31, 71, 129, 194, 226, 343, 367
  oculodentodigital (Meyer-Schwickerath-Weyers), 30, 70, 78, 192, 194, 225, 268
  oculomandibulodyscephaly (Hallerman-Streiff), 27, 28, 43, 112, 129, 192, 203, 211, 225, 268, 343
  ophthalmorhinostomatohygrosis, 90
  optic atrophy ataxia (Behr's disease), 487
  oral facial digital, 26
  orbital apex sphenoidal (Rollet's), 9, 51, 148
  orofaciodigital, 79
  otomandibular dysotosis (hemifacial microsomia), 113, 225, 316, 317
  oto-palato-digital, 26, 42
  Pancoast's (superior pulmonary sulcus), 17, 50, 55
  paratrigeminal, 56
  Parinaud's (paralysis of vertical movements), 50, 58, 106, 123, 128, 152, 169
  Pelizaeus-Merzbacher, 434
  Pierre-Robin, 113, 192, 268, 346
  pineal, 137

606

Syringobulbia, 121, 122, 125, 144
Syringomyelia, 97, 115, 241

Takayasu's syndrome (aortic arch syndrome; pulseless disease), 279, 318, 322, 395, 520
Tangier's disease, 223
Tapetoretinal degeneration, 253
Tarsalis epicanthus, 70
Tartar emetic, 480
Tay-Sachs disease (familial amaurotic idiocy), 130, 374, 383, 400, 428, 487
Tears, bloody, 87
  excessive, 89
  hypersecretion of, 89
  paucity of, 92, 93, 94
Telangiectasis of retina, 380
Telecanthus, 24, 100, 380
Temporal arteritis (cranial arteritis; giant cell arteritis), 6, 134, 318, 383, 395, 400, 477, 488, 522
Temporal syndrome (Gradenigo's), 218
Teniae, 332
Terrien's marginal degeneration of cornea, 248
Terson's syndrome, 363
Tetanus, 62, 65, 143
Tetany, 63, 341
Tetracycline, 486
Tetralogy of Fallot, 288
Thalamic hyperesthetic anesthesia (Dejerine-Klumpke syndrome), 17, 49
Thalidomide, 63, 140, 192, 256, 316
Thallium, 82, 478, 499
Thiamine (vitamin B_1), 499
Thickened eyelids, 77-78
Thioglycolates, 480, 499
Third nerve (oculomotor nerve), 47, 53, 134, 136, 296, 526
Thorazine (chlorpromazine), 133, 255, 296, 340, 421, 537
Thromboangitis obliterans, 363
Thrombocytopenia purpura, 180, 363, 532
Thrombosis, 13, 14, 15, 67, 122
Thyroid, 6, 12, 14, 59, 90, 145, 155, 214, 271, 453
Tobacco, 478, 499, 529
Tolbutamide, 180
Tolosa-Hunt syndrome, 22, 30, 51, 122, 148
Tortuosity of retinal vessels, 392
Torula, 477
Tournoy's reaction, 306
Toxemia of pregnancy (eclampsia), 54, 92, 236, 344, 470, 531
Toxic epidermal necrolysis (Lyell's disease; scalded skin syndrome), 231, 246
Toxocara, 443, 460, 462, 478

610